Linking Quality of Long-Term Care and Quality of Life

Linda S. Noelker, Ph.D., is the Director of the Margaret Blenkner Research Center and Associate Director for Research at The Benjamin Rose Institute. She is also an Adjunct Professor of Sociology at Case Western Reserve University where she received her graduate degrees. She has researched and published extensively on family caregiving, relationships between informal and formal helpers, long-term care, case management, and stress on nursing staff in skilled care facilities. Dr. Noelker is a fellow of the Gerontological Society of America and a member of the Board of the American Society on Aging.

Zev Harel, Ph.D., is Professor and former Chair of the Department of Social Work at Cleveland State University. He was the founding Director of the CSU Gerontological Studies Program. He has conducted research and written extensively on extreme stress and aging, ethnicity and aging, and vulnerable older populations. His latest co-edited books include: *An Adaptation and Coping: From the Holocaust to Vietnam; The Black Aged: Understanding Diversity and Service Need; The Vulnerable Aged: People, Services and Policies; The Jewish Aged in the U.S. and Israel;* and *Matching People and Services in Long-term Care* (the last three with Springer Publishing Company). Dr. Harel has been serving in leadership roles with local, state, and national organizations in aging.

Linking Quality of Long-Term Care and Quality of Life

Linda S. Noelker, PhD and
Zev Harel, PhD, Editors

 Springer Publishing Company

Springer Publishing Company, Inc.
536 Broadway
New York, NY 10012-3955

Acquisitions Editor: Helvi Gold
Production Editor: Jeanne W. Libby
Cover design by Susan Hauley

01 02 03 04 05 / 5 4 3 2 1

Library of Congress Cataloging-in-Publication Data

Linking quality of long term care and quality of life / Linda A. Noelker
and Zev Harel, editors
       p.cm.
    Includes bibliographical references and index.
    ISBN 0-8261-1381-8
    1. Long-term care facilities—Administration.   2. Aged—Long-term
care.   3. Quality of Life.   I. Noelker, Linda S.   II. Harel, Zev.

    RA997 .L565 2000
    362.1'6'068—dc21

                                                            00-045024

Printed in Canada

Contents

Part III   Design and Delivery of Long-Term Care

Contributors

Georgia J. Anetzberger, Ph.D.
Associate Director for Community
Services Division
The Benjamin Rose Institute
Benjamin Rose Center at Margaret
Wagner House
Cleveland Heights, OH

Neena L. Chappell, Ph.D., FRSC
Director, Centre on Aging;
Professor, Department of
Sociology
Centre on Aging
University of Victoria
Victoria, British Columbia,
Canada

J. Kevin Eckert, Ph.D.
Department of Sociology &
Anthropology
University of Maryland Baltimore
County
Baltimore, MD

Farida Kassim Ejaz, Ph.D., L.I.S.W.
Senior Coordinator for Residential
Care Research
Margaret Blenkner Research Center
The Benjamin Rose Institute
Cleveland, OH

**Barry J. Gurland, F.R.C.
(Psychiatry), F.R.C.
(Physicians)**
Sidney Katz Professor of
Psychiatry & Director
Stroud Center on Science of
Quality of Life and Aging
Columbia University
College of Physicians
and Surgeons
New York, NY

Sidney Katz, M.D., M.A.
Professor Emeritus of Geriatric
Medicine & Senior Consultant
and Program Evaluator of
Stroud Center on Science of
Quality of Life and Aging,
Columbia University;
Distinguished Scholar, The
Benjamin Rose Institute
Stroud Center on Science of Life
and Aging
Columbia University
New York, NY

Alice J. Kethley, Ph.D.
Executive Director
The Benjamin Rose Institute
Cleveland, OH

**Gerri S. Lamb, Ph.D., R.N.,
F.A.A.N**
Associate Dean, Clinical and
  Community Services
College of Nursing
University of Arizona
Tuscon, AZ

M. Powell Lawton, Ph.D.
Senior Research Scientist
Philadelphia Geriatric Center
  (TCCC)
Philadelphia, PA

Wendy Lustbader, M.S.W.
Affiliate Assistant Professor,
  University of Washington
  School of Social Work;
  Mental Health Counselor,
  Pike Market Medical Clinic
Seattle, WA

Vincent Mor, Ph.D.
Chairman, Department of
  Community Health; Professor,
  Medical Sciences
Department of Community
  Health
Brown University
Providence, RI

Leslie A. Morgan, Ph.D.
Professor and Chair
Department of Sociology and
  Anthropology
University of Maryland,
  Baltimore County
Baltimore, MD

Charles D. Phillips, Ph.D., M.P.H.
Director and Senior Research
  Scientist
Meyers Research Center
Menorah Park Center for the Aging
Beachwood, OH

Philip D. Sloane, M.D., M.P.H.
Elizabeth and Oscar Goodwin
  Distinguished Professor
Department of Family Medicine
University of North Carolina
Chapel Hill, NC

Sheryl Itkin Zimmerman, Ph.D.
Co-Director and Senior Research
  Fellow, Program on Aging,
  Disablement, and Long-Term Care
Cecil G. Sheps Center for Health
  Services Research
University of North Carolina
Chapel Hill, NC

Foreword

In his book *Zen and the Art of Motorcycle Maintenance*, Robert Pirsig attracted almost cultlike interest in his search for quality. Since then consumer groups and advertisers have continually reminded consumers about the importance of quality. One cannot be exposed to any form of media without being overwhelmed by advertisements promoting the quality of a product or service. What is this thing we call quality and how do we know when we have it in the field of long-term care? Although our efforts to improve the quality of life and care for people experiencing a chronic disability have been considerable, the success of these efforts has been modest. Long-term care remains heavily criticized on both the quality of life and quality of care fronts. As we continue to struggle with these quality issues, this book represents yet another important step in our efforts to make quality in long-term care the norm, rather than the exception.

Why is quality so hard to achieve and regulate in long-term care? In some ways the answer to this question is straightforward. Despite the recent increase in high-tech medical services provided in nursing homes and by home health care agencies, long-term care primarily involves personal assistance. The work is hard, the pay is generally low, the benefits are limited, the majority of workers have little flexibility over their work lives, and competition for workers creates staffing shortages and increased workloads. In most communities teenagers working in fast food establishments earn more than home care, assisted living, or nursing home workers.

In addition to the challenges of recruiting and retaining employees, long-term care providers face intense scrutiny from consumers, regulators, and the media. Some regulatory efforts, such as the OBRA 1987 nursing home reform, have increased quality in some arenas, especially reduced restraint use or reductions in the use of psychotropic drugs. However, there is consensus that quality challenges abound in each of the long-term care settings. Despite a complex regulatory world, and the often repeated statement that nursing homes are second only to nuclear power in their regulatory requirements, few argue that any sector of long-term care is well regulated.

And yet despite these challenges, there are model home care agencies, assisted living facilities, and nursing homes that do not experience the traditional quality problems. Despite facing the aforementioned problems, these agencies have been able to achieve high quality care on a consistent basis. Whether it involves restructuring the environment, changing the nature of the work provided, empowering staff to improve service delivery, increasing resources allocated to workers, training staff in a different manner, or rethinking the paradigm of service delivery, somehow these agencies have figured it out. Our challenge in long-term care is to create a system in which the overwhelming majority of providers can deliver high quality services, rather than a select few.

To achieve this goal, change needs to occur both within individual organizations and within the system. Many of the individual- and system-level change areas are discussed in this volume. For example, long-term care providers in any setting have traditionally lacked good comparative information to assist in making decisions about how to improve practice. Yet the groundwork for quality improvement efforts in any organization involves the development of benchmarks and comparative data to compare one's agency or facility to like organizations over time. The majority of agency, state, and federal policy decisions in long-term care have been made in the absence of such information. With the advent of the MDS in nursing homes and OASIS in home health care we have taken some steps forward to meet this information challenge.

Perhaps the most disturbing criticism is that long-term care has, by and large, ignored consumers. Because of the frailty of many who receive long-term care and the dominance of the health care model, we have received very little input from consumers on the design and overall quality of long-term care services. If we have learned anything from the successes of the total quality management efforts being implemented throughout the world, it is that you must hear the voices of consumers if you are to have a quality product or service.

A final challenge for long-term care concerns the mismatch in the definition of quality between those experiencing a chronic disability compared to informal caregivers and the regulatory environment. Consumers of long-term care consistently tell us that quality for them is having control, choice, and autonomy over the environment they live in and the services they receive. Informal caregivers and regulatory personnel are much more concerned about issues of health and safety. Although we cannot ignore the safety components of people's lives, these are not the issues that dominate the day-to-day lives of most people needing long-term assistance. A better intersection between what is important to consumers and what the regulatory system emphasizes would make quality issues more relevant to both groups.

These and many other important issues are addressed in this volume. We have a great deal of work to do to make long-term care better. This book provides guidance on moving us closer to the goal of making high quality of care and quality of life the norm rather than the exception in long term care .

ROBERT APPLEBAUM
Scripps Gerontology Center
Miami University
Oxford, Ohio

Preface

The primary intent of this book is to promote an emphasis on quality of life as the focal outcome in long-term care services and research and to further understanding of the relationship between quality of care and quality of life. The motivation for the book comes from the challenging mission of The Benjamin Rose Institute, which has been and continues to be "to promote quality of life for older people, their families, and their caregivers through community-based and residential care, research, education, and advocacy." The editors, both of whom have served as Director of Research at the Institute, collaborated for more than 20 years on research projects designed to enhance knowledge about quality of life for long-term care users, especially those who are most vulnerable: minorities, the severely impaired, impoverished, and socially isolated.

The book's first section provides an overview of pivotal issues related to quality of care and quality of life in long-term care. It begins with our chapter that posits that the ultimate goal in long-term care is to ensure the maintenance and, whenever possible, the enhancement of the self for older persons whose care is so closely intertwined with their daily lives. Despite the ravages of chronic illnesses such as Alzheimer's disease, Parkinson's, and Multiple Sclerosis, it is our belief that the persons affected can be cared for in ways that help to preserve what remains of their unique selves. The chapter also sets forth a conceptual model that links preservation of the self to essential qualities of life such as security and autonomy, and how these qualities tie to qualities of caring such as individualized care and respectful treatment. Environmental, structural, organizational, and interpersonal features necessary to ensure that care is provided in ways that contribute to qualities of life in long-term care are identified and elaborated.

The second chapter in this section reviews efforts of regulatory and accrediting bodies to improve the quality of nursing home care and how federally mandated assessment tools and procedures now in place are beginning to lend themselves to examining quality of life. The section's concluding chapter addresses conceptual and methodological approaches to provide quality across the continuum of care. It highlights the limitations of single-setting approaches and offers strategies for a continuum-based approach in outcome assessment. The efficacy of this approach is clear when consideration is given to the multiple transitions between acute and long-term care that occur throughout the course of chronic illnesses as well as different acuity levels in long-term care settings.

The charge set forth to authors of the book's second section was to explore the dimensions of quality of care and quality of life and their interrelationship in specific long-term care settings. Our thinking was that the points of convergence would identify core qualities that crosscut settings and thus serve as the basis for conceptual and measurement advances focused on quality of life. Authors of these chapters highlight the complexities of the issue: the heterogeneity of the population served; the prominence of the nursing home as the locus for long-term care; where authority and responsibility should lie for ensuring quality; and workable methods for evaluating quality that are valid, do not impose intolerable burdens on providers, and are financially viable. These chapters also offer directions for advancing conceptual and measurement efforts for assuring and monitoring quality of care and quality of life in various long-term care settings.

The chapters in the concluding section raise intriguing questions about major shifts in thinking that are needed about the design and delivery of long-term care if we are to achieve the goal of promoting quality of life. These include the importance of removing disciplinary straightjackets that prevent us from implementing a holistic approach to care; listening to and affirming what older persons and their families have to say about their long-term care needs and how they can best be met; and how to implement changes that challenge regulatory and reimbursement restrictions but hold promise of improving quality of life for both the providers and consumers of long-term care.

The Benjamin Rose Institute serves as a case example of the continuous quest by a long-term care provider over the last century to adhere to its mission to improve the quality of life for those whom it serves and the methods it has used to achieve this mission. Lastly, not to be forgotten in this effort to improve the quality of life in long-term care are those whom fewer and fewer acute and long-term care providers willingly serve, the vulnerable elderly, because "without margin there is no mission."

Acknowledgments

We are grateful to the authors for their contributions and patience as we encouraged them to extend their thinking to focus on quality of life and its relationship to quality of care. Their timely responsiveness to our requests reaffirms our belief in collegiality. The Cleveland Foundation and, in particular, its Senior Program Officer, Dr. Robert Eckardt, deserve our thanks for continued support over the past 20 years as we pursued a variety of projects designed to lead to improvements in the quality of life for older persons using long-term care services. Lastly, Sue Miranda graciously took up the task of keeping our work organized and attending to the myriad details involved in assembling the book.

LINDA NOELKER AND ZEV HAREL

PART I

Pivotal Issues

1

Humanizing Long-Term Care: Forging a Link Between Quality of Care and Quality of Life

Linda S. Noelker
Zev Harel

This chapter begins with a review and discussion of long-term and chronic care to place quality of care and quality of life issues in a historical context. It then discusses the concepts of quality of care and quality of life and how they are linked through the process of providing care to the maintenance and enhancement of the self. Third, environmental, structural, organizational, and interpersonal factors that support the process of caring and the enhancement of qualities of care and life are covered. The chapter concludes with the implications of this linkage for efforts to improve the quality of life for older persons with chronic illnesses and impairments requiring long-term care services.

LONG-TERM CARE: AN OVERVIEW

Long-term care refers to the provision of a range of services to individuals who require assistance with daily activities because of chronic illnesses and functional impairments. About 12.8 million Americans require long-term care, most (57%) are aged 65 or older, and 2.4 million are institutionalized (National Academy on Aging, 1997). Historically, family members, predominately wives, daughters, and daughters-in-law, have done the yeoman's share of long-term care. More recently, concerns have been raised about whether this trend will continue in view of changes in family structure and labor force participation that are likely to limit women's ability and willingness to serve as unpaid caregivers (Binstock, Cluff, & von Mering, 1996). Should this occur, as recent research suggests (Pezzin & Schone, 1999), future generations of older and chronically impaired persons will rely to a greater extent on formal providers of long-term care.

When families or other informal caregivers were unable or unwilling to provide assistance, those in need of long-term care have typically entered institutions, primarily nursing homes. The close tie between nursing homes and long-term care inadvertently resulted from the evolution of institutional care in this nation, leading to the steady growth in the nursing home industry over the last 40 years. As Holstein and Cole (1996) point out, some knowledge about the historical evolution of long-term care is necessary to understand its current state and how it continues to affect the quality of care and quality of life for its users. According to their analysis, long-term care began with almshouses and poor farms established during the last century to shelter the impoverished who had no informal caregivers. Eventually, these institutions became home for all needing long-term care, including the aged, those with physical and mental illnesses, and the developmentally disabled.

Societal values and norms during this period equated poverty and frailty, even in old age, with personal failure. As a result, those in need of ongoing assistance were devalued and viewed as requiring surveillance, discipline, and reform. Religious institutions, fraternal organizations, and private charities also constructed homes for the aged during this period. However, this care was intended only for deserving older persons of good character and members of their own associations and organizations. Thus, publicly funded care and charitable care was colored by moral disapproval and a paternalistic stance that expected passivity and submissiveness from recipients. To this day, issues of autonomy and personal choice continue to dominate discussion and debate about ways to improve the quality of care and quality of life for users of long-term care (Gamroth, Semradek, & Tornquist, 1995).

Other events in this century further strengthened the tie between long-term care services and nursing homes (Holstein & Cole, 1996). The signal event was the passage of the Social Security Act in 1935 that provided economic benefits but not health security for older Americans. A key provision of the act was that Old Age Assistance funds could not be used to pay for the support of older persons in public institutions which had come to be seen as a deplorable end of life for the long-lived. The intent was that these public institutions, formerly almshouses, would become obsolete when indigent elderly were provided with economic support enabling them to remain in their own homes. This provision addressed poverty as the reason why older persons were admitted to public institutions, yet it did not address the impact of chronic illness and infirmity as a cause. Thus, frail residents in public institutions who needed personal assistance were forced into proprietary or philanthropic nursing homes in order to receive both financial and personal care assistance.

The growth of the nursing home industry as the locus for long-term care was further advanced by federally authorized loans made available for their construction as well as direct federal loans and loan guarantees. The bulk of these dollars for the construction of new facilities went to for-profit providers through loans authorized by the Small Business Administration and Federal Housing Authority. Furthermore, the enactment of Medicare and Medicaid offered reimbursement for institution-based long-term care but not for home or community-based care. As a result, proprietary nursing homes came to dominate the long-term care landscape, resulting in the development of strong nursing home lobbies at both state and federal levels. Their influence is still evident from the disproportionate expenditures made by many states for nursing home care compared to home- and community-based care, although in some states there has been a shift toward greater support for home- and community-based care (Kane, Kane, & Ladd, 1998).

Holstein and Cole's analysis (1996), as well as those by others (Applebaum, 1998; Chassin, Galvin, & The National Roundtable on Health Care Quality, 1998; Kane et al., 1998; Morris, Caro, & Hansan, 1998), lead to the conclusion that long-term care in this nation has been neither carefully planned nor deliberately designed. Rather, it has evolved haphazardly subject to changing political, economic, governmental, and market forces. Although billions of dollars have been spent on it and the amount continues to increase, there is widespread agreement that its quality has continued to be compromised by a host of factors. Some of these include the bias toward nursing home care by elected officials, effective lobbying by the nursing home industry, poor regulation, inequities in access and reimbursement, and a lack of responsiveness to user preferences. Perhaps equally important is the lack of leadership at federal and state levels in crafting long-term care policy and linking it with housing policy to ensure the development of a system of integrated health, social, and personal care services with a variety of residential options.

An examination of factors that pose threats to the quality of long-term care would not be complete without addressing issues related to the integration of acute and long-term care across the continuum of care settings. Acute care generally refers to hospital care and medical care provided by physicians and other health care practitioners. Long-term care, as defined earlier, refers to ongoing assistance with daily activities due to chronic illness and disability. It has been argued, however, that this is a false dichotomy and a more appropriate term is "chronic care" which encompasses both acute and long-term care (Kane, 1999). In fact, older persons in need of long-term care are major users of acute care as well, hence the need for their integration.

Integration refers to the connections that exist between care settings around information transfer, care plan design and implementation, service delivery, and outcome monitoring to ensure that there is no under, over, or misuse of services. There are several obstacles that challenge the integration of care and thus have the potential to compromise both the quality of care and quality of life. Throughout the course of long-term care, acute episodes occur due to illness or injury. These episodes result in transfers between long-term and acute care settings, more specifically, from nursing home to hospital. After hospitalization, care recipients are often transferred to another setting for post-acute or rehabilitative care before returning to their more permanent residence (e.g., board and care home, assisted living facility, nursing home). The length of time spent in these settings tends to be brief, making it difficult to pinpoint exactly where less than adequate care occurred and who is directly responsible when there are negative outcomes. Thus, accountability for the outcomes of care is more problematic when long-term care users move through various care settings or levels of care that are not integrated. Furthermore, there are as yet no agreed on core measures of quality of care across the continuum of care settings to determine variations from setting to setting (Kane & Kane, 1988; Mor, chapter 3).

The establishment of effective transitions between acute and long-term care settings is further complicated because one professional discipline (medicine) dominates in acute care, while long-term care by its nature demands interdisciplinary teams of professionals. Furthermore, most professionals have relatively little contact with the users of long-term care compared to nursing assistants and home care workers who provide virtually all the direct care. The outcomes of interest in acute and long-term care also differ in that the focus in acute care is on narrowly defined health-related outcomes. In long-term care, a broader focus on quality of life is required since these settings provide the locale for ongoing experiences of life along with the provision of long-term care. The differences in the philosophy, structure, organization, and delivery of acute and long-term care pose obstacles to bridging the two systems. Leutz (1999) points out that the lack of integration poses the greatest peril for a particular segment of the long-term care population, and this segment should be singled out for inclusion in fully integrated systems. The segment includes vulnerable older individuals who have more unstable and severe conditions, more urgent needs for intervention, and limited capacity for self-direction.

QUALITY OF CARE

Despite the prevalent state of fragmentation between chronic and long-term care and other obstacles, significant efforts have been made during the last 2 decades to advance the conceptualization and measurement of quality of care and, to a lesser extent, quality of life. Research and practice attention to quality of care has a lengthier history than attention to quality of life, a concept seen as less amenable to scientific investigation (Birren & Deutchman, 1991). Efforts to develop quality assurance techniques and health-related quality of care measures have been pursued more aggressively in the acute care sector (Kane & Kane, 1988). In the 1950s, for example, research began to focus on the process of health care and the evaluation of physician practice, often finding major deficiencies (Wagner, 1988). More rigorous scientific work that developed quality indicators for the care process and related quality outcome measures for acute care has been underway for 25 years, producing a growing inventory of useful measures (Chassin et al., 1998).

Much of the work on quality of care has been guided by Donabedian's framework (1980) emphasizing the components of structure, process, and outcomes. Early attempts to assess and regulate quality of care focused on structural features, that is, characteristics of the setting in which care was provided such as room size, training and credentialing of staff, and staff to resident ratios. These features have come to be viewed as relatively crude measures of quality (Donabedian, 1988; Romeis & Coe, 1991). Subsequent efforts have been directed to the care process and outcomes of care. The care process refers to what is done (appropriateness of care), when it is done (its timeliness), and how well it is done (technical proficiency). Significant efforts have been expended to develop process measures, such as care pathways in hospital settings, to manage the care of patients with specific chronic diseases such as chronic obstructive pulmonary disease or diabetes who were experiencing an acute episode and in need of more intensive and highly technical care.

The current emphasis in integrated delivery systems is on the development of extended care pathways (ECPs) that cut across settings for the purpose of providing "seamless" care (Buckle, 1997). This means that all necessary care is properly provided in a timely manner regardless of transitions across settings in order to optimize the patient's recovery and minimize iatrogenic effects. Considerable time and expense are required to develop and implement these tools for seamless care because they require cross-functional, interdisciplinary teams that span all the services involved in the care process throughout its entirety (Buckle, 1997).

To date, care indicators and outcomes have received the lion's share of attention for monitoring the quality of long-term care. Care indicators are widely regarded as key to quality assurance and regulatory practices (Sainfort, Ramsay, & Monato, 1995). They also appear to lend themselves to relatively straightforward measurement (Romeis & Coe, 1991). The emphasis on quality of care was strengthened by the implementation of the Patient Care and Services system in 1986 (Zimmerman, 1991) and by the Omnibus Budget Reconciliation Act (OBRA-87) requiring routine and uniform assessments of residents, with this information serving as the basis for the development of quality outcomes (Phillips, chapter 8). It should be noted, however, that Donabedian's (1988) original intent was to consider the three components of structure, process, and outcomes when assessing quality, as well as the amenities and interpersonal dimensions of care.

Attention to care outcomes in the area of home-based services was spurred by implementation of the prospective payment system for hospitals, followed by an increase in "quicker and sicker" discharges to home, and by the provision of more highly technical care in the home. A conceptual framework for assessing quality in home health care has been proposed based on Donabedian's model that includes focused process and outcome measures related to the care delivered to similar groups of patients (Shaughnessy et al., 1994). The diversity of home care service users and the environments in which they reside result in a wide variety of factors that can affect outcomes apart from the home care services themselves. For these reasons, the model links process and outcome measures in order to determine which aspects of care are problematic. Most home care providers have developed problem-specific standards or guidelines for comparison with the actual care given to determine where greater technical proficiency is needed to improve the care process. Furthermore, all Medicare-certified home care agencies are currently required to collect routine assessment information using the Outcome and Assessment Information Set (OASIS) for standardized risk-adjusted outcome reporting, similar to the use of Minimum Data Set (MDS) reporting by skilled nursing facilities (Shaughnessy, Crisler, & Schlenker, 1998).

It is apparent that the model developed for nursing homes dominates conceptual and empirical approaches to quality of care in long-term care settings. This has resulted from their major role in long-term care and the federal mandate to improve the quality of nursing home care by tightening regulatory standards, the review process, and enforcement procedures. Yet, some have argued that despite the sophisticated tools and measurement procedures developed to assess and monitor quality of care in nursing homes, the concept of quality and its relationship to organizational characteristics remains unclear (Sainfort et al., 1995). Questions also have been raised about the appropriateness of applying models and techniques developed for evaluating the quality of acute care to long-term care in view of the narrowness of outcomes used in acute care. As noted earlier, differences in the philosophy, structure, organization, and delivery of acute and long-term care suggest that new paradigms and models are needed that take a far broader, multidimensional approach to quality, in contrast to the medically based focus on physical health and functioning. The application of acute care models for quality assurance and quality indicators and outcomes to long-term care, even when modified or adapted, is likely to be ineffectual especially when the larger purpose of improving quality of care is to optimize quality of life. Additionally, their application may continue to thwart the creative thinking required to reengineer long-term care services and settings into "development-enhancing and age-friendly environments" in which older persons can flourish (Baltes & Baltes, 1990).

QUALITY OF LIFE

In 1987, Levine argued in a seminal article that quality of life was emerging as the major criterion for evaluating health interventions. The basis for this stance was that medicine has failed to respond to the social dimension in health and illness that takes on overriding significance in the case of chronic illness. More specifically, social meanings and the social context of health and illness, competing definitions of the situation, social roles and networks, and individual lifestyles shape the outcomes of health care. He defined the forces driving this paradigm shift as the tremendous increase in persons with chronic illnesses that can be managed but not cured, new technologies that present ethical questions about the quality of end-of-life care, and social movements (consumerism, feminism) that have challenged health care providers to humanize health care.

In their overview of quality of life, Birren and Deutchman (1991) note that attention to this concept continues to increase because of the threats that later-life frailty poses to quality of life, especially in residential long-term care settings. Quality of life becomes a key issue in the case of chronic illnesses, particularly when dementing disorders are involved, because of their potential to rob the individual of his or her sense of self by forcing unwanted changes in living environment, lifestyle, social relationships, and interaction with others. Consequently, researchers and clinicians are continuing to advance new conceptualizations of quality of life in later years, distinguishing among those that are global, health-related, and disease-specific (Brod, Stewart, & Sands, 1999).

More global conceptualizations of quality of life include Lawton's (1991) multidimensional view involving both subjective and objective evaluations of the person-environment system of an individual in past, present, and future time. His framework includes two central sectors of quality of life: behavioral competence and perceived quality of life. Behavioral competence is viewed as hierarchial, moving from the dimensions of health, functioning, and time use to social behavior. This component requires objective assessment by performance or observation. In contrast, perceived quality of life is inherently subjective, involving evaluation of functioning in the behavioral competence dimensions. The two other sectors of quality of life include environment and psychological well-being. Environment has a necessary but not sufficient influence on behavioral competence and perceived quality of life by providing the external context in which interactions occur between a person and the environment. Psychological well-being is defined as the ultimate outcome or the "weighted" evaluation of all competencies and perceived quality of life. The weighting process is the self or the schema that is formed proactively and reactively, providing a template for interpreting all experiences.

In contrast to global conceptualizations of quality of life, health-related quality of life refers to how various health conditions, treatment regimens, and projected outcomes affect patient preferences for care and their desire to live. The consistent finding from research in this area is that people prefer to trade off more years of life for fewer years of higher quality (Lawton et al., 1999). Wieland, Rubenstein, and Hirsch (1995) have identified clinical quality of life as one type of health-related quality of life construct that is key to improving the quality of life in nursing homes. Investigation of clinical quality of life requires a thorough diagnostic assessment of the resident's health status and functioning, prognosis (suffering a particular health outcome and experience of treatment), and evaluation of the resident's preferences for outcome and process. One method used to investigate residents' treatment choices are time trade-offs (TTOs) that weigh the resident's preferences for trading off a shorter but better life for a more extended but compromised life. They contend that the application of this approach is essential to making quality of life the focal outcome in nursing homes. It would do so by ensuring that the basis for care planning is determining and enacting residents' preferences and values, thereby broadening care plans to include individualized social, spiritual, and other activities that enhance quality of life.

More recently, Lawton et al. (1999) have introduced another concept, valuation of life, that appears to clarify the relative influence of more global constructs of quality of life and health-related constructs on desired years of life. Valuation of life (VOL) is seen as a mediator between the multidimensional construct, quality of life, and years of desired life. It is defined as a dynamic cognitive-affective thought process in which a variety of external factors (environment, social networks, status) and intrapersonal factors (health, competence, cognition, mental pathology) are weighed and influence decision making about how long one wishes to live. Their research on the quality of life concept suggests that it represents an important intrapsychic process by which individuals assess a complex variety of health- and non-health-related factors that result in strong or weak valuations of life. Their findings also underscore the potency of *non-health-related* sources of quality of life that equal health-related sources as influences on the wish to live.

Disease-specific quality of life constructs have been developed in response to the diverse course and outcomes of a wide variety of diseases and to better assess the effects of specific treatments and interventions (Logsdon & Albert, 1999). Within the last decade, substantially more conceptual and empirical attention has been given to quality of life for older persons with Alzheimer's disease. Prior to the current decade, questions were raised as to whether it were even possible for persons with this disorder to experience quality of life (Brod et al., 1999). Because the subjective component is essential to quality of life, it poses a particular challenge in dementia quality of life research since persons with the disease eventually lose the ability to communicate their perceptions. Another challenge is that throughout the course of the illness the person often moves through different care settings (independent, assisted, skilled nursing care), and the impact of environmental change as well as effects of each environment must be taken into consideration when evaluating quality of life (Logsdon & Albert, 1999).

One proposed dementia quality of life model focuses on the individual's subjective experience and evaluation of life circumstance in five domains including aesthetics, positive affect, negative affect, self-esteem, and feelings of belonging that can be assessed using the Dementia Quality of Life (D-QoL) Instrument (Brod et al., 1999). It is premised on the assumption that although objectively measurable mental, social, and financial factors affect dementia-specific quality of life, it is the individual's evaluation of personal circumstances that ultimately defines quality of life. Preliminary research on the model indicates the instrument adequately assesses the five domains, each of which demonstrates acceptable internal consistency.

A different conceptual approach that evolved from research on special care units for residents with Alzheimer's disease set forth by Lawton (chapter 6) proposes that a new approach and methods are needed to assess resident quality of life. This approach focuses on relationships between positive and negative affect expressed by residents and environmental features of the facility. It employs a wide variety of data collection methods to represent subjective and objective aspects of quality. Similar to others cited in this chapter, Lawton maintains that quality of life rather than quality of care should be the primary focus in long-term care, and he defines quality of care as the quality of operations that meet the residents' basic needs (cleanliness, nutrition, elimination).

Glass (1991), however, distinguishes quality of *caring* from quality of *care* as key to quality of life in nursing homes. Traditional quality of care approaches focus on the skill levels of staff, the appropriateness of medical and physical care, and adherence to standard guidelines and procedures for providing this care. Quality of caring, in contrast, refers to the nature of staff and resident interaction that is as important to quality of life as the quality of care received. The traditional emphasis on technical proficiencies in care as they relate to health and functional outcomes stands in contrast to the fact that most chronic care involves routine, non-technical, and time-consuming assistance with personal care tasks and activities of daily living.

Most of this care is given by nursing assistants and home care workers who receive minimal training and the lowest pay in health care, yet they are the backbone of long-term care services. As an older person becomes frailer and more dependent on these workers, the manner in which they interact with the person as they provide care can enhance or undermine the self, thereby affecting quality of life. Kahana (in press) has incorporated this emphasis on interaction as the core of the "Patient Responsive Model of Care," which is predicated on systematic and empathetic discernment of residents' preferences and perspectives by staff. Older service consumers and their family members also emphasize qualities of interaction, such as being treated with dignity and respect, as the most important features of long-term care services (Cohn & Sugar, 1991; Harrington et al., 1999; Kane et al., 1998; National Citizens' Coalition for Nursing Home Reform, 1985). However, the environment, structure, and organization of work in nursing homes often do not support the qualities of caring that affirm and maintain the older person's sense of self.

LINKING QUALITY OF CARE AND QUALITY OF LIFE

Tobin (1999) has written extensively about preservation of the self in later life and the challenges to this process presented by adverse life events and losses, including changes in residence. In long-term care settings where older persons cannot control where and with whom they live, social interaction with others, and their daily schedule and activities, the self becomes increasingly vulnerable. His research on preservation of the self among residents in nursing homes led him to conclude that the psychosocial quality of care is paramount to the successfulness of this process. The four components of quality psychosocial care include: the warmth of staff and resident relationships; the availability of personally meaningful activities and stimulation; tolerance for resident deviance such as aggression, wandering, and incontinence; and the extent to which residents are perceived and treated as individuals, or individuation (Tobin, 1999).

These components relate to the eight types of coping techniques Tobin observed in residents struggling to maintain the integrity of the self in later life. He defined four types as rational based on their relationship to reality, while the other four "less rational" types are the ones likely to present significant challenges for staff. The more rational ones include: 1) involvement in meaningful activities that affirm the core self; 2) control over daily activities and interactions; 3) contracting one's personal space, sense of future time, and range of relationships for better personal management; and 4) downward social comparisons. The latter refers to the cognitive process of selectively seeking out others in the environment that can be defined as worse off in order to protect or enhance the self. Heidrich and Ryff (1993) hypothesized that this and other cognitive processes utilized by the self system mediate between the actual losses experienced in later life and psychological functioning (morale, life satisfaction, subjective health). Hence, even elderly persons with severe health and functional impairments can demonstrate unexpectedly high levels of subjective well-being. The mediation process also helps to explain why physicians and other health care providers rate ill older persons as having a poorer quality of life than older persons themselves (Birren & Deutchman, 1991).

The four less rational coping techniques are 1) magical mastery in which reality is ignored or denied; 2) verbal and physical aggressiveness under stress; 3) functional paranoia or blaming others to reduce feelings of vulnerability; and 4) acceptance of repressed material that helps to clarify the core self. These techniques, particularly aggressiveness, blaming others, and denial of reality, can tax the patience of long-term care staff and ultimately demoralize them if they do not comprehend their role in the older individual's quest to preserve the self. Yet, the limited training given to long-term care staff, especially direct care staff (nursing assistants and home care workers), emphasizes the technical proficiencies of care rather than the psychosocial aspects of caring.

Inadequate training is just one feature of the structure, organization, and delivery of long-term care that compromises the quality of caring and thus quality of life. The planning, organization, and delivery of services that promote quality of life for older persons using these services at home, in the community, or in long-term-care settings have to be seen as the over-riding goal by public officials, decision makers, and professionals. Enhancing quality of life entails enabling the older person to remain in his or her environment of choice or, if this is not possible, providing high quality alternative living environments and the gratification of basic and higher level needs to ensure the maintenance and enhancement of the self.

While this orientation is equally applicable across chronic care settings, it is formulated in the following pages for nursing homes because of their greater potential as total institutions to undermine the self (Goffman, 1961).

Figure 1.1 depicts the relationships between some environmental, structural, organizational, and interpersonal features necessary for care providers to embody the key qualities of caring. The qualities of caring are linked to qualities of life for residents that enable them to maintain and enhance the self. The care provider requirements under the four domains are not comprehensive but meant to illustrate how these domains can affect the qualities of caring exhibited by staff that in turn promote qualities of life for residents to help preserve and enhance the self. Although the qualities of caring refer to all care providers, the narrative focus is on care provided by nursing assistants because they have the most direct and extensive involvement with residents. The first two domains, environmental and structural, and the qualities of caring to which they relate (safe, timely, and technically proficient care) have been given the most attention by regulators, accrediting bodies, and legislators. The organizational and interpersonal domains have a significant influence on the provision of individualized and respectful care that enhances resident autonomy, well-being, and affirmation of self, qualities essential for maintenance and enhancement of the self.

Environmental Requirements for Quality Care and Quality of Life

The environmental domain includes three features necessary for care to be delivered in a safe and timely manner, thereby enhancing the residents' sense of security. A hazard-free environment and adequate and accessible supplies are important for minimizing injuries to staff. According to the Bureau of Labor Statistics, nursing home workers have the second highest rate of non-fatal, job-related injuries after automobile manufacturers (Buss, 1995). In 1994, nursing home workers experienced more than 221,000 injuries or about 16.9 per 100 workers. When nursing assistants have to search for supplies, do not have equipment such as a Hoyer lift readily available, or do not know how to use it properly, the safety and timeliness of resident care is compromised, diminishing residents' sense of security. Research also shows that the availability of supplies is associated with higher job satisfaction and lower rates of burnout and demoralization (Ramirez, Teresi, Holmes, & Fairchild, 1998). This suggests that available supplies can help to reduce burnout and promote job satisfaction among nursing assistants and, correspondingly, result in greater continuity in the relationships between residents and those who care for them.

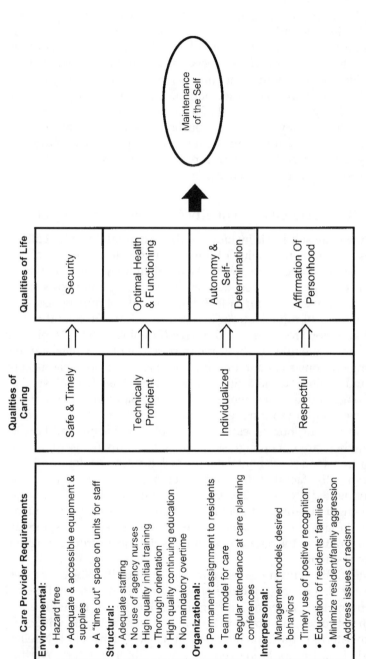

Care Provider Requirements

Environmental:
- Hazard free
- Adequate & accessible equipment & supplies
- A "time out" space on units for staff

Structural:
- Adequate staffing
- No use of agency nurses
- High quality initial training
- Thorough orientation
- High quality continuing education
- No mandatory overtime

Organizational:
- Permanent assignment to residents
- Team model for care
- Regular attendance at care planning conferences

Interpersonal:
- Management models desired behaviors
- Timely use of positive recognition
- Education of residents' families
- Minimize resident/family aggression
- Address issues of racism

Qualities of Caring

Safe & Timely

Technically Proficient

Individualized

Respectful

Qualities of Life

Security

Optimal Health & Functioning

Autonomy & Self-Determination

Affirmation Of Personhood

Maintenance of the Self

FIGURE 1.1   Relationships between requirements for care providers, quality of caring and quality of life for residents in long-term care.

15

The third feature in this domain, a time-out space for staff, affords those working in residential care a private space to which they can retreat for a few minutes when they feel overwhelmed or losing control of their feelings or behavior. This feature is especially important when staff are caring for older persons with dementing disorders manifested by aggressive behaviors that may lead to retaliation. The availability of time-out space can significantly reduce the staff's negative reactions to disruptive residents and, hence, may result in less burnout and resident abuse. Taken together, these three environmental features can help to create a work setting that is safer for both direct care providers and residents, thereby enhancing residents' sense of security.

Structural Requirements for Quality Care and Quality of Life

Although adequate staffing is included in the structural domain, it affects all qualities of caring and quality of life. Qualitative research shows that nursing assistants have more work to do than they can accomplish (Bowers & Becker, 1992). A seven-state study of nursing home costs found that residents receive an average of 77 minutes daily of nursing assistant care, compared to 16 minutes from licensed practical nurses and only 8 minutes of attention from registered nurses (Friedlob, 1993). Despite the wealth of empirical evidence about the importance of adequate staffing, short staffing is a consistent and uniform complaint by nursing assistants, residents, and families (Cohn & Sugar, 1991; Cohen-Mansfield & Noelker, 2000). Although nurse to resident ratios are regulated by state government, the levels require routine reexamination as the acuity level continues to rise in nursing homes, especially in sub-, post-acute and hospice units. When there are not enough staff available, a nursing assistant may try to lift or transfer a resident alone if the task needs to be done and time is short, despite the fact that the resident requires a two-person lift. This practice undoubtedly contributes to the high rate of job-related injuries among nursing assistants and places the safety and security of residents in jeopardy. In fact, the most common injuries to nursing assistants are sprains and strains to the back and shoulders that result from lifting and transferring residents.

Adequate staffing encompasses more than meeting nursing staff to resident ratios. It also refers to the use of staff who are not overly fatigued and thus in greater danger of injuring themselves or residents. It is not uncommon for nursing assistants to be asked to work a double shift, come in early, stay late, or come in on their day off (Cohen-Mansfield & Noelker, 2000; Teresi et al., 1993a). Moreover, the practice of mandatory overtime in skilled nursing facilities is not uncommon. This practice requires nursing assistants to work over shift and, if they refuse, they are disciplined, including dismissal for repeated refusals. Mandatory overtime can create havoc with one's personal life, especially if the staff member has child care or transportation plans in place that fall apart when required to work a second shift. Mandatory overtime is one work-related stress that, along with personal sources of stress from family and financial worries common among nursing assistants, compromise their ability to engage in the qualities of caring necessary for resident quality of life (Chappell & Novak, 1992; Cohen-Mansfield & Noelker, 2000; Foner, 1994; Tellis-Nyak & Tellis-Nyak, 1989).

Reasons for mandatory overtime are the high rates of tardiness, absenteeism, and turnover among staff in skilled nursing facilities. Turnover among nursing staff is one of the most serious problems in nursing homes and can run as high as over 100% annually among nursing assistants (Helmer, Olsen, & Heim, 1993; Wagnild, 1988). Some nursing assistants welcome the overtime work to supplement their meager wages, while others take a second job or are on call with an agency in their off hours in addition to their full-time job. The long work hours increase nursing assistants' vulnerability to injury as they provide care to residents and perform other strenuous physical labor. Yet, the overtime work and additional jobs are necessary for many of these workers, especially those who are single female heads of households with dependents to support on an inadequate wage.

Another feature in the structural domain related to adequate staffing is to avoid or minimize use of agency nurses. These licensed nurses and nursing assistants from temporary placement agencies enable facilities to meet staffing requirements but at an excessively high cost. Temporary nurses are not familiar with the facility's physical plant, the location of supplies and equipment, care procedures and routines, the other staff, and, most importantly, the residents. They have little reason to be committed to the residents and qualities of caring since they have no future at the nursing home. Because they are unfamiliar with the residents and their conditions, the care they give may be technically proficient but certainly not individualized. Moreover, their presence engenders resentment among the other nursing assistants who are well aware that temporary nurses earn a higher hourly wage, in addition to the fee the facility pays to the temporary agency.

There is substantial research indicating that both the initial training and continuing education of frontline workers are inadequate, particularly in the area of care for cognitively impaired elderly (Hallberg & Norberg, 1995; Moss, Swanson, Specht, & Buckwalter, 1994; Stevens, Burgio, Bailey, Burgio, Paul et al., 1998; Teresi et al., 1993a). The initial 75 hours of training mandated by OBRA-87 are insufficient to prepare frontline staff to provide technically proficient care with bathing, dressing, feeding, and elimination, much less prepare them to provide the psychosocial care necessary to enhance quality of life and preservation of the self. In the state of Ohio as in other states, cosmetologists are required to receive more training (1,500 hours) than frontline workers before they can be licensed. The mandatory 12 hours of annual continuing education repeatedly covers safety and security issues such as fire safety and universal precautions, resulting in complaints that the sessions are "boring" and "have nothing to do with the work" (Schur, Noelker, Looman, Whitlatch, & Ejaz, 1998). As a result, frontline workers feel unsure about the adequacy of their training in managing behavior problems (Burgio & Burgio, 1990). In fact, one team of researchers investigating nursing assistant training on special and non-special care units described the picture with respect to training as "dismal" (Teresi et al., 1993a).

An additional requirement to foster the desired qualities of caring is an adequate orientation process for newly hired frontline workers, especially those who are new to this work. Some agencies and facilities do not provide a formal orientation program, while others conduct orientation sessions that emphasize policies and procedures. A thorough orientation ensures that new workers are oriented to the environment in which they will work, including the background, life histories, coping styles, and current conditions of older persons who will be in their care. They will be also properly oriented to the facility's operational procedures, equipment, and supplies, and the work styles of their peers and supervisor. In the event that nursing assistants will be working on other units rather than permanently assigned to certain residents on one unit, an orientation to all other units on which they will work is necessary.

Organizational Requirements for Quality Care and Quality of Life

The three organizational features included in Figure 1.1 are permanent assignment of frontline workers to residents or clients, a team model for care, and the presence of all providers who care for the older person, including frontline workers, at care planning conferences. These features maximize the workers' opportunities to establish ongoing relationships with those in their care, thereby learning about their backgrounds, lifestyles, and preferences, and current conditions, and sharing this information with other staff involved in the care. By implementing these organizational features, frontline workers and other team members are enabled to provide individualized care that is responsive to the older person's personal style and preferences, which promote personal autonomy.

The basis of the team model for care is enhanced communication among staff, older consumers, and members of their families to enrich the personal information available to staff that can be used to individualize care. The team model also levels the traditional nursing staff hierarchy in skilled nursing facilities by getting the licensed nurses out from behind their desks and onto the units where they work along with nursing assistants on resident care, especially when there are call-offs and staff are "working short." A key feature of the team's operation is that nursing assistants are regularly included in care planning conferences at which their input is solicited and its importance is acknowledged. Their regular inclusion also reinforces the fact that they have the most contact with residents and hence their observations and opinions about resident preferences, functioning, and needs are essential to the formulation and revision of care plans.

The model also can be used to incorporate family members into the team because they can provide staff with the most extensive and detailed information about the resident. For this reason, family members should be encouraged to attend care planning conferences at which their suggestions for individualizing care can be explored since many served as the resident's caregiver prior to nursing home entry. Care planning conferences, however, are typically scheduled during normal working hours thus employed family members often find it impossible to attend. In addition to bringing in family photos, furnishings, mementos, and other objects to personalize the resident's space, family members should be encouraged to visit and interact constructively with nursing staff to help them better understand and appreciate the resident as an individual. Research on the team or primary care model in nursing homes that incorporates the practice of permanent assignment and team meetings suggests that it is associated with less burnout among nursing assistants (Teresi et al., 1993b).

Interpersonal Requirements for Quality Care and Quality of Life

It has been widely acknowledged in the literature that the nursing home environments are highly interactive. Yet, research suggests that the interaction among staff, residents, and their families is not affectively neutral but that expressions of negative rather than positive affect can come to dominate the socioemotional milieu (Noelker & Poulshock, 1982; Pillemer & Moore, 1989). Evidence suggests that at all levels of staffing, there are consistent complaints about a lack of recognition and respect for the work done. These circumstances place added burdens on staff who are expected to provide individualized and respectful care for residents and their families when they themselves do not feel recognized and respected for their work.

One consequence of the lack of recognition and respect is unacceptably high rates of turnover in nursing homes at all staffing levels. Findings from a survey of nursing home administrators in Michigan and Indiana revealed a 40% annual turnover rate; administrators' perceptions that their supervisor did not view them as performing well, treated them unfairly, and did not value their opinions were related to greater turnover (Singh & Schwab, 1998). Similarly, a study of registered nurses, licensed practical nurses, and nurses aides in North Carolina nursing facilities revealed annual turnover rates of 36%, 54%, and 69%, respectively (Halbur & Fears, 1986), while another cited the annual turnover rate for nurses at 65% (Huey, 1990). Conversely, nursing staff in long-term care who report greater cohesiveness, teamwork, coworkers as friends, and feel those in their care recognize their work, are more committed to the facility, and satisfied with their job (Fisher-Robertson & Cummings, 1991; Francis-Felsen et al., 1996).

Unfortunately, interaction among persons in nursing homes often goes beyond lacking respect and involves aggression. Because 60 to 90% of the residents in nursing homes have Alzheimer's disease or other types of dementia, they experience perceptual distortions and misinterpret cues in the environment. The stimulation surrounding personal care activities such as bathing can elicit feelings of helplessness that may escalate to catastrophic reactions and violent behaviors that are directed at nursing staff (Berg, 1991; Dougherty, Bolger, Preston, Jones, & Payne, 1992; Everitt, Fields, Soumerai, & Avorn, 1991; Lusk, 1992). Some of these behaviors include yelling, swearing, hair pulling, scratching, kicking, hitting, and spitting, the latter being viewed by nursing assistants as the most offensive.

These behaviors by residents, however, tend to be understood by nursing assistants as a consequence of the resident's disease or disorder rather than as personal attacks. Mistreatment by residents' families is less easily explained. When residents have dementia, family members are more involved in making decisions about and monitoring care, and nursing assistants are frequently a target for family members' frustrations when care does not meet their expectations (Tellis-Nyak & Tellis-Nyak, 1989; Zarit & Whitlatch, 1992). In fact, one investigation of aggression toward nursing staff in 70 Florida facilities showed that administrators reported 1,193 acts of verbal aggression and 13 acts of physical aggression over a 6-month period (Vinton & Mazza, 1994). Even less flagrant behaviors by family members can have damaging effects on nursing assistants' enjoyment of and commitment to their job. One study showed that nursing assistants' perceptions of disrespect by residents' families, manifested by a lack of understanding of their workload, unrealistic expectations, and inappropriate requests, had a strong relationship to job dissatisfaction and thus potentially to turnover (Noelker, Schur, Looman, Ejaz, & Whitlatch, in revision). Tobin (1999, p. 210) concluded that it is impossible to develop a "home" for residents unless underpaid and unappreciated nursing assistants are themselves individualized and insulated from disrespect and verbal abuse by residents' families.

Another cause of negative interaction in residential care facilities is racism expressed as racial slurs and stereotyping (Dougherty et al., 1992; Holmes, Ramirez, & Fairchild, 1994; Tellis-Nyak & Tellis-Nyak, 1989). Research by Ramirez and her colleagues (1998) found that significant predictors of nursing assistant job burnout included stress related to ethnic and racial conflict. This source of stress refers to nursing assistants' perceptions that residents were biased toward them based on the nursing assistant's ethnic background. For example, nursing assistants who perceived that the residents thought they would not do a good job or unjustly accused them of things because of the nursing assistant's race were more likely to report burnout. Their work underscores previous findings by Grau and Wellin (1992) that nursing home subcultures develop based on differences in occupational status and ethnic background, and the subcultures cause tensions in the facility's interpersonal climate when administration fails to address them.

The irony of this situation is that many of the care provider requirements listed in Figure 1.1 are not costly or time-consuming with the exception of adequate staffing and staff training. The team model for care described above as an approach for individualizing care can also serve to promote respectful interaction among staff. Studies of staff relations in residential care facilities indicate that poor staff cohesiveness, lack of recognition, and being criticized and not praised are linked to job-related stress and dissatisfaction (Carr & Kazanowski, 1994; Dunn, Rout, Carson, & Ritter, 1994). Another investigation found that the quality of work relationships in both acute and long-term care settings was the strongest predictor of burnout (Hare, Pratt, & Andrews, 1988). Moreover, a lack of cohesion among coworkers and a lack of support from supervisors resulting in burnout have a cyclical effect by causing further deterioration in staff relationships and greater burnout.

CONCLUSIONS

As indicated in earlier pages of this chapter, health and human service scholars and researchers consistently conclude that long-term care in this nation has been neither carefully planned nor deliberately designed. Rather, it has evolved haphazardly subject to changing political, economic, governmental, and market forces. The cost of long-term care has steadily increased during the second half of the twentieth century, and the amount will continue to increase in the future. There is widespread agreement, however, that the quality of care will continue to be determined by several factors.

Primary among these are the bias toward nursing home care by elected officials, lobbying by the nursing home industry, insufficient regulation and quality assurance, and a lack of responsiveness to user preferences. Perhaps equally important is the lack of leadership at federal and state levels that precludes the development of a comprehensive long-term care policy and thus an integrated system of long-term care services including a variety of housing options with supportive services responsive to individual choice.

There have been considerable advancements in the conceptualization, measurement, and enforcement of quality of care in nursing homes. Efforts to develop quality assurance and health care–related quality of care measures have led to the gradual development and application of nursing home regulations implemented at the state level. Most of the work has been guided by Donabedian's conceptual approach encompassing structural features of the settings, service delivery process, and outcomes, although empirical attention has not been given to all components simultaneously.

While considerable conceptual efforts have been made to model and measure quality of life in long-term care, these have not yet been included in long-term regulatory practices. Quality of life measures need to include maintenance and enhancement of the self, emphasizing its preservation and the gratification of basic and higher level needs. The ultimate goal is to ensure the beneficial effects of quality of care practices on quality of life, thereby enhancing the living experiences of older persons in their later years when they are dependent on members of their informal system and service providers for long-term care.

Comprehensive and integrated long-term care services that promote quality of life and enhance the living experiences of older persons using such services need to be the dominant theme in political, academic, and professional associations and organizations. This orientation needs to permeate all levels, involving federal and state legislators making policy decisions, planners of long-term care services, administrative, and professional staff organizing and delivering the services. It also needs to involve the care recipients themselves as active consumers along with members of their informal support system.

REFERENCES

Applebaum, R. (1998). Long-term care policy: Lots of smoke, not many mirrors, and little progress. *Gerontologist, 38,* 135–138.

Baltes, P. B., & Baltes, M. M. (1990). In P. B. Baltes & M. M. Baltes (Eds.), *Successful aging: Perspectives from the behavioral sciences.* New York: Cambridge University Press.

Berg, M. D. (1991). Special care units for persons with dementia. *Journal of the American Geriatrics Society, 39*, 1229–1236.

Binstock, R. H., Cluff, L. E., & von Mering, O. (1996). Issues affecting the future of long-term care. In R. H. Binstock, L. E. Cluff, & O. von Mering (Eds.), *The future of long-term care* (pp. 1–18). Baltimore: The Johns Hopkins University Press.

Birren, J. E., & Deutchman, D. E. (1991). Concepts and content of quality of life in the later years: An overview. In J. Birren, J. Lubben, J. Rowe, & D. Deutchman (Eds.), *The concept and measurement of quality of life in the frail elderly* (pp. 344–360). San Diego: Academic Press.

Bowers, B., & Becker, M. (1992). Nurse's aides in nursing homes: The relationship between organization and quality. *Gerontologist, 32*, 360–366.

Brod, M., Stewart, A. L., & Sands, L. (1999). Conceptualization of quality of life in dementia. *Journal of Mental Health and Aging, 5*(1), 7–19.

Buckle, J. (1997). Care management and clinical decisions across settings: Measuring outcomes and cost. In *Minnesota Senior Health Options 1997 Annual Educational Forum: Innovations and issues in clinical integration: Improving systems for MSHO clients* (pp. 12–13).

Burgio, L. D., & Burgio, K. L. (1990). Institutional staff training and management: A review of literature and a model for geriatric, long-term care facilities. *International Journal of Aging and Human Development, 34*(4), 287–302.

Buss, D. (1995, April). Nursing homes rank high in workplace injuries. *Contemporary Long Term Care, 11*.

Carr, K. K., & Kazanowski, M. K. (1994). Factors affecting job satisfaction of nurses who work in long-term care. *Journal of Advanced Nursing, 19*, 878–883.

Chappell, N. L., & Novak, M. (1992). The role of support in alleviating stress among nursing assistants. *Gerontologist, 32*, 351–359.

Chassin, M. R., Galvin, R. W., & The National Roundtable on Health Care Quality (1998). The urgent need to improve health care quality: Institute of medicine national roundtable on health care quality. *Journal of the American Medical Association, 280*(11), 1000–1005.

Cohen-Mansfield, J., & Noelker, L. (2000). Satisfaction of nursing staff in long term care: An overview. In J. Cohen-Mansfield, F. K. Ejaz, & P. Werner (Eds.), *Satisfaction surveys in long-term care* (pp. 52–75). New York: Springer Publishing.

Cohn, J., & Sugar, J. (1991). Determinant of quality of life in institutions: Perceptions of frail older residents, staff, and families. In J. Birren, J. Lubben, J. Rowe, & D. Deutchman (Eds.), *The concept and measurement of quality of life in the frail elderly* (pp. 28–49). San Diego: Academic Press.

Donabedian, A. (1980). *Explorations in quality assessment and monitoring.* Ann Arbor, MI: Health Administration Press.

Donabedian, A. (1988). Quality assessment and assurance: Unity of purpose, diversity of means. *Inquiry, 25*, 173–192.

Dougherty, L. M., Bolger, J. P., Preston, D. G., Jones, S. S., & Payne, H. C. (1992). Effects of exposure to aggressive behavior on job satisfaction of health care staff. *Journal of Applied Gerontology, 11*(2), 160–172.

Dunn, L. A., Rout, U., Carson, J., & Ritter, S. A. (1994). Occupational stress amongst care staff working in nursing homes: An empirical investigation. *Journal of Clinical Nursing, 3*, 177–183.

Everitt, D. E., Fields, D. R., Soumerai, S. S., & Avorn, J. (1991). Resident behavior and staff distress in the nursing home. *Journal of the American Geriatric Society, 39*(8), 792–798.

Fisher-Robertson, J., & Cummings, C. C. (1991). What makes long-term care nursing attractive? *American Journal of Nursing, 91*(11), 41–46.

Foner, N. (1994). Nursing home aides: Saints or monsters? *Gerontologist, 34*(2), 245–250.

Francis-Felson, L. C., Coward, R. T., Hogan, T. L, Duncan, R. P., Hilker, M. A., & Horn, C. (1996). Factors influencing intentions of nursing personnel to leave employment in long term care settings. *Journal of Applied Gerontology, 15*(4), 450–470.

Friedlob, A. (1993). *The use of physical restraints in nursing homes and the allocation of nursing resources.* Minneapolis: University of Minnesota, Health Services and Resources Administration.

Gamroth, L. M., Semradek, J. A., & Tornquist, E. M. (1995). *Enhancing autonomy in long-term care: Concepts and strategies.* New York: Springer Publishing Co.

Glass, A. P. (1991). Nursing home quality: A framework for analysis. *Journal of Applied Gerontology, 10*(1), 5–18.

Goffman, E. (1961). *Asylums: Essays on the social situation of mental patients and other inmates.* Garden City, NY: Doubleday.

Grau, L., & Wellin, E. (1992, February). The organizational cultures of nursing homes: Influences on responses to external regulatory controls. *Qualitative Health Research, 2*(1), 42–60.

Halbur, B. T., & Fears, N. (1986). Nursing personnel turnover rates turned over: Potential positive effects on resident outcomes in nursing homes. *Gerontologist, 26*(1), 70–76.

Hallberg, I. R., & Norberg, A. (1995). Nurses' experiences of strain and their reactions in the care of severely demented patients. *International Journal of Geriatric Psychiatry, 10,* 757–766.

Hare, J., Pratt, C. C., & Andrews, D. (1988). Predictors of burnout in professional and paraprofessional nurses working in hospitals and nursing homes. *International Journal of Nursing Studies, 25*(2), 105–115.

Harrington, C., Mullan, J., Woodruff, L. C., Burger, S. G., Carrillo, H., & Bedney, B. (1999). Stakeholders' opinions regarding important measures of nursing home quality for consumers. *American Journal of Medical Quality, 14*(3), 124–132.

Heidrich, S. M., & Ryff, C. D. (1993) Physical and mental health in later life: The self-system as mediator. *Psychology and Aging, 8*(3), 327–338.

Helmer, F. T., Olson, S. F., & Heim, R. I. (1993, Summer). Strategies for nurse aide job satisfaction. *Journal of Long-Term Care Administration,* 10–14.

Holmes, D., Ramirez, M., & Fairchild, S. (1994). *Racial and ethnic differences among staff and between staff and residents: Preliminary findings of a pilot study.* Paper presented at the Fifth Annual Health Services Research Symposium.

Holstein, M., & Cole, T. R. (1996). The evolution of long-term care in America. In R. H. Binstock, L. E. Cluff, & O. von Mering (Eds.), *The future of long-term care* (pp. 19–47). Baltimore: The Johns Hopkins University Press.

Huey, F. L. (1990, November/December). Shocking staffing statistics. *Geriatric Nursing,* 265.

Kahana, E. (In press). Long term care facilities. *Encyclopedia of Gerontology*. New York: Macmillan.

Kane, R. A., & Kane, R. L. (1988, Spring). Long-term care: Variations on a quality assurance theme. *Inquiry, 25*, 132–146.

Kane, R. A., Kane, R. L., & Ladd, R. C. (1998). *The heart of long-term care*. New York: Oxford University Press.

Kane, R. L. (1999, Summer). A new model of chronic care. *Generations: Journal of the American Society on Aging, 23*(2), 35–37.

Lawton, M. (1991). A multidimensional view of quality of life in frail elders. In J. Birren, J. Lubben, J. Rowe, & D. Deutchman (Eds.), *The concept and measurement of quality of life in the frail elderly* (pp. 3–27). San Diego: Academic Press.

Lawton, M. P., Moss, M., Hoffman, C., Grant, R., Have, T. T., & Kleban, M. H. (1999). Health, valuation of life, and the wish to live. *Gerontologist, 39*(4), 406–416.

Leutz, W. N. (1999). Five laws for integrating medical and social services: Lessons learned from the United States and the United Kingdom. *The Milbank Quarterly, 77*(1), 77–110.

Levine, S. (1987). The changing terrains in medical sociology: Emergent concern with quality of life. *Journal of Health and Social Behavior, 28*(1), 1–6.

Logsdon, R. G., & Albert, S. M. (1999). Assessing quality of life in Alzheimer's disease: Conceptual and methodological issues. *Journal of Mental Health and Aging, 5*(1), 3–6.

Lusk, S. L. (1992). Violence experienced by nurse's aides in nursing homes: An exploratory study. *American Association of Occupational Health Nurses, Inc., 40*(5), 237–241.

Morris, R., Caro, F. G., & Hansan, J. E. (1998). *Personal assistance: The future of home care*. Baltimore, Johns Hopkins University Press.

Moss, M. L., Swanson, E., Specht, J., & Buckwalter, K. C. (1994). Alzheimer's special care units. *Nursing Clinics of North America, 29*(1), 173–194.

National Academy On Aging (1997, September). *Facts on long-term care*. Washington, DC: Author.

National Citizens' Coalition for Nursing Home Reform (1985, April). *Consumer perspective on quality care: The residents' point of view*. Washington, DC: Author.

Noelker, L. S., & Poulshock, S. W. (1982). *The effects on families of caring for impaired elderly in residence*. Final report to the Administration on Aging. Cleveland: The Benjamin Rose Institute.

Noelker, L. S., Schur, D., Looman, W., Ejaz, F. K., & Whitlatch, C. J. (In revision). Impact of stress and support on nursing assistants' satisfaction with supervision. *Journal of Applied Gerontology*.

Pezzin, L. E., & Schone, B. S. (1999). Parental marital disruption and intergenerational transfers: An analysis of lone elderly parents and their children. *Demography, 36*(3), 287–297.

Pillemer, K., & Moore, D. (1989). Abuse of patients in nursing homes: Findings from a survey of staff. *Gerontologist, 29*, 314–320.

Ramirez, M., Teresi, J. A., Holmes, D., & Fairchild, S. (1998). Ethnic and racial conflict in relation to staff burnout, demoralization, and job satisfaction in SCUs and Non-SCUs. *Journal of Mental Health and Aging, 4*(4), 459–479.

Romeis, J. C., & Coe, R. M. (Eds.) (1991). *Quality and cost containment in care of the elderly.* New York: Springer Publishing Co.

Sainfort, F., Ramsay, J. D., & Monato, J. (1995). Conceptual and methodological sources of variation in the measurement of nursing facility quality: An evaluation of 24 models and an empirical study. *Medical Care Research and Review, 52*(1), 60–87.

Schur, D., Noelker, L. S., Looman, W., Whitlatch, C. J., & Ejaz, F. K. (1998, Jan/Feb). 4 steps to more committed nursing assistants. *Balance, 2*(1), 29–32.

Shaughnessy, P. W., Crisler, K. S., & Schlenker, R. E. (1998). Outcome-based quality improvement in the information age. *Home Health Care Management and Practice, 10*(2), 11–19.

Shaughnessy, P. W., Crisler, K. S., Schlenker, R. E., Arnold, A. G., Kramer, A. M., Powell, M. C., & Hittle, D. F. (1994, Fall). Measuring and assuring the quality of home health care. *Health Care Financing Review, 16*(1), 35–67.

Singh, D. A., & Schwab, R. C. (1998). Retention of administrators in nursing homes: What can management do? *Gerontologist, 38*(3), 362–369.

Stevens, A. B., Burgio, L. D., Bailey, E., Burgio, K. L., Paul, P., Capilouto, E., Nicovich, P., & Hale, G. (1998). Teaching and maintaining behavior management skills with nursing assistants in a nursing home. *Gerontologist, 38*(3), 379–384.

Tellis-Nyak, V., & Tellis-Nyak, M. (1989). Quality of care and the burden of two cultures: When the world of the nurse's aide enters the nursing home. *Gerontologist, 29*, 307–313.

Teresi, J., Holmes, D., Benenson, E., Monaco, C., Barrett, V., Ramirez, M., & Koren, M. J. (1993a). A primary care nursing model in urban and rural long-term care facilities: Attitudes, morale, and satisfaction of residents and staff. *Research on Aging, 15*, 414–432.

Teresi, J., Holmes, D., Benenson, E., Monaco, C., Barrett, V., Ramirez, M., & Koren, M. J. (1993b). A primary care nursing model in long-term care facilities: Evaluation of impact on affect, behavior, and socialization. *Gerontologist, 33*(5), 667–674.

Tobin, S. S. (1999). *Preservation of the self in the oldest years.* New York: Springer Publishing Co.

Vinton, L., & Mazza, N. (1994). Aggressive behavior directed at nursing home personnel by residents' family members. *Gerontologist, 34*(4), 528–533.

Wagner, D. M. (1988). *Managing for quality in home health care: Effective business strategies.* Rockville, MA: Aspen Publishers, Inc.

Wagnild, G. (1988). A descriptive study of nurse's aide turnover in long-term care facilities. *Journal of Long-Term Care Administration, 17*, 19–23.

Wieland, D., Rubenstein, L. V., & Hirsch, S. H. (1995). Quality of life in nursing homes: An emerging focus of research and practice. In P. R. Katz, R. L. Kane, & M. D. Mezey (Eds.), *Quality care in geriatric settings: Focus on ethical issues* (pp. 149–194). New York: Springer Publishing Co.

Zarit, S. H., & Whitlatch, C. J. (1992). Institutional placement: Phases of the transition. *Gerontologist, 32*, 665–672.

Zimmerman, D. R. (1991). Impact of new regulations and data sources on nursing home quality of care. In National League for Nursing, *Mechanisms of quality in long-term care: Service and clinical outcomes* (pp. 29–42). New York: National League for Nursing Press.

2

Assessing Quality Across the Care Continuum

Gerri S. Lamb

Today, the majority of older adults rely on multiple providers and settings to meet their acute and chronic care needs. In the course of recuperating from an acute event, such as a stroke or fractured hip, an individual can traverse across as many as four or five settings, including hospital, transitional, or sub-acute care, home care, and outpatient rehabilitation care. Similarly, the day-to-day management of chronic conditions such as heart failure or Alzheimer's disease often requires primary and specialty care as well as various home- and community-based services, including home care, day care, and/or residential care.

Health care, and in particular, long-term care for older adults, is best characterized as longitudinal and continuous and by necessity, must deal effectively with chronic health conditions. Kane (1999, p. 35) commented "A chronic care model starts from a different premise. Encounters with patients are just part of a total scenario. One is playing for long-term results."

To effect improvements in the quality of long-term care, numerous professionals and community organizations must come together in a well-orchestrated sequence that may play out over months or years. Consequently, no single provider or setting can take sole credit or blame for quality or cost outcomes. An outcome captured at one single point in time, in one setting is rarely a true measure of meaningful impact. To paraphrase a well-known saying, the hip surgery and immediate post-surgical rehabilitation may be a success, but if the patient stops walking 3 months later, what has been achieved? What *is* the measure by which quality of long-term care should be assessed?

To date, much of the work on outcome assessment in long-term care has been limited to outcomes of care in single settings. This is not surprising in light of the significant regulatory and administrative pressures to use site-specific indicators and demonstrate site-specific profitability. Yet, setting specific outcomes reflect only a piece of the performance of the long-term care system. Growth of knowledge about effective health care for older adults indicates that setting specific outcomes are not sufficient to evaluate the quality and financial performance of the system of long-term care services (Castle, 1999). More often, organization and integration across settings are required in order to achieve outcomes in critical areas for the elderly, including quality of life, functional performance and independence, and satisfaction with health care services.

This chapter addresses the imperative for a continuum-based approach to outcome assessment. Factors that support and impede this approach are identified. Strategies and tools to support this broader approach to quality and cost assessment are offered.

CONTINUUM-BASED CARE

A continuum-based approach to outcome assessment is based on a framework of integration and coordination. The operative premises of continuum-based performance are that (1) there is greater value in optimization of the whole rather than the parts, and (2) participants in the continuum have shared responsibility for cumulative outcomes in addition to specific programmatic outcomes.

Continuum-based outcome assessment is concerned with the incremental and cumulative effects of multiple providers and services on quality and cost outcomes. For a defined sequence of care, effective quality and fiscal performance for each setting is a necessary, but not sufficient contributor to overall system performance (Young & Barrett, 1997). It is possible that a single setting may be profitable and have good quality outcomes, but due to transition failures or poor coordination, the ultimate clinical and fiscal outcomes for the patient and his/her family are not optimal. Integration has been identified as an important vehicle to improve quality of care particularly for vulnerable and high-risk elderly, reduce fragmentation, and save significant dollars.

In the seminal work on integration, Shortell, Gillies, Anderson, Erickson, and Mitchell (1996) characterized integrated or organized systems as those that share knowledge and skill across settings and in doing so, reduce duplication and fragmentation of services. The Health System Integration Study of 11 health care systems (Gillies, Shortell, Anderson, Mitchell, & Morgan, 1993; Shortell, Gillies, Anderson, Mitchell, & Morgan, 1993) identified three components of integration: (1) functional integration of financial, human resources, information, and quality services; (2)

physician integration; and (3) clinical integration or coordination of patient services across providers, settings, and time. Clinical integration is viewed as pivotal to achieving quality and cost outcomes. There is still considerable debate about the extent to which other types of integration are necessary for accomplishing clinical integration (Leutz, 1999).

In long-term care, clinical integration requires coordination across complex networks of acute and chronic care. Coffey, Fenner, and Stogis (1997) propose the concept of a "virtually integrated health system" to capture the dynamic interplay between the many components of our current health care delivery system. Within the virtually integrated system, traditional and non-traditional providers interact with community agencies and formal and informal patient supports. Together, they are responsible for achieving targeted outcomes for the patients and family who enter their systems of care.

Continuum-based outcome assessment is an integral component of clinical integration (Young & Barrett, 1997). Structures and processes must be put in place in order to evaluate the combined impact of multiple players and settings on short- and long-term outcomes. Built on a foundation of effective communication and coordination of care, outcomes of continuum-based care address whether integration has achieved the targeted quality and cost goals.

Much of the early descriptive research on integration and continuum-based care emerged during a rapid growth period in managed care and capitated payment. Not surprisingly, attention rapidly turned to demonstrating the feasibility and benefits of integrating services and outcomes across the acute and long-term care (Branch, 1999; Kane, 1998; Nerenz & Zajac, 1996).

THE CASE FOR CONTINUUM-BASED OUTCOMES

Support for a continuum-based approach to outcome assessment comes from the various constituencies of health care. Patients want and expect coordination of care and continuity (Gerteis, 1999). Gerteis, Edgman-Levitan, Daley, and Delbanco (1993, p. 46) observed that "at the end points of delivery systems, patients are eyewitnesses to how those systems work." Providers, too, recognize the shortcomings of disconnected and fragmented services on patient quality of life and social and functional outcomes. Many have called for a more coherent and organized system (Hoffman & Rice, 1996; Howe, 1999; Kane, 1999). Payers seek the quality and cost advantages of reduced fragmentation and coordination.

Numerous authors, concerned about the impending growth of populations with chronic illness, have called for a new way of organizing health care (Kane, 1999; Sandy & Gibson, 1996). The majority of the proposed models require comprehensive system changes, rather than redesign of individual components. Integrative processes, including coordination and collaboration, have been identified as essential to improved health-care for older adults (Coleman, Grothaus, Sandhu, & Wagner, 1999). Boult, Boult, and Pacala (1998) emphasize the importance of reducing fragmentation, "the Achilles heel" (p. 504) of the current system of care for people with chronic and complex health care needs.

Studies of patient expectations of health care and long-term care indicate that the patient, the primary customer of health care services, places great value on continuity and integration. In the Picker/Commonwealth study of patient-centered care, patient expectations included sharing of information across providers and settings, as well as appropriate discharge planning and transitional care (Gerteis et al., 1993). Similarly, in interviews conducted by the Foundation for Accountability (Lansky, 1998), patients considered communication and coordination basic to their satisfaction with health care services.

Research has shown that for patients, the health care experience is a continuous process, not a series of discrete episodes. Patients resent being asked the same questions repeatedly. They expect professionals to talk to each other and create a unified plan of care. They expect their providers to care about them as complete and unique individuals and to take interest in their progress over time.

Managed care and capitated financing have offered the most direct incentives for providers and payers to integrate care and look at the combined outcomes of multiple services (Della-Penna, 1999). The hallmark of managed care systems is to create the optimum service package at the lowest cost. This typically is translated into service plans that closely manage transitions between settings and substitute equally effective and lower cost services whenever possible.

Under capitated payment, significant cost-savings are associated with preventing or reducing the use of higher cost acute care services. Numerous combinations of services and settings may be arranged in order to balance quality and costs of care across acute and chronic care settings. To be successful, it is essential for managed care plans to demonstrate acceptable outcomes at each point of service and at the end points of completed episodes of care.

While hypotheses about the benefits of integration on outcomes abound, research on integration is still in its infancy. Despite substantial anecdotal support for the impact of integration on quality and cost, Branch (1999) suggests that we would be hard pressed to make a strong case in its favor. There is little empirical evidence that integration of acute and chronic care results in better health status or lower costs. Branch (1999) has pointed out thorny methodological issues, such as determining complete expenses for integrated care, which will need to be resolved to move the field ahead.

Early findings related to the outcomes of integrated care are mixed, but point researchers in some promising directions. When Boult, Kane, Pacala, and Wagner (1999) went to experts to identify innovative health care programs for older adults, the majority of the programs put forward were ones that had developed sophisticated systems for coordination of care and case management.

In a recent study of patient and facility correlates of quality of care in long-term care facilities, Bravo, DaWals, Dubois, and Charpentier (1999) found that the number of external collaborators was one of the few facility-level variables associated with quality of care as measured by the QUALCARE Scale. The QUALCARE Scale is an instrument composed of 54 items that assess six areas of care including environmental, physical, psychosocial, medical management, financial, and human rights. Long-term care facilities that had more regular contact with other providers and settings along the continuum of care, including primary care, home health, hospitals, and local community agencies, had higher QUALCARE scores.

In their review of research on the relationship between organizational structure and processes and mortality, complications and adverse events, Mitchell & Shortell (1997) noted that collaboration and coordination are among the limited set of process variables that consistently show a relationship to lower mortality. They hypothesized that reciprocal interdependence, the sharing of professional expertise and resources, within and across settings may be a crucial link between organizational factors and important outcomes of care.

In a provocative analysis of the state of integrated health care in the United States and the United Kingdom, Leutz (1999) summarized lessons from the many projects and demonstrations conducted in both countries. He looked at what we have learned to date about target populations for integrated services, the costs of integration, the competencies and time requirements, and the boundaries of what is possible to integrate in health care today. While he acknowledges the lack of empirical data supporting his resulting "laws" of integration, he suggests that years of national experimentation with public and private programs offer some important areas for model development and testing. He proposes, for example, that we look at how to increase participation of users and providers in the design and evaluation of integrated systems and how to enhance the synergy between medical and nonmedical systems.

Support for continuum-based care and outcomes tracking comes from many sectors. Clearly, patients tell us that they want coordinated and continuous care. Theoretically, at least, providers and payers benefit from integration between the acute and chronic care systems. Strong empirical evidence of the benefits of integration is lacking, but our national experiences with integrated care and the results of early research point to promising areas for future development.

OBSTACLES TO CONTINUUM-BASED OUTCOME ASSESSMENT

Although the arguments in favor of continuum-based outcomes can be compelling, there continue to be significant obstacles to moving outcome assessment to the system level. Roadblocks come in multiple forms including financial, regulatory, administrative, and operational/methodological.

Perhaps the greatest barrier to a continuum-based model of outcome assessment is financial. Current financing in long-term care reinforces a narrow, single site perspective. Recent changes in Medicare reimbursement for hospitals, home health, and skilled facilities, for example, have reduced payment and many of the previous financial benefits associated with coordinating care across settings (National Chronic Care Consortium, 1999). As a result, these organizations have become more focused on their own financial survival than the performance of the health care system as a whole. In delivery systems that serve large Medicare markets, there is diminishing incentive to shift care to other levels of service, even when another level of service may be more appropriate or cost-effective.

Even in managed care, where the incentive for integration is greatest, recent trends in contracting have detracted from the movement toward integrated outcomes. Complex combinations of fee-for-service and capitated reimbursement for long-term care service providers create conflicting incentives for coordination of care and substitution of services across settings. Although there has been considerable discussion about how to achieve aligned incentives across providers and services, a successful model has yet to be identified. Some of the more promising steps are the development of risk adjusters that create incentives to provide care for people with chronic illness and the re-examination of bundling of payments across service settings.

Regulatory requirements for site-specific outcome measurement also reduce the likelihood of moving toward continuum-based assessment. Several long-term care settings, including home health and skilled facilities, already must complete and submit extensive site-specific outcome data via OASIS or the Resident Assessment Instrument (RAI) for Medicare certification and funding. Unfortunately, many of the key outcome indicators for older adults included in these data are not measured using the same questions or instruments across settings. Under traditional Medicare funding, there is minimal incentive for each long-term care setting to add questions to already burdensome data collection tools or to share disparate data across settings.

At present, the performance of each long-term care setting tends to be judged according to its own quality outcomes and profitability. Indeed, it is not uncommon for multi-service organizations to discontinue programs if they are not profitable as stand-alone services, rather than to examine the contribution of the service to overall system profitability.

Distinguishing the unique contributions of each setting to continuum-based outcomes is complex from a methodological standpoint. How do we assign value to each component of the long-term care system? For the patient with a stroke who has reached target indicators for quality of life, functional status, satisfaction with care, and costs at 6 months, how much "credit" do we allocate to the sub-acute unit, the home health agency, the day care program, the meal program (see Figure 2.1)? How do we account for synergy between settings and interaction effects? The conceptual and analytic problems associated with this scenario are more difficult than most delivery systems are willing or able to address.

Even if long-term care settings were collecting common outcome indicators, few have information systems that permit easy access to data or tracking of data over time. The lack of common data platforms restricts integration within and across settings. Efforts to bring together financial and clinical data within single settings have been shown to be extremely labor-intensive, much less across settings and systems.

So, while patients and providers call for new integrated approaches to deal with the shortcomings of both acute and long-term care systems, there is still a long way to go in developing, refining, and demonstrating the effectiveness of integrated systems. Many factors mediate against getting the needed clinical innovation and research done in this area. Boult and colleagues (Boult, Boult, & Pacala, 1998; Boult, Kane, & Pacala, 1999) have drawn attention to the powerful role that market factors play in decisions about and resources allocated to clinical innovation, including many of the programs focused on improving service integration and reducing fragmentation of care.

MODELS AND MEASURES FOR CONTINUUM-BASED OUTCOME ASSESSMENT

Selection of models and measurement tools for assessing continuum-based outcomes clearly will be influenced by a variety of factors, including financial incentives for integration and shared outcome measurement and organizational structure and capacity for data management and sharing. Several authors, including Lamb (1997) and Wojner and MacCutcheon

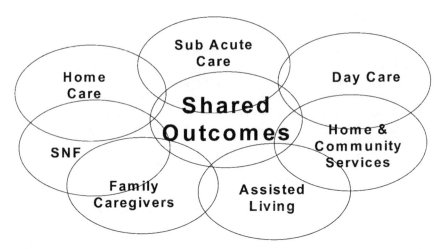

FIGURE 2.1   Shared and unique contributions to long-term care outcomes: Who gets the credit?

(1998) have proposed an incremental approach to assessing continuum-based outcomes.

Organizations interested in building toward system-level outcomes may begin with "snapshots" of performance in each setting (Lamb, 1997). While this approach has numerous obvious shortcomings in achieving continuum-based outcome assessment, it does begin to place setting-specific outcomes in the context of larger system goals. Wojner and MacCutcheon (1998) noted that intermediate outcomes collected at the completion of each phase of care should be monitored closely due to their obvious contribution to the achievement of long-term outcomes.

As a next step, organizations may focus on outcome markers associated with movement across systems, such as maintenance of functional performance between subacute care and home care or unplanned returns to a previous level of care. Lezzoni et al. (1999), for example, recently introduced a new tool, the Complications Screening Program for Outpatient data (CSP-O), to retrospectively identify hospital complications from postdischarge events in primary care, outpatient, home care, and hospice settings.

More comprehensive attempts at continuum-based outcome assessment track outcomes of targeted patient populations at the end of an episode or common sequence of care. This approach may be used to compare quality and cost outcomes of different models of service use for high-volume/high-cost clinical conditions. For example, Figure 2.2 shows two common trajectories of care for individuals who experience a stroke. In

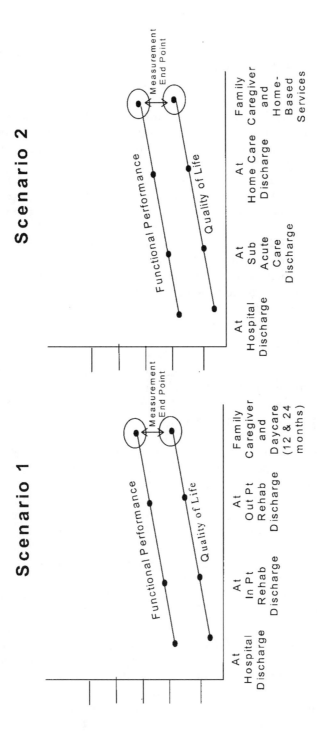

FIGURE 2.2 Comparing quality outcomes of different service trajectories.

one scenario, individuals proceed from hospital to inpatient rehabilitation to outpatient rehabilitation to home with family and day care support. In a second scenario, the care path goes from subacute to home and community-based care. Assuming the outcomes are adjusted for the appropriate factors reflecting clinical risk, in this third level of continuum-based assessment, the endpoints of both scenarios might be evaluated and compared using measures of quality of life, functional status, satisfaction, service use, and cost.

Evaluations of the Medicare long-term care demonstrations from the 1970s to the present provide several excellent examples of the next stage of outcome evaluation: continuum-based outcome assessment. The majority of long-term care demonstrations sponsored by the Health Care Financing Administration (HCFA) including Channeling, PACE, the Social HMOs, and the Medicare Alzheimer's Disease Demonstration covered various combinations of acute and chronic care services. They incorporated financial incentives for integration and effective use and substitution of services across settings (Brown, 1999). Different strategies for clinical integration and coordination were tested across the demonstrations with case management and interdisciplinary teams predominating.

Several of these demonstrations were evaluated using randomized control designs and measurement of quality, service use, and cost indicators over time. Many, particularly the later demonstrations, used the Andersen model of predisposing, enabling, and need factors to adjust for differences in risk for various quality and service use outcomes (Andersen, 1995). While the same outcome instruments were not used across demonstrations (and in some cases, not even across the participating sites in the same demonstration), all of the demonstrations have looked at some combination of common outcomes of interest in long-term care.

Together, the evaluations of the long-term care demonstrations suggest the beginnings of a shared model for continuum-based evaluation (Figure 2.3). Many of the demonstrations have built-in sampling and statistical techniques to identify and control for level of risk for use of health services and costs. Figure 2.3 incorporates some of the common risk variables that have been used in long-term care demonstrations grouped according to Andersen's three major dimensions of predisposing, enabling, and need factors.

In many of the demonstrations, service integration is a key moderating link between patient risk factors and targeted quality and cost outcomes. Several of the demonstrations have incorporated qualitative and/or quantitative methods to describe core clinical integration processes, such as case management or interdisciplinary teams. Financial integration, commonly examined in terms of the payment and incentive structures in the demonstrations, has been an important element of the evaluations. Most

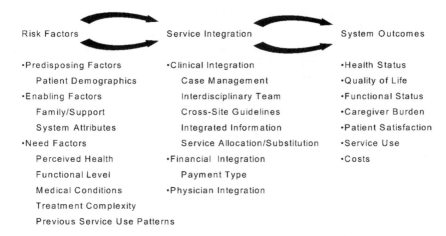

Risk Factors	Service Integration	System Outcomes
•Predisposing Factors	•Clinical Integration	•Health Status
Patient Demographics	Case Management	•Quality of Life
•Enabling Factors	Interdisciplinary Team	•Functional Status
Family/Support	Cross-Site Guidelines	•Caregiver Burden
System Attributes	Integrated Information	•Patient Satisfaction
•Need Factors	Service Allocation/Substitution	•Service Use
Perceived Health	•Financial Integration	•Costs
Functional Level	Payment Type	
Medical Conditions	•Physician Integration	
Treatment Complexity		
Previous Service Use Patterns		

FIGURE 2.3   Model for assessing quality across settings and time.

recently, the amount of physician integration within the demonstrations has been scrutinized more closely for its contribution to quality and cost outcomes.

Each subsequent evaluation has added valuable methodological lessons (Lamb, 1999). The evaluation of the Channeling and the other long-term care demonstrations of the 1970s and 1980s highlighted the importance of using common outcome indicators across settings and targeting at-risk populations for participation (Kemper, 1988; Kemper, Applebaum, & Harrigan, 1987; Weissert, Lesnick, Mushliner, & Foley, 1997). PACE and the S/HMOs advanced understanding about risk assessment, case management, and interdisciplinary teams (Eng, Pedulla, Eleazer, McCann, & Fox, 1997; Hansen, 1999; Kane et al., 1997). The evaluation program for the Alzheimer's Disease demonstration showed the feasibility of testing separate analytic models for each outcome variable (Newcomer, Spitalny, Fox, & Yordi, 1999). In addition, this evaluation provided important new insights about risk adjustment and case management through a combination of qualitative and quantitative methodologies.

In recent years, the outcome tools used in the long-term care demonstrations have paralleled those required in clinical settings and managed care. For example, health status is most commonly measured with the MOS Short-Form 36. Service use outcomes are looked at in terms of use per defined population. Although the designs of the demonstrations are more complex than most organizations will want or need to carry out for ongoing outcome assessment, they incorporate the key elements that are integral to continuum-based outcome assessment:

- Risk adjustment or measurement of risk factors expected to influence differences in quality and financial outcomes;
- Longitudinal measurement of outcomes at critical change points;
- Common outcome indicators across providers and settings; and
- Capture of a minimum set of process indicators considered integral to achievement of targeted outcomes.

As models for continuum-based outcome assessment such as shown in Figure 2.3 evolve, a number of new measurement tools have been proposed to differentiate levels of integration, track outcomes over time, and capture system-level outcomes. Leutz (1999) provided a typology of three levels of integration each of which has unique clinical markers. Kane (1998) proposed clinical glidepaths to document outcomes across a sequence of care. The Consortium for Research on Indicators of System Performance (CRISP) developed and tested a preliminary set of performance measures for integrated delivery systems (Nerenz & Zajac, 1996). CRISP, like the Health Plan Employer Data and Information Set (HEDIS) and the Foundation for Accountability (FAcct) measurement set, is intended to provide a systematic, clinically and consumer-relevant set of indicators to evaluate system-level performance.

Each of these conceptual models and tools represent important efforts to advance outcome assessment from site-specific to continuum-based measurement over time. Glidepaths attempt to capture changes in individual outcomes over time. Kane (1998) suggests that they can be used to adjust treatment to better approximate targeted outcomes for chronic conditions like diabetes or heart failure. In contrast, CRISP and HEDIS-type indicators measure system-level performance on key elements of preventive and chronic illness care.

In an important development, researchers are beginning to explore how various outcomes and measurement tools behave across various care settings. Murdaugh (1997), for example, described both conceptual and methodological issues associated with health-related quality of life research across populations, service settings, and time. She suggests that with refinement, health-related quality of life measures will be critical indicators of the performance of new and more integrated care delivery processes and models.

Today, in light of the significant financial and regulatory constraints, incremental approaches to continuum-based outcome assessment seem most promising. Although each successive step toward full continuum-based assessment has unique strengths and weaknesses, movement along the sequence of outcome measurement assures attention to and recognition of other players in achieving short-term and long-term goals.

There are numerous exciting areas of research underway: risk adjustment, interaction effects between interventions across settings, and more precise measurement of the core processes of integration. Our ability to optimize outcomes across services and settings will require the refinement of past research and the development of new conceptual and measurement models for clinical integration.

CONCLUSION

Judgment about the quality of care for older adults, by necessity, transcends assessment of process and outcomes in a single setting. Ultimately, quality of care will be determined by the sequence of care across settings that results in an older person's ability to achieve targeted goals in self-care performance, function, safety, and quality of life.

Today, due to a variety of constraints, few long-term care settings link their outcomes to services and settings that precede or follow them in the usual flow of care. Assessments of quality are limited to single snapshots along the trajectory of acute and chronic care. Assessments of system-level performance are still uncommon.

In spite of the obstacles, the science of continuum-based outcome assessment continues to move forward. Shortell (Shortell et al., 1993; Shortell et al., 1996), Leutz (1999), and others continue to explore the significant conceptual issues associated with the definition and explication of integration. New models and measurement tools are emerging. Critical analyses of various outcomes highly relevant to the older adult population, such as quality of life (Murdaugh, 1997), consistently raise provocative questions about how these outcomes behave conceptually and operationally across systems of care.

Numerous conceptual and methodological issues remain. New models are needed to explain how diverse systems and services come together to produce quality and cost outcomes. In today's financially driven markets, it is essential to capture and allocate distinct contributions of each provider and setting to cost outcomes.

Finally, it is clear that the development of the science and tools for continuum-based outcome assessment will require new incentives that reinforce shared accountability for outcomes for targeted populations and outcomes. Leutz (1999, p. 83) notes in his first law of integration, "You can integrate all of the services for some of the people, some of the services for all of the people, but you can't integrate all of the services for all of the people." The promise of developing the field of continuum-based outcome assessment is to guide the development of systems and services for long-term care that reach the most appropriate populations, coordinate and integrate the most appropriate services, and achieve essential goals for a growing population of older adults.

REFERENCES

Andersen, R. M. (1995). Revisiting the behavioral model and access to medical care: Does it matter? *Journal of Health and Social Behavior, 36*, 1–10.

Boult, C., Boult, L., & Pacala, J. T. (1998). Systems of care for older populations of the future. *Journal of the American Geriatrics Society, 46*(4), 499–505.

Boult, C., Kane, R. L., Pacala, J. T., & Wagner, E. H. (1999). Innovative healthcare for chronically ill older persons: Results of a national survey. *American Journal of Managed Care, 5*(8), 1–11.

Branch, L. G. Integrating acute and chronic care. (1999). *Generations, xxiii*(2), 5–8.

Bravo, G., DeWals, P., Dubois, M. F., & Charpentier, M. (1999). Correlates of care quality in long-term care facilities: A multilevel analysis. *Journal of Gerontology, 54B*(3), 180–188.

Brown, T. E. (1999). Integration of acute and chronic care: Lessons learned from South Carolina. *Generations, xxiii*(2), 15–20.

Castle, N. G. (1999). Outcomes measurement and quality improvement in long-term care. *Journal for Healthcare Quality, 21*(3), 21–25.

Coffey, R. J., Fenner, K. M., & Stogis, S. L. (1997). *Virtually integrated health systems.* San Francisco: Jossey-Bass Publishers.

Coleman, E. A., Grothaus, L. C., Sandhu, N., & Wagner, E. H. (1999). Chronic care clinics: A randomized controlled trial of a new model of primary care for frail older adults. *Journal of the American Geriatrics Society, 47*(7), 775–783.

Della-Penna, R. D. (1999). Integrating nursing home care in managed care. *Generations, 23*(2), 29–34.

Eng, C., Pedulla, J., Eleazer, G. P., McCann, R., & Fox, N. (1997). Program of All-inclusive Care for the Elderly (PACE): An innovative model of integrated geriatric care and financing. *Journal of the American Geriatrics Society, 45*, 223–232.

Gerteis, M. (1999). Through the patient's eyes: Improvement strategies that work. *Journal on Quality Improvement, 25*(7), 335–342.

Gerteis, M., Edgman-Levitan, S., Daley, J., & Delbanco, T. L. (1993). *Through the patient's eyes.* San Francisco: Jossey-Bass.

Gillies, R.R., Shortell, S. M., Anderson, D. A., Mitchell, J. B., & Morgan, K. L. (1993). Conceptualizing and measuring integration: Findings from the Health Systems Integration Study. *Hospital and Health Services Administration, 38*(4), 467–489.

Hansen, J. C. (1999). Practical lessons for delivering integrated services in a changing environment: The PACE model. *Generations, xxiii*(2), 22–28.

Hoffman, C., & Rice, D. P. (1996). *Chronic care in America: A 21st century challenge.* Princeton, NJ: Robert Wood Johnson Foundation.

Howe, R. (1999). Case management in managed care. *Case Manager, 10*(5), 37–40.

Kane, R. L. (1998). Managed care as a vehicle for delivering more effective chronic care for older persons. *Journal of the American Geriatrics Society, 46*, 1034–1039.

Kane, R. L. (1999). A new model of chronic care. *Generations, xxiii*(2), 35–38.

Kane, R., Kane, R. A., Finch, M., Harrington, C., Newcomer, R., Miller, N., & Hulbert, M. (1997). S/HMOs, the second generation: Building on the experience of the first social health maintenance organization demonstration. *Journal of the American Geriatrics Society, 45*(1), 101–107.

Kemper, P. (1988). The evaluation of the national long-term care demonstrations: Overview of the findings. *Health Services Research, 23,* 161–174.

Kemper, P., Applebaum, R., & Harrigan, M. (1987). Community demonstrations: What have we learned? *Health Care Financing Review, 8,* 87–100.

Lamb, G. S. (1997). Outcomes across the care continuum. *Medical Care, 35*(11, Supplement), NS106–114.

Lamb, G. S. (1999). Case management for older adults. In F. Chan & M. J. Leahy (Eds.), *Health care and disability case management* (pp. 639–662). Lake Zurich, IL: Vocational Consultants Press.

Lansky, D. (1998). Measuring what matters to the public. *Health Affairs, 17*(4), 40–41.

Leutz, W. N. (1999). Five laws for integrating medical and social services: Lessons from the U.S. and U.K. *Milbank Quarterly, 77*(1), 77–110.

Lezzoni, L. I., MacKiernan, V. D., Cahalane, M. J., Phillips, R. S., Davis, R. B., & Miller, K. (1999). Screening inpatient quality using post-discharge events. *Medical Care, 37*(4), 384–398.

Mitchell, P. W., & Shortell, S. M. (1997). Adverse outcomes and variations in organizations of care delivery. *Medical Care. 35*(11, Supplement), NS19–32.

Murdaugh, C. (1997). Health-related quality of life as an outcome of organizational research. *Medical Care, 35*(11, Supplement), NS41–NS48.

National Chronic Care Consortium (1999). *Health networks for the chronically ill in turmoil: Unintended consequences of the Balanced Budget Act of 1997.* Bloomington, MN: The National Chronic Care Consortium.

Nerenz, D. R., & Zajac, B. M. (1996). *Assessing performance of integrated delivery systems.* New York: Faulkner & Gray, Inc.

Newcomer, R., Spitalny, M., Fox, P., & Yordi, C. (1999). Effects of the Medicare Alzheimer's Disease Demonstration on the use of community-based services. *Health Services Research, 34*(3), 645–668.

Sandy, L.G., & Gibson, R. (1996). Managed care and chronic care: Challenges and opportunities. *Managed Care Quarterly, 4*(2), 5–11.

Shortell, S. M., Gillies, R. R., Anderson, D. A., Erickson, K. M., & Mitchell, J. B. (1996). *Remaking healthcare in America.* San Francisco: Jossey Bass Publishing.

Shortell, S. M., Gillies, R. R., Anderson, D. A., Mitchell, J. B., & Morgan, K.L. (1993). Creating organized delivery systems: The barriers and facilitators. *Hospital and Health Services Administration, 38*(4), 447–466.

Weissert, W. G., Lesnick, T., Mushliner, M., & Foley, K. A. (1997). Cost savings from home and community-based services. *Journal of Health Politics, Policy & Law, 22*(6), 1329–1357.

Wojner, A. W., & MacCutcheon, M. A. (1998). *Critical Care Nursing Clinics of North America, 10*(1), 33–40.

Young, D. W., & Barrett, D. (1997). Managing clinical integration in integrated delivery systems: A framework for action. *Hospital and Health Services Administration, 42*(2), 255–279.

3

Approaches to Quality of Care by Regulatory and Accreditation Organizations

Vincent Mor

This chapter reviews the basis for the measurement of long-term care quality relying upon patient information to create aggregated measures characterizing provider performance. This approach is now at the core of HCFA's and the Joint Commission's revised vision of how to monitor and regulate the quality of long-term care providers (Joint Commission on Accreditation of Healthcare Organizations [JCAHO], 1998–1999). For all the potential weaknesses inherent in using data about patients that is generated by facility staff, these data are currently readily available in both the institutional and the home health arena. Substantial research effort has been devoted to the use of individual level data to create aggregated performance measures.

Following a brief review of the Omnibus Budget Reconciliation Act of 1987, which mandated the development of a comprehensive resident assessment instrument for use in all U.S. nursing homes, this chapter goes on to discuss the differences between individual resident assessment and the use of aggregated resident assessment information to "assess" the performance of a nursing facility. This is followed by a review of the various policy applications to which the mandated nursing home resident assessment instrument has been applied, including monitoring the quality of care provided by nursing homes. After explaining the various models currently being used to calculate the quality of care and quality of life provided in nursing, the chapter reviews the various complexities and methodological challenges facing those who want to apply these kinds of data to groups of nursing facilities.

Over the last decade long-term care has moved to develop and implement uniform, universally required, individual level data collection systems that can form the basis for measures of quality performance. This occurred in the long-term care field for several reasons. First, the 1986 Institute of Medicine Report recommended a uniform minimum data set (MDS) for nursing home resident assessment. This would never have been recommended without a general consensus that nursing home quality was poor and that the provider community was neither willing nor able to make the changes needed to improve the quality of care without specific direction. The perceived success of the nursing home resident assessment system, particularly the adoption of case-mix reimbursement based upon the patient data, prompted the Health Care Financing Administration to mandate a multipurpose client measurement system for Medicare reimbursed home health care.

Uniform patient assessment systems and quality measurement is possible in the long-term care sector because of the relative homogeneity of the patients (relative to hospitals and ambulatory care settings).[1] The advantages of having a common language to characterize nursing home residents was not lost on the home health industry, particularly since they, too, were becoming increasingly inundated with acutely ill patients and wanted some systematic way to describe this in order for them to be compensated accordingly. Other long-term care settings, such as Assisted Living Facilities, Senior Centers, and non-Medicaid Home Care providers, have sporadically introduced patient-based information systems that include data on the individual recipients of care for a variety of reasons. No national standards exist, although, numerous states are now struggling with the adoption of common clinically relevant data elements pertinent to all long-term care clients regardless of the setting in order to facilitate and track Medicaid Managed Care Reforms tentatively being applied to the long-term care population. The nursing home is the paradigm for other long-term care sectors. Although some feel what is needed is an integrated setting independent patient assessment system, this vision is a long way off.

THE EMERGENCE OF OBRA '87

The landmark Institute of Medicine Study (IoM, 1986) on the quality of care in nursing homes led to the passage of the Omnibus Budget Reconciliation

---

[1] While it is true that patients entering nursing homes increasingly resemble hospitalized patients in their complexity and heterogeneity, nursing homes do not handle pediatrics, obstetrics, nor post-surgical recovery. Thus, they are relatively more homogeneous than are acute hospital patients.

Act of 1987 (OBRA '87) one year later. This legislation was the most far-reaching revision to the standards, inspection process and enforcement system since the passage of Medicare and Medicaid in 1965 (Hawes, 1998). The structure and content of the OBRA nursing home reforms were heralded as a model for a regulatory system by simultaneously altering three fundamental elements of the existing structure: 1) the standards; 2) the process for determining compliance; and 3) the enforcement system. As recommended by the IoM Committee, these reforms were predicated upon a shift in focus from the structural features of the care environment to one directed toward the patient. In contrast to the focus on "paper compliance," new inspection procedures were to focus on process and outcome quality, incorporating interactions with residents, families, and ombudsmen about daily experience in the home by requiring direct observation of the resident. Enforcement was to be focused on outcomes, and the new standards mandated that states apply a wide array of sanctions tailored to the nature of the quality problem observed ranging from fines to "holds" on admissions to facility closure.

Because of documentation of past abuses and overuse, some specific provisions related to the processes of care were also contained in OBRA '87. Facilities had to extensively justify and document the use of physical restraints and psychotropic drugs, particularly neuroleptics and benzodiazepines. The role of consultant pharmacists reviewing the appropriateness of residents' prescribed medications was mandated under OBRA.

A major feature of OBRA, that the IoM saw as tying many of the other regulatory components together, was the introduction of a uniform, comprehensive resident assessment instrument (RAI) to guide the clinical care planning process in order to systematically document residents' needs. The RAI was not only to be used to systematically assess the resident and generate a comprehensive care plan to document clinical progress as that plan was implemented, but it was to be used by regulators to focus on resident outcomes and by facilities to improve their performance. Thus, elements of reform were supposed to support both external and internal quality assurance and improvement (Hawes et al., 1997).

Throughout this chapter, the term *assessment tool* is used in various ways. First, assessment is used as a clinical activity designed to assess a patient's condition in order to determine and then prescribe treatments needed by the patient. Second, assessment can be used as a measurement system to evaluate and monitor (assess) the quality of care clients receive. Finally, assessing assessment instruments is undertaken as a means of systematically contrasting the strengths and weaknesses of various resident level, but particularly provider assessment systems. This differentiation is important since it is possible for a clinically adequate patient assessment tool to be translated into an inadequate quality monitoring system. On the other hand, quite limited clinical assessment tools can have powerful applications to quality monitoring. In the paragraphs below, each of these applications as well as their interrelationships are described.

PATIENT SPECIFIC ASSESSMENT

Clinical assessment tools generally have a set of operational definitions and procedures for their application in the clinical setting. These instructions may stipulate the sources of information to be examined and how the examination is to be done. The Geriatric Assessment literature has repeatedly shown that having such explicit directions for clinicians to follow in assessing patients' needs results in identifying clinical conditions and problems that might otherwise have been missed (Rubenstein, Wieland, & Bernabei, 1995). Once identified, these can be acted upon to the benefit of the frail, elderly patient with multiple co-morbid conditions (Stuck et al., 1995). Additionally, explicit instructions and training in how to assess patients has been found to result in greater data reliability (Bernabei, Murphy, Frijters, DuPaquier, & Gardent, 1997).

The comprehensive assessment instrument mandated by OBRA '87 was, by law, to include concepts such as quality of life and not just aspects of clinical care or symptom management. Consequently, the designers of the instrument tried to incorporate concepts such as psychosocial well-being, usual and customary behaviors prior to nursing home entry, activities preferences and interpersonal conflicts with roommates, staff, and family members (Morris et al., 1990). While not always easy to measure operationally, by the time Version 2.0 of the RAI was promulgated, even these complex ideas had been defined in such a way as to result in reasonable levels of inter-rater reliability when trained assessors were compared (Morris et al., 1997).

Patient assessment data, like clinical data from hospital discharge records, have direct clinical utility for care planning and to document the patient's clinical history in such a way as to assist in future prognostication that affects treatment decisions. As in the case of hospital discharge data, patient assessment information can be aggregated to the level of the provider to describe the population served and how it is treated. Providers use such aggregated clinical data to monitor changes in the mix of patients admitted, or discharged, by season or year, and to compare the diagnostic profile of discharges from one provider versus another. Similarly, in the acute care sector these patient level clinical data have been used to conduct "pattern of care" studies, epidemiological investigations and to document geographic variation in medical practices for distinct clinical procedures. As the long-term care sector increasingly becomes computerized, similar phenomenon are occurring. In light of the multidimensional nature of the items in the assessment, however, monitoring of services rendered in facilities can include activities programs as well as the well-being of the residents and not just the infection or pressure ulcer incidence rate.

APPLICATIONS OF CLINICAL DATA FOR PROVIDER MONITORING

In developing and refining quality monitoring systems, one starting point is to define the goals or objectives of the quality measurement activity. Information about the quality of care has several possible constituents. The *provider* needs aggregated information regarding the quality of care provided and the resident outcomes experienced in order to target efforts to improve the care rendered. The *regulator* needs this information to target the on-site inspection and quality monitoring process and to document observed deterioration in care provided. The *purchaser* of care, such as Medicare, Medicaid, or even a Managed Care insurer, might want the results of quality monitoring systems in order to contract with the "best" provider for their patients and subscribers. Finally, the *consumer* and her advocates will want the information both in order to guide selection of a long-term care provider and to focus political pressure for system wide improvements in care and/or reimbursement rates.

Consistent with these different goals and constituents, particular approaches to the measurement of quality can vary in a number of ways (see, e.g., Donabedian, 1996; IoM, 1986; Blumenthal, 1996). Assessments may focus on individuals receiving care or on those providing care. They may be used to rate performance (e.g., by judging it acceptable or unacceptable, or better or worse than for a comparable organization), or to improve performance (e.g., by linking outcomes to processes of care) or both. They may be undertaken internally (e.g., by those providing or directly supervising care) or externally (e.g., by regulators, accreditors, or purchasers). They may be implicit (e.g., rated by a physician or someone else without reference to defined standards) or explicit (e.g., based on written criteria).

The use of quality monitoring systems may be voluntary or mandatory. The case for voluntary use is that it allows an organization to match measures to its priorities and resources (including existing information systems) and to adapt quickly as circumstances change, or better measures are introduced. Mandatory use of specific measures promotes valid cross-organizational comparisons based on standardized data and responds to consumer's, purchaser's, and regulator's interest in making informed choices. Obviously, a mixture of both voluntary and mandatory approaches is possible. For example, providers could be required to generate certain core measures but would be encouraged to also use others for their own quality improvement purposes.

The different purposes for which quality measurement is done may imply different levels of measurement. For example, information may be used at the level of the individual recipient to track changes in that patients' status over time. This is the basis of patient-based "outcome" measurement as used by several extant measurement systems ranging from the Functional Impact Measure (FIM) which is commonly used in rehabilitation and was the basis for the creation of the OASIS (Granger, 1998; Shaughnessy & Kramer, 1990). Both measurement tools were explicitly designed to look at change in a single patient's functioning over the course of their treatment. The OBRA mandated Resident Assessment Instrument (RAI) in its MDS form was designed as an individual level care planning tool that allowed for the monitoring of a single patient's change in status between assessment intervals. Indeed, the initial purpose of the quarterly assessment update as stipulated in the original RAI manual in 1991 was to allow for tracking changes in patient functioning: physical, cognitive, and emotional. Indeed, in light of the multidimensional nature of the items in the RAI that are repeated on a quarterly basis, one could readily say that it facilitates monitoring of changes in nursing home residents' health-related quality of life (Lawton et al., 1999).

As noted earlier, these person specific data may also be aggregated at different levels. Much aggregation of information operates at the organizational level for purposes of internal management or external assessment. Accordingly, regulators or purchasers of care may aggregate data to monitor organizational performance, to develop comparative information, to guide choices among providers of care, and to feed back summary and comparative information that helps providers set priorities for improvement. Data aggregated to the level of communities, states, or nations can be used to identify broader differences in practice patterns or resource use, which might be helpful in characterizing regional differences in practice patterns.

STANDARDS AND COMPARISONS

A component of most regulatory strategies is establishing minimal standards of acceptable performance. Minimum regulatory standards usually are not based on explicit comparisons. That is, someone does not necessarily fail an inspection by virtue of being in, say, the bottom 20% of providers on a set of quality parameters. Minimum standards are often defined as based on expert clinical criteria (e.g. specified staffing level, a maximum number of certain types of "violations," or the presence of a single instance of identifiable egregious care). Under HCFA's State

Operations Manual for skilled nursing facilities, each potential area in which a deficiency can be applied has an explicit set of criteria against which the performance (based on records, observation, or aggregated data) of the provider is compared.

Standards are generally fixed, not relative. They are based on assumed performance criteria generally based on structural (e.g., staffing) or process (e.g., percent of patients in restraints) domains of care. All such standards are predicated on a "commandment" that one *should, or should not* provide care in a particular way. Standards may apply to a wide variety of different domains of organizational functioning, ranging from the extensiveness of chart documentation to the kind of infection control program in place.

Performance measures often include a comparative component, usually called benchmarking. Organizations identify—through their own analyses and by accepting findings of others—some level of demonstrated positive performance that they will aim to achieve. These others may be perceived as "best" performers if excellence in that area is the goal. Alternatively, if tradeoffs among different areas of performance are considered necessary, then the standard may be set at, say, the 50th or 75th percentile.

Increasingly, individual level data are used in aggregate form to identify providers performing below acceptable standards and/or which are below, or above, some established set of absolute or normative benchmarks. In the case of nursing homes, the computerized MDS data formed the basis for the development of "quality indicators" which have been used on a demonstration basis to identify instances of problematic care or to rank facilities in terms of their performance. This is the relevance of the "cross-walk" between the individual level data and its aggregated form. Indeed, the application of these data for this quality monitoring purpose may blur the distinction between standards and benchmarks and between norms and average rankings.

POLICY APPLICATIONS OF THE M.D.S.

HCFA created the RAI in response to a Congressional mandate, but found that its universality made it possible to consider expanded applications. First, building upon Medicaid prospective payment systems and practices in a number of states, an expanded set of Resource Utilization Groups (RUGS-III) was developed. A multi-year demonstration project conducted in six states tested the feasibility of introducing this case-mix reimbursement system for paying facilities for their Medicaid patients (Fries et al., 1997). Most recently, the Balanced Budget Act of 1997 mandated the phased introduction of patient specific case-mix reimbursement for all Medicare beneficiaries entering skilled nursing facilities under the Medicare benefit. Second, under the same large demonstration project, HCFA created a set of Quality Indicators by aggregating patient level data to characterize each facility (Zimmerman et al., 1995). In some states, regulators responsible for surveying the quality of nursing home care were given data on the performance of the home they were about to inspect based on such quality indicators. As described in greater detail below, HCFA plans are to expand this use now that transmittal of computerized data is a requirement for all nursing homes in the United States (Vladeck, 1995).

ESTIMATES OF THE IMPACT OF OBRA '87

By 1992, most OBRA provisions were to have been instituted, although certain aspects of the implementation of the changes in the approach to conducting facility surveys had yet to be introduced. A number of studies have documented changes in a variety of different indicators of the quality of nursing home care that have appeared over the past half decade. Some have focused on specific provisions and found that the rate of restraint use, psychotropic drug use, and catheterization have all dropped (Borson & Doane, 1997; Castle, Fogel, & Mor, 1996; Kane, 1993; Mosley, 1996; Shorr, Fought, & Ray, 1994; Snowden & Ray-Byrne, 1998). Others have solicited the opinions of facility staff and others in the long-term care field to determine whether quality has improved since the introduction of the OBRA provisions. They found that, by and large, there is agreement that things have improved, although there is still considerable room for improvement (Hawes et al., 1997; Marek, Rantz, Fagin, & Krejci, 1996).

A large, quasi-experimental study of the nursing home reform provisions of OBRA, in a random sample of some 250 nursing homes in 10 states, found that the accuracy and comprehensiveness of resident assessments improved with the introduction of the MDS. Furthermore, processes of care in several areas improved and residents were found to be less likely to decline functionally and were less likely to be hospitalized than was the case prior to OBRA implementation (Fries et al., 1997; Hawes et al., 1997; Mor et al., 1997; Phillips et al., 1997). Although tested, no positive effects were noted for several quality of life related outcomes, ranging from mood disturbance to well-being; indeed there was some suggestion that following the introduction of the OBRA reforms and the RAI, these more qualitative aspects of residents' lives were less likely to improve (Phillips et al., 1997).

In spite of these generally positive empirical findings stating that OBRA has had a positive effect on the quality of nursing home care, there is limited evidence that states are taking advantage of the new enforcement provisions of OBRA to more aggressively regulate nursing facilities. Industry and Congressional efforts to undermine important provisions of

OBRA '87 during 1996, generated considerable concern among advocates that still colors the debate about the appropriateness of designing an out-comes-based quality monitoring system since existing enforcement mechanisms have not been consistently introduced (Latimer, 1998; Weisskopf, 1998). Some commentators have expressed concern that reliance on the distribution of "report cards" and quality improvement initiatives is too reminiscent of the failed "collaborative approach" to improving the quality of nursing home care (Nursing Home Law Letter, May 16, 1995). Furthermore, they distrust the market-based approach implicit in provid-ing consumers and advocates with information on which they can make informed choices about which facility to use (Latimer, 1998).

Recent newspaper exposes, a raft of civil torts, and cases of criminal fraud as well as the rise of civil suits seeking, and being awarded, dam-ages for poor care in nursing homes, have all contributed to a renewed sense of concern about the quality of care nursing homes provide (Do your hospital . . ., 1998; State moves . . ., 1998). Add to this a report from the GAO regarding the quality of care in California nursing homes and it would appear, to the educated lay person, that OBRA has been only mar-ginally effective in improving nursing home care because it was so poorly implemented and enforced (Government Accounting Office (GAO), 1997). Indeed, based on recent news reports from the White House, it would appear that HCFA may be charged with the responsibility for stimulating more stringent state level enforcement actions (Clinton orders . . ., 1998).

A NEW PARADIGM FOR DATA-BASED QUALITY MONITORING

In keeping with the original vision of how RAI data might be used, HCFA has developed a new paradigm for regulating the quality of nursing home care by targeting inspections based on and aided by ongoing data obtained from facilities. The paradigm assumes that clinical data from the resident assessment and care planning process, data assembled during the regula-tory survey and certification process, along with service utilization data from claims and other sources can be used to characterize the "perfor-mance" of nursing facilities on key measures of quality. In light of the host of available clinical information and the existence of longitudinal data on many nursing home residents, data are available to "risk adjust" these indicators to ensure comparison of the performance of facilities with com-parable patients. Optimally, state surveyors can use performance mea-sures to guide their on-site inspections to focus on those clinical areas in which the home appears to be most deficient. This same source of data can be used by the facility as a way to target certain care problems for continuous quality improvement efforts. HCFA's paradigm postulates that the resulting information will stimulate both more effective regulatory action and internal quality improvement efforts.

One goal of further systematizing the protocol used by surveyors through the use of aggregated data about the homes' past performance is to reduce state variation in when and how many and what types of "violations" are cited as deficiencies. Analyses of the data generated by state inspectors regarding the number and type of deficiencies found during an inspection revealed nearly a 10-fold difference across all states in the median number of deficiencies. These apply to both health-related care problems and structural factors. This enormous effect of geography (presumably surveyor team) was observed by Rudder and Phillips (1998) within New York. In the New York City area, which has the most facilities, the fewest deficiencies were cited following inspections. The importance of deficiency citations is that they are a necessary prelude to enforcement actions, since New York City instituted the fewest such actions.

CREATION AND USE OF QUALITY INDICATORS

Measures of nursing home quality have frequently been proposed and used by researchers in the past, but generally only for a small number of facilities or in select groups of facilities. Until recently, most such measures have been based on aggregate data obtained about a home in order to compare the rate of "events" between facilities with various characteristics. Zinn and Mor (1994) used facility level survey data to test the effect of facility staffing and market factors on indicators of quality of care. Nyman (1989) also relied on aggregate data to examine the effect of different types of facility characteristics on selected quality indicators. These studies are limited, in that risk adjustment is restricted without patient level data. As researchers have repeatedly pointed out, the heterogeneity of patients served by facilities due to strategic choices, the need to adjust the patient mix is paramount (Banaszak-Holl, Zinn, & Mor, 1996; Zinn & Mor, 1994). Existing aggregated data available nationally was able to identify the existence of "special care units" as a sign of heterogeneity, but measures of staffing or case-mix were not specific to unit. This is one of the reasons that so many of the early studies of the determinants of quality of care in nursing homes led to contradictory findings (Davis, Sebastian, & Tschetter, 1997).

Use of individual level data to conduct studies of nursing home quality require large numbers of nursing homes and data on large proportions of their residents and these almost always come from administrative data. The National HealthCorp, a chain of approximately 100 facilities located in the South Central United States, maintained longitudinal, resident level assessment data on all patients in the facilities since the early 1980s. Numerous studies using these data have been conducted investigating organizational determinants of the quality of care, the impact of Medicare policies, and the clinical determinants of falls and hospitalization (Kiel, O'Sullivan, Teno, & Mor, 1991; Mor, Intrator, & Laliberte, 1993; Morris, Hawes, Murphy, & Nonemaker, 1995; Ooi, Morris, Brandeis, Hossain, & Lipsitz, in press). Medicaid data, particularly available hospitalization and medication use information, has been a good source of patient specific information for creating indicators of the quality of care residents receive (Lipowski & Bigelow, 1996). Canadians in Manitoba have also been able to use linked administrative data to examine the effect of organizational factors on how long between a resident's admission and when she experiences a negative outcome (Shapiro & Tate, 1995).

While few nursing facilities across the country currently have the sophistication to use the MDS for institutional planning, staff loading, or outcome monitoring, some facilities are actively using the MDS for one or more of these functions. Some states, particularly those which began statewide computerization of their MDS data prior to the HCFA mandate in June 1998, began rudimentary efforts to report aggregated quality indicators from a variety of different domains. These efforts are designed to make facilities aware of the potential uses of the MDS and to show them where they stand relative to statewide averages in terms of the quality of care provided.

DEVELOPMENT AND APPLICATION OF THE CHSRA QIs

Under HCFA's Nursing Home Case-Mix and Quality Demonstration, Wisconsin's Center for Health Systems Research and Analysis (CHSRA), was charged with developing an array of readily useable facility and resident quality indicators based on computerized data from the RAI (Zimmerman et al., 1995). Numerous versions of these indicators were proposed and reviewed by various clinical and industry panels for appropriateness, meaningfulness, and potential identified for attributing problems to the care of the facility. Indicators ranged from the prevalence of pressure ulcers, to the prevalence of use of antipsychotics, the incidence of late loss ADLs, and the use of high dose benzodiazapines in those states where detailed drug data were available. Following creation of the algorithms used to identify individual residents and their aggregation to the level of the facility, reports were designed for facilities as well as for surveyors who were to use this information to help them in the survey process.

Various efforts to develop and test quality indicators focused on quality of life issues such as mood or well-being generally ended up with a clinical expression simply because it was easier to gain the consensus of experts on the meaning of clinically pertinent QIs than broader quality of life measures. The development process for most, if not all QIs, was to generate potential measures based on routinely collected MDS items. A QI was generally specified in detail, complete with a specification of which patients were in the denominator and what combination of items and clinical conditions constituted membership in the numerator, all of the CHSRA QIs were developed as dichotomous, indicating the presence or absence of a condition or circumstance that might be suggestive of problems in the associated domain of care. Given this logic, it is not surprising that all QIs have a strong clinical focus and tend not to encompass measures suggesting that residents' quality of life is not what it should be because there is little agreement about an indicator that cannot be readily operationalized.

Abt Associates evaluated the Nursing Home Case-Mix and Quality (NHCMQ) demonstration and interviewed state surveyors to determine how the (CHSRA) quality indicators (QIs), were implemented in the survey process, and how surveyors and providers reacted to their use (Moore & White, 1998). Only three of the five demonstration states were found to be using the QIs in the survey process. Maine and South Dakota had fully implemented them. Due to improper programming of the indicators and inaccurate peer group data, there was only limited implementation in Kansas.

In states using the indicators, their role in the survey process appeared to be exclusively in the pre-survey preparation phase, at which point QI reports are reviewed to aid in the resident sample selection process. None of the states included in the Abt Associates study were utilizing the QIs to alter survey schedules based on periodic review of reports or to alter survey team staffing based on issues flagged in the QI reports.

In spite of limited implementation of QIs in the survey process, interviewees in some states were positively inclined toward their use and felt that with greater experience they could expand the range of uses of the data. For example, reports comparing QIs flagged at one period in time with those flagged at another period might be helpful in tracking changes. South Dakota surveyors noted that QIs helped them identify issues they may not otherwise have detected. QIs reportedly increased surveyors' confidence by reinforcing their observations. Furthermore, QIs were reported to assist the team both in focusing on problem areas and thinking broadly about what is going on in the facility on a systemic level.

ORYX: THE NEXT EVOLUTION OF ACCREDITATION

The Joint Commission on Accreditation of Healthcare Organizations (JCAHO) is integrating the use of outcomes and other performance measurement data into the accreditation process (JCAHO, 1998a). Under the ORYX initiative, accredited organizations (over 2,500 long-term care organizations as of July, 1999) are being required to regularly furnish outcome and performance measurement data to JCAHO, through a contracted JCAHO certified ORYX vendor. Data submitted is being used by JCAHO to monitor performance and to focus surveys (JCAHO, 1998b). Certified ORYX vendors must have performance measurement systems with the following *Attributes of Conformance:*

- Includes appropriate performance measures focusing on organization performance or on patient care processes or outcomes;
- Has an automated, operational database;
- Ensures the accuracy and completeness of performance data;
- Uses risk adjustment or stratification methods to reduce or clarify the influence of confounding patient factors;
- Provides timely feedback of comparative data to participating organizations; and
- Is useful and relevant to the accreditation process (JCAHO, 1998a).

Evaluation criteria for these attributes are being implemented incrementally. For example, key criteria, such as risk adjustment and establishment of reliability across health care organizations, were not required until January 2000. There are presently over 70 certified ORYX vendors with clinical measures relevant to long-term care organizations, and 51 of these vendors are "the vendor of choice" for at least one accredited long-term care organization (documented choice required as of March, 1998 (JCAHO, 1998b). By March 31, 1999, accredited long-term care organizations, via their chosen ORYX vendor, are required to submit to JCAHO third-quarter 1998 data for at least two clinical measures relating to at least 20% of their resident populations. Ultimately, at least eight clinical measures relating to at least 35% of their resident populations will be required (JCAHO, 1998b).

Q-METRICS® AND OTHER NURSING HOME QUALITY MODELS

Since the availability of computerized clinical data on nursing home residents, several organizations have developed and are applying alternate sets of performance measures for nursing facilities. Q-Metrics® offers 18 different performance measures which compare how well a given facility is doing at, for example, preventing cognitive decline, as compared with other facilities with a similar mix of residents. Each performance measurement is risk adjusted using multivariate models, relies upon several quarters of longitudinal data to maximize the stability of the performance measure, and comes with a set of quality improvement suggestions in the form of a "care plan" for the facility (Mor, Morris, Lipsitz, & Fogel, 1997, 1998). The Q-Metrics® system is applied in voluntary Quality Care Consortia whose members compare their performance against national benchmarks and one another and share best practices concerning how to improve performance in selected outcome domains.

In contrast to the CHSRA indicators, the Q-Metrics® system includes several measures characterizing aspects of the quality of life of residents. One of these is based upon the Social Engagement Scale embedded in the MDS that was developed by Mor and colleagues. Another addresses the extent to which residents are experiencing conflicted relationships with staff and roommates. The meaningfulness of such aggregated quality of life measures, obviously have not been validated.

Other systems have been developed by, and are now being used by, elements of the industry associations, either at the national or the state level. For example, AHCA has developed a variation of the CHSRA quality indicators report called "Facilitator" for use by its members. The American Association of Homes and Services for the Aged is working with CHSRA to institute state association level projects that can provide quality indicators for its members.

There are several other commercial "nursing home" finder programs available on the Internet now being marketed for consumers and their family members contemplating the choice of a nursing home. Few of these have quality indicator data available based on aggregated resident information. Rather, they are based on publicly available data such as the results of HCFA's regulator surveys or even the coded results of state surveys (for some states). Nonetheless, it is these more readily useable sources of information which might have the greatest impact on consumers' knowledge since they are most readily and universally available at this time. Indeed, the Health Care Financing Administration has its own Internet-based "Web page" containing information obtained from the annual facility surveys pertinent to the quality of all facilities in the country, particularly the number and types of deficiencies identified by the state surveyors at the last inspection.

MONITORING PRESCRIPTION DRUG APPROPRIATENESS IN NURSING HOMES

Regulations issued pursuant to OBRA '87 that pertained to prescription medications for the first time required physicians to justify the use of a class of drugs based on specific diagnoses. Moreover, nursing homes, and not the prescribing physician, are held responsible for regulatory sanctions for undocumented and unjustified use of psychotropic drugs (Medicaid State Operations Manual, 1989). Studies of the impact of these regulations, on psychotropic prescribing patterns in several states using different study designs, reveal a significant reduction in prescriptions for neuroleptics with no sustained increase in use of physical restraints, or in prescriptions for sedative/hypnotics (Garrard, Chen, & Dowd, 1995; Rovner, Edelman, Cox, & Shmuely, 1992; Shorr et al., 1994; Wollstadt & Porter, 1992). Because none of these studies evaluated the appropriateness of drug use for an individual, the assumption is that this decrease does not represent a decline in use of needed medications by nursing home residents with mental illness.

In spite of the evidence for improved prescribing, recent studies from the Office of the Inspector General on prescription drug use in nursing homes continue to raise concern over the state of prescribing in nursing homes (Office of Inspector General 1,2,3, 1997). Using data from three separate data sources: 1) the Texas Medicaid drug claims; 2) a national survey of consultant pharmacists; and 3) an independent review of medical records and drugs for a sample of nursing home residents, the studies found that 20% of patients were receiving at least one drug deemed inappropriate for their diagnosis and 20% were receiving at least one medication deemed inappropriate for use by the elderly. The Inspector General states that improvements are needed in the prescribing, administration, and monitoring practices in nursing homes and recommends that medication reviews be strengthened.

With two-thirds taking between 5 and 12 drugs per day (Baum, Kennedy, & Knapp, 1997), elderly people receive nearly a third of all drugs prescribed in the United States. Given the physiologic changes associated with aging (i.e., alterations in pharmacokinetics and pharmacodynamics) (Hume & Owens, 1995; Kurfees & Dotson, 1987) and the co-morbid conditions, concomitant drug use and interactions, nutrition and environmental factors, drugs may contribute to functional decline among the elderly. Yet, the potential for maximizing physical functioning or prolonging the time until decline in physical functioning given optimal prescribing is substantial as has been shown in the few clinical trials which enrolled frail elderly individuals.

A recent study by Abt Associates investigating the potential effects of prospective payment system (PPS) on prescribing, found that nursing home residents in New York under a state-based PPS reimbursement system were less likely to receive optimal therapy for medical conditions (e.g., congestive heart failure and osteoporosis) than residents in states without PPS (Moore & White, 1998). These data highlight the need to consider, not only the absence of inappropriate drug use as an indicator of quality, but also the presence of good prescribing practices. Analyses undertaken at Brown support these findings, extending them to the broader, long-stay, Medicaid nursing home resident (Teno, Bird, & Mor, 2000).

Relying upon several simple, but highly reliable data elements, Zimmerman et al. (1995) developed a number of quality indicators to identify facilities with high rates of psychotropic drug use. Both antipsychotic agents, often cited as being used as "chemical restraints," and hypnotics which have been associated with increased falls and hip fracture (Ray, Federspiel, & Schaffner, 1980) are included in these drug-based quality indicators. Substantial interfacility and interstate variation in the use of these drugs has been documented (Bernabei et al., 1998). However, to effectively use prescription drug use as quality indicators, the multidimensional nature of prescribing must be considered. Defining inappropriate drug use, the Beers criteria were developed specifically for very frail residents as a means to evaluate quality prescribing in nursing homes (Beers et al., 1991). These criteria have been updated to incorporate clinical criteria and to assign a relative rating of the potential negative effects (Beers, 1997). Considering not only effectiveness of agents and potential for serious side effects, these criteria also considered co-morbid conditions and dose, frequency, and duration of the drugs.

Indicators of prescription quality may be sensitive to inappropriate prescribing for elderly inpatients. While the occurrence of therapeutic duplication is rare (Oborne, Batty, Maskrey, Swift, & Jackson, 1997) and drugs at high risk for adverse effects are prescribed more appropriately than drugs at low risk (Schmader et al., 1994), consideration of less severe side effects deserves attention as well. For example, drugs may have anticholinergic effects including decreased secretions, slowed gastrointestinal motility, blurred vision, increased heart rate, heat intolerance, and sedation (Goodman & Gilman, 1996). While anticholinergic effects may only be an issue of mild discomfort in healthy, younger patients, these effects can impair physical functioning in the frail elderly patient (Feinberg, 1993). Consider the example of dry mouth. In addition to reducing the ability to communicate, this anticholinergic effect may predispose the frail elderly patient to malnutrition, promote mucosal damage, denture misfit, dental caries, and increase the risk of serious respiratory infection secondary to loss of antimicrobial activity in saliva (Feinberg, 1993). Furthermore, elderly patients are at increased risk of anticholinergic effects owing to polypharmacy and the potential for pharmacodynamic and pharmacokinetic drug interactions. Unfortunately, these effects are often quickly attributed to old age, eliminating the opportunity for alleviating them by altering the drug regimens that may be causing them.

While prescribing indicators may be sensitive to inappropriate pre-scribing for elderly inpatients, evaluating quality prescribing on the basis of this alone is insufficient. Consideration of the underuse of some med-ications is also important (Avorn, Dreyer, Connelly, & Soumerai, 1989; Avorn & Gurwitz, 1995; Beers et al., 1988; Beers et al., 1992; Larrat, Spore, Mor, Hiris, & Hawes, 1995; Lindley, Tulley, Paramsothy, & Tallis, 1992; Owens, Sherburne, Silliman, & Fretwell, 1990; Ray et al., 1980; Soumerai et al., 1997; Wilcox, Himmelstein, & Woodhandler, 1994). The evaluation of the use of proven therapy in the elderly reveals a complimentary, yet sometimes contradictory picture to the evaluation of inappropriate med-ication use. For example, only 22% of patients with atrial fibrillation who are on digoxin also received warfarin or aspirin (300mg) to prevent stroke (Schmader et al., 1994). In a study of elderly patients with acute myocar-dial infarction, the elderly patients were three times more likely to receive the medication not proven to increase survival instead of beta-blockers (Soumerai et al., 1997). Analysis of detailed drug data on nursing home residents under HCFA's Case Mix demonstration, reveal underuse of anti-hypertensives, ACE inhibitors among CHF patients and analgesics for pain, particularly narcotic analgesics for dying cancer patients (Bernabei, Gambassi, & Mor, 1998; Gambassi et al., 1998). Thus, indicators of the quality of drug prescribing can focus both on the prevalence of inappropriate drug use as well as the prevalence of inadequate drug use. Examination of data from nursing homes in multiple U.S. states suggests that both constitute significant quality problems in nursing home care.

THE MISSING QUALITY OF LIFE MEASURES

In spite of all the effort that has been devoted to developing quality indi-cators that capture the multidimensional nature of quality in the long-term care facility, little progress has been made in adding measures that explic-itly attempt to introduce the "patient's voice." Measures of clinical quality or even the "appropriateness" of drug prescribing ignore patients' per-spectives regarding what it is like to live in the facility. Numerous struc-tural and process measures have been proposed, ranging from whether patients and families attend care planning conferences to the frequency of meetings of residents' councils. While many facilities have attempted to assess residents "satisfaction" with care, even those investigators that have used very loose requirements for being cognitively intact have found relatively low response rates to such surveys. The Health Care Financing Administration has issued a contract to the Kanes, who, togeth-er with Powell Lawton are trying to develop and test resident specific as well as facility specific quality indicators that specifically focus on residents' quality of life. The biggest barrier to this and similar efforts is that a high proportion of long stay residents of nursing homes are unable to respond to satisfaction questionnaires nor even to reliably respond to personal interviews about their preferences and their perception of life in the facility. This quality of the resident population complicates efforts to measure the quality of life of all but a select few residents of nursing homes.

IMPLEMENTING THE NEW PARADIGM FOR QUALITY MONITORING

HCFA is now working to implement its vision for quality monitoring now that transmittal of computerized data is a requirement for all nursing homes in the United States. In the short term, HCFA plans to introduce quality indicator software into states' existing systems for uploading computerized MDS data from all facilities in the state. The plan is that the software will generate quality indicator reports describing the proportion of the residents of the facility that, based on the most recent MDS assessment, meet criteria for potential quality problems ranging from having pressure ulcers to taking antipsychotic medications in the absence of specific psychiatric diagnoses. The observed rate of a quality indicator in each facility is contrasted to some "benchmark" that has yet to be determined. These reports will be generated, both for the surveyors scheduled to inspect a facility, as well as the facility itself.

In order to guide the actual surveyor inspection protocol, the software will generate a listing of the actual facility residents who, as of the last MDS assessment, met the quality indicator criteria as possibly having quality problems in how care is provided. This "roster" of residents will, according to current plans, serve as the starting point for the surveyors' sampling of records to determine whether the particular quality problems identified in the aggregated MDS data are actually indicative of a verifiable quality of care problem.

The image of state facility inspectors arriving at the door of a facility armed, not only with the facilities' own history of deficiencies from earlier years, but also statistical data and lists of potential problem cases, must give providers nightmares. However, this approach could pervert the whole process. Once the lists of residents on these rosters become the basis for the quality review, it is very easy to forget that the coded MDS data are not, nor can they ever be, perfectly valid. It is easy to forget that the simple algorithms, labeled as "quality indicators," are merely suggestive, and not definitive. Indeed, in many respects resident lists constitute an official enumeration of people with ostensible quality problems even though the true patient specific sensitivity and specificity of the validity of these quality indicators has not been established, nor is it likely to be established.

The long-range goals for HCFA in moving toward a more information intensive approach is an outgrowth of the short-term plans enumerated above. HCFA has awarded four major contracts to advance past work on quality indicators in the nursing home field. All are designed to further HCFA's goal of using the MDS, in both aggregated and individual level form to bolster and systematize the quality monitoring process. HCFA's vision of this process is that the MDS data constitute the basis for directing survey and certification activities, setting payment levels, and to promulgate information about the quality of long-term care providers to consumers and purchasers. One contract is developing explicit protocols for facility surveys which will target particular areas of patient care performance based on the facilities' ranking with respect to established quality indicators. This protocol is to include the identification of individual resident records which, based upon their MDS data, appear to manifest quality performance problems. These "rosters," based on the most recently reported computerized MDS data, represent the first line of inquiry about the validity of an aggregated quality indicator.

Another contract is identifying which existing quality indicators have sufficient validity to be used in the state survey process and which need additional validation and modification. This contract also is charged with developing new quality indicators for special patient populations such as those receiving "post-acute" care for a short-term period in nursing homes and those residents requiring "palliative" care.

Another contract seeks to develop analytic algorithms and on-site audit protocols to identify facilities whose MDS data, as reported, appear to be inconsistent, fallacious, or even fraudulent. Finally, one contract seeks to develop a whole new set of measures of facility quality that take into consideration the "voice" and values of the resident and her advocates. Emanating from this contract may be new approaches to measuring resident satisfaction with care as well as residents' perceptions of the adequacy of care received in terms of meeting their needs. The contractors charged with developing, testing, and validating existing and new quality indicators are to consider more than the state facility inspectors as the consumers of this information. They are considering the application of different types of quality indicators for the different audiences for that information outlined earlier in this chapter. In addition to the regulators focused on holding the facility accountable for their performance, either in absolute or relative terms, other audiences include, "value purchasers" and consumers and their advocates. The use of quality indicators by facilities may be most appropriate as a means of targeting internal quality improvement activities. If facilities are held immediately accountable for the results of the data for their own internal comparisons rather than against some external benchmark, they are less likely to "game" the coding instructions to maximize reimbursement or minimize the appearance of quality problems. However, if purchasers are deciding to contract with a facility based on these data, or if consumers decide to select a facility based on indicators of quality performance, data quality issues become paramount and the validity standards for such "actionable" applications need to be more stringent.

In addition to the technical measurement problems, as well as the problems of adverse coding incentives, quality-based performance measurement implies that the observed disparities are attributable to differences in treatment input. Obviously, some differences in observed quality are due to differences in patient mix, and some differences are due to patient preferences and treatments the facility does not control. Not only does the validity of interfacility comparisons depend on the adequacy of risk adjustment for clinical and patient preference differences but also on the degree of control the provider has over the care provided to the patient. No matter how good the nursing care, poor medical care of complex nursing residents may not be overcome.

ORGANIZATIONAL DETERMINANTS OF VARIATION IN QUALITY INDICATORS

Considerable research in geriatrics has investigated the clinical factors associated with various outcomes experienced by nursing home residents. Falls, pressure ulcers, incontinence, infection, and hospitalization have all been investigated leading to the development of resident risk factor profiles. These are quite useful in designing and implementing preventive interventions within a facility but have generally ignored the considerable variation in outcomes between study facilities. Nonetheless, considerable evidence suggests that facility characteristics, such as ownership status (Cohen & Dubay, 1990; Fottler & Crawford, 1985; O'Brien, Saxberg, & Smith, 1983; Riportella-Mueller & Slesinger, 1982), size (Riportella-Mueller & Slesinger, 1982), staffing (Lee, 1983), occupancy (Nyman, Levey, & Rohrer, 1987), and resident payor mix (Nyman, 1989) bear on nursing home quality of care whether defined in terms of process or outcomes. Since 80% of nursing home beds are in investor-owned facilities, the quality of care provided their residents has frequently been compared to that given to residents of not-for-profit facilities. Whereas for-profit status has been associated with lower expenditures and staffing levels (Cohen & Dubay, 1990; Fottler & Crawford, 1985; O'Brien et al., 1983; Riportella-Mueller & Slesinger, 1982), lower resource use could signify greater efficiency rather than superior quality (Davis et al., 1997; O'Brien et al., 1983), and quality outcomes do not always covary with higher resource inputs (Gottesman & Bourestom, 1974; Greene & Monahan, 1981; Lee, 1983; Linn & Lewis, 1977; Nyman, 1989; Nyman et al., 1987; Spector, 1991). Indeed, recent research by Mukamel and Bower (1998) using data from the state of New York suggest that the relationship between the level of resource inputs and the quality outcomes as measured by several different indicators is curvilinear.

Ooi and his colleagues (in press) examined the incidence of pressure ulcers in facilities that had a poor record in preventing pressure ulcers in the prior year as compared to homes that had low rates in the prior year. After adjusting for up to 12 different risk factors at the resident level, they still found a three-fold increase in the incidence rates of residents in homes with poor prevention records relative to those with good records. Mor and his colleagues have examined the effect of facility staffing and resource characteristics on the likelihood of hospitalization among nursing home residents (Intrator, Castle, & Mor, 1999). After considering numerous resident characteristics, the risk of hospitalization was significantly increased as a function of facility resources and ownership. State variation in hospital use rates has also been documented, controlling for resident characteristics, suggesting that state Medicaid policy or geography plays as great a role in long-term care as it does in acute care (Castle & Mor, 1996; Murtaugh & Frieman, 1995; Mor et al., 1997; Teno et al., 1997).

All these findings confirm the importance of facility factors in helping to understand variation in residents' quality of care and outcome experience. The problem is that, to date, there have been few studies that have been able to successfully understand the myriad causes of this variation. The well-known Donebedian model, which hypothesizes that the structural characteristics of a provider (the capacity to provide care) determines the way in which the processes of care are actually implemented and undertaken, which, in turn, determine the outcomes of care, has rarely been tested. Few studies in the long-term care arena have been able to formally test this model, although numerous studies have approximated testing it (see Zinn & Mor, 1998 for a review of this literature). A recent attempt to formally test the model was undertaken using MDS data from all facilities in a single state (Ramsey, Sainfort, & Zimmerman, 1995). This study was unable to confirm the specified path analysis model. Some have suggested that executive leadership and organizational commitment to quality improvement are really the salient characteristics rather than the structural factors (Castle, Fogel, & Mor, 1996). Zinn and Brannon have observed considerable variation in the prevalence and use of quality improvement approaches in populations of nursing homes, suggesting the potential explanatory power of this factor (Dansky & Brannon, 1996; Zinn, Brannon, & Mor, 1995).

Facilities' own past performance is also a predictor of the future. Not only have analyses of MDS data across multiple states revealed the importance of prior rates of pressure ulcers in predicting individual residents' risk of acquiring a pressure ulcer, but similar results have been observed with deterioration of behavioral problems and functional decline. However, the past does not condemn all facilities to continued poor performance nor does it guarantee continued good performance. Real changes such as turnover in key positions occur in the life of a facility that alter the way in which structural resources are organized to deliver care processes, which in turn, under proper circumstances, may affect the outcomes experienced. This means that all predictions based on history, even quite contemporaneous data, are probabilistic and have some potential for being incorrect.

THE FEASIBILITY OF USING AGGREGATED PATIENT DATA FOR QUALITY MONITORING PURPOSES

While the universal availability of the MDS and its current use under Medicare SNF PPS facilitates HCFA's new regulatory paradigm, there are numerous conceptual and technical challenges that may compromise the effective implementation of the vision.

First, case-mix difference in the types of residents living in facilities make direct comparisons difficult. Research by Zimmerman and his colleagues (Arling, Karon, Sainfort, Zimmerman, & Ross, 1997; Zimmerman et al., 1995) as well as Morris and his colleagues (Mor et al., 1998; Morris et al., 1997; Ooi et al., in press) strongly point to the need to risk adjust most outcomes in order to make adequate between facility comparisons. A recent paper by Mukamel and Bower (1998) used pre-MDS data from New York (the PRI which was used to risk adjust Medicaid payment levels) on 550 facilities over a 4-year period. They found very large differences in the quality rankings that emerged from the three major quality indicators that they used as a function of the type and extent of risk adjustment. In spite of the importance of risk adjustment, there are reasonable concerns about over-adjusting by taking into consideration past clinical problems. Indeed, in general, which factors to consider in creating adjustment models is a complex issue that could backfire if not done properly. Whether the field is ready for this remains to be seen.

Second, facilities with many new admissions per quarter have patients whose clinical problems may reflect conditions acquired in acute hospitals. Gillen and his colleagues observed very different outcome rates as a function of admission status and payer source (Gillen, Spore, Mor, & Freiberger, 1996). Maxwell, Zimmerman, Karon, Sainfort, and Purnell

(1998) applied the CHSRA QIs to new admissions and long stay residents and found very different rates across many measures. Rehospitalization rates were found to be much higher in hospital-based nursing facilities than freestanding skilled nursing facilities even after controlling for numerous clinically relevant variables precisely because of the influence of length of stay and the purpose of admission (recovery, rehabilitation, and return home) which are more prevalent in hospital-based settings (Intrator et al., 1999).

Third, many relevant QIs in the nursing home are relatively rare, making estimates of their rate necessarily imprecise in all but the largest nursing facilities. This is even more true for incident or change markers, such as acquiring a pressure ulcer or an infection, as only those "at-risk" of newly acquiring the condition are included in the denominator. This promotes great instability in the relative position (quality rank) of the nursing facilities because the number of patients acquiring new pressure ulcers per quarter might easily vary from 0 to 3, even in an excellent facility. While risk adjustment may reduce the fluctuation somewhat, a longer time period of observation, or some form of averaging, might be necessary to smooth out the large shifts. Using Massachusetts' Management Minutes Questionnaire, which is resident level longitudinal data used to reimburse facilities, Porell and Caro (1998) examined longitudinal changes in quality indicators across some 500 facilities throughout the state. They found that several of the quality indicators that they were examining revealed only minimal to poor correlations over time. This was particularly true for outcomes like changes in ADL functioning as opposed to the prevalence of restraint use.

Fourth, certain domains of outcome may be more reliably measured using a combination of different MDS items, rather than relying upon a single indicator. To date, most quality indicators reported in the literature (Mukamel, 1997; Mukamel & Bower, 1998; Porell & Caro, 1998; Zimmerman et al., 1995) have relied upon single item indicators rather than looking at changes on some form of ordinal, or linear, summary scale. However, measures such as Activities of Daily Living Cognitive Performances (Morris et al., 1994), social engagement (Mor et al., 1995), and distressed mood (Phillips, Zimmerman, Bernabei, & Jonsson, in press) have been shown to be internally consistent, summary scales that discriminate among different types of patients in expected ways. These measures can provide a more reliable means of documenting other degrees of deterioration a nursing home resident experiences. They form the basis for several quality performance measures used by private companies doing risk adjusted ranking of facilities (Mor et al., 1998).

Finally, the multiplicity of long-term care outcomes that are relevant to our understanding of quality of care are necessarily multidimensional, meaning that no single indicator is likely to capture facility quality. This means that facilities that may perform extremely well on one type of indicator do not necessarily perform as well on another. Indeed, recently two papers confirmed this hypothesis, one using New York state data and the other data from Massachusetts (Mukamel & Brower, 1998; Porell & Caro, 1998). Thus, the notion that these data will make it easier for purchasers or consumers to identify the "best" long-term care provider is not borne out. Nursing home ratings will have to consider the many values and preferences that influence one's perception of quality, rather than selecting a single "gold star" provider.

SUMMARY

The emergence of HCFA's Resident Assessment Instrument as the *Lingua Franca* of long-term care, replete with code sets, definitions, and new "language" to describe the long-term care resident has made it possible to surmount the "Tower of Babel" that has heretofore reigned. While designed to try to improve the performance of the many long-term care providers that did only rudimentary comprehensive resident assessments (if they were done at all), the universality and uniformity of code sets for describing and classifying resident needs made it possible to use the same information for many different purposes. Thus, standardized care planning guides have been applied, hopefully resulting in more residents getting some treatment or service which they would not have received had they not been more systematically assessed. For better or for worse, standardized care protocols augment (or replace) clinical skill and discretion. A dozen years ago few facilities systematically asked about mood, interpersonal conflict, or psychosocial well-being—now it is required and some residents may benefit. Thus, the rudimentary tools to begin to ask about quality of life in a meaningful way are now present, however inadequately, for the first time.

Whether the policy-related applications of the MDS lexicon actually pervert or amplify the initial clinical intent remains to be seen. Many have noted that using clinical assessment information to classify residents in terms of their average care resource requirements will result in an overstatement of residents' needs in the same way that the introduction of Diagnosis Related Groups as the prospective payment system for hospitals resulted in "upcoding" of medical records to maximize reimbursement. Similarly, how the original purpose of the assessment information will change as providers realize that the data are being used to specifically monitor the quality of care remains to be seen.

All in all, this last decade has seen the emergence of myriad opportunities in long-term care assessment and quality monitoring. It may be another decade before we know whether those opportunities will be realized.

REFERENCES

Arling, G., Karon, S., Sainfort, F., Zimmerman, D., & Ross, R. (1997). Risk adjustment of nursing home quality indicators. *Gerontologist, 37*(6), 757–766.

Avorn, J., Dreyer, P., Connelly, K., & Soumerai, S. B. (1989). The use of psychoactive medication and quality of care in rest homes: Findings and policy implications of a statewide study. *New England Journal of Medicine, 320,* 227–232.

Avorn, J., & Gurwitz, J. H. (1995). Drug use in the nursing home. *Annals of Internal Medicine, 23,* 195–204.

Banaszak-Holl, J., Zinn, J. S., & Mor, V. (1996). The impact of market and organizational characteristics on nursing care facility service innovation: A resource dependency perspective. *Health Services Research, 31*(1), 97–117.

Baum, C., Kennedy, D. L., & Knapp, D. E. (1997). *Drug utilization in the US—1986.* Rockville MD: Department of Health and Human Services, Food and Drug Administration.

Beers, M. H. (1997). Explicit criteria for determining potentially inappropriate medication use by the elderly: An update. *Archives of Internal Medicine, 157,* 1531–1536.

Beers, M., Avorn, J., Soumerai, S. B., Everitt, D. E., Sherman, D. S., & Salem, S. (1988). Psychoactive medication use in intermediate-care facilities. *Journal of the American Medical Association, 260,* 3016–3020.

Beers, M. H., Ouslander, J. G., Fingold, S., Morgenstern, H., Reuben, D., Rogers, W., Zeffren, M. J., & Beck, J. C. (1992). Inappropriate medication prescribing in skilled-nursing facilities. *Annals of Internal Medicine, 117,* 684–689.

Beers, M. H., Ouslander, J. G., Rollingher, I., Brooks, J., Reuben, D., & Beck, J. C. (1991). Explicit criteria for determining inappropriate medication use in nursing homes. *Archives of Internal Medicine, 151,* 1825–1832.

Bernabei, R., Gambassi, G., Lapane, K., Landi, F., Gatsonis, C., Dunlop, R., Lipsitz, L., Steel, K., & Mor, V., for the SAGE Study Group (1998). Management of pain in elderly patients with cancer. *Journal of the American Medical Association, 279*(23), 1877–1882.

Bernabei, R., Gambassi, G., & Mor, V. (1998). Introducing functional outcomes in geriatric pharmaco-epidemiology: The SAGE database. *Journal of the American Geriatric Society, 46,* 250–252.

Bernabei, R., Murphy, K., Frijters, D., DuPaquier, J. N., & Gardent, H. (1997). Variation in training programs for resident assessment instrument implementation. *Age and Aging, 26*(2), 31–35.

Blumenthal, D. (1996). Effects of market reforms on doctors and their patients. *Health Affairs Millwood, 15*(2), 170–184.

Borson, S., & Doane, K. (1997). The impact of OBRA-87 on psychotropic drug prescribing in SNF's. *Psychiatry, 48*(10), 1289–1296.

Castle, N. G., Fogel, B., & Mor, V. (1996). Quality of care in nursing homes administered by members of the American College of Health Care Administrators. *Journal of Long Term Care Administrators, 24*(2), 11–16.

Castle, N. G., & Mor, V. (1996). Hospitalization of nursing home residents: A review of the literature, 1980–1995. *Medical Care Research and Review, 53*(2), 123–148.

Clinton orders better nursing home care; more oversight, worker registry urged. (1998, July 22). *Washington Post*, p. A03.

Cohen, J. W., & Dubay, L. C. (1990). The effects of Medicaid reimbursement method and ownership on nursing home costs, case mix, and staffing. *Inquiry, 27*(2), 183–200.

Dansky, K. H., & Brannon, D. (1996). Using TQM to improve management of home health aides. *Journal of Nursing Administration, 26*(12), 43–49.

Davis, M., Sebastian, J., & Tschetter, J. (1997). Measuring quality of nursing home services: Residents' perspective. *Psychological Reports, 81*(2), 531–542.

Do your hospital and physician make the grade? Hospital checkup. (1998, July 27). *Los Angeles Times*.

Donabedian, A (1996). The effectiveness of quality assurance. *International Journal of Quality of Health Care, 8*(4), 401–407.

Feinberg, M. (1993). The problems of anticholinergic adverse effects in older patients. *Drugs and Aging, 3*(4), 335–348.

Fottler, M., & Crawford, M. (1985). The impact of diagnosis related groups and prospective pricing systems on health care management. *Health-Care-Manage-Review, 10*(4), 73–84.

Fries, B. E., Hawes, C., Morris, J. N., Phillips, C. D., Mor, V., & Park, P. S. (1997). Effect of the national resident assessment instrument on selected health conditions and problems. *Journal of the American Geriatrics Society, 45*(8), 994–1001.

Gambassi, G., Landi, F., Peng, L., Brostrup-Jensen, C., Calore, K., Hiris, J., Lipsitz, L., Mor, V., & Bernabei, R. (1998). Validity of diagnostic and drug data in standardized nursing home resident assessments: Potential for geriatric pharmacoepidemiology. *Medical Care, 36*(2), 167–179.

Garrard, J., Chen, V., & Dowd, B. (1995). The impact of the 1987 federal regulations on the use of psychotropic drugs in Minnesota nursing homes. *American Journal of Public Health, 85*, 771–776.

Gillen, P., Spore, D., Mor, V., & Freiberger, W. (1996). Functional and residential status transitions among nursing home residents. *Journal of Gerontology: Medical Sciences, 51A*(1), M29–M36.

Goodman, L. J., & Gilman, G. S. (1996). *The pharmacological basis of therapeutics* (9th ed.). McGraw-Hill: International Edition.

Gottesman, L. E., & Bourestom, N. C. (1974). Why nursing homes do what they do. *Gerontologist, 14*(6), 501–506.

Government Accounting Office (1997). *Long term care: Diverse, growing population includes millions of Americans of all ages.* Washington, DC: Author.

Granger, C. V. (1998). The emerging science of functional assessment: Our tool for outcomes analysis. *Archives of Physical Medicine and Rehabilitation, 79*(3), 235–240.

Greene, V. L., & Monahan, D. J. (1981). Inconsistency in level of care assignment decisions in skilled nursing facilities. *American Journal of Public Health, 71*(9), 1036–1039.

Hawes, C. (1998). Regulation and the politics of long-term care. *Generations: Journal of the American Society on Aging, 21*(4), 5–9.

Hawes, C., Mor, V., Phillips, C. D., Fries, B. E., Morris, J. N., Steele-Friedlob, E., Greene, A. M., & Nennstiel, M. (1997). The OBRA '87 nursing home regulations and implementation of the resident assessment instrument: Effects on process quality. *Journal of the American Geriatrics Society, 45*(8), 977–985.

Hume, A. L., & Owens, N. J. (1995). Drugs and the elderly. In *Care of the elderly. Clinical aspects of aging* (4th ed.). Baltimore, MD.

Institute of Medicine (1986). *Improving the quality of care in nursing homes.* Washington, DC: National Academy of Sciences Press.

Intrator, O., Castle, N., & Mor, V. (1999). Facility characteristics associated with hospitalization of nursing home residents: Results of a national study. *Medical Care, 37*(3), 228–237.

Joint Commission on Accreditation of Healthcare Organizations (1998a). Internet site.

Joint Commission on Accreditation of Healthcare Organizations (1998b). *Performance measurement.*

Joint Commission on Accreditation of Healthcare Organizations (1998–1999). *Comprehensive accreditation manual for long term care.* Oakbrook Terrace, IL.

Kane, R. (1993). Restraining restraints: Changes in a standard of care. *Annual Review of Public Health, 14,* 545–584.

Kiel, D. P., O'Sullivan, P. O., Teno, J., & Mor, V. (1991). Health care utilization and functional status in the aged following a fall. *Medical Care, 29,* 221–228.

Kurfees, J. F., & Dotson, R. L. (1987). Drug interactions in the elderly. *Journal of Family Practice, 25*(5), 477–488.

Larrat, E. P., Spore, D., Mor, V., Hiris, J., & Hawes, C. (1995). Medication utilization in board and care facilities. *Consultant Pharmacist, 10,* 1263–1277.

Lawton, M. P., Moss, M., Hoffman, C., Grant, R., Ten-Have, T., & Kleban, M. H. (1999). Health, valuation of life and the wish to live. *Gerontologist, 39*(4), 406–416.

Latimer, J. (1998). The essential role of regulation to assure quality in long-term care. *Generations: Journal of the American Society on Aging, 21*(4), 10–14.

Lee, A. (1983). How nursing homes behave: A multi-equation model of nursing home behavior. *Social Science Medicine, 17*(23), 1897–1906.

Lindley, C. M., Tulley, M. P., Paramsothy, V., & Tallis, R. C. (1992). Inappropriate medication is a major cause of adverse drug reactions in elderly patients. *Age and Aging, 21,* 294–300.

Linn, L. S., & Lewis, C. E. (1977). The content of care provided by family nurse practitioners. *Journal of Community Health, 2*(4), 259–267.

Lipowski, E., & Bigelow, W. (1996). Data linkages for research on outcomes of long-term care. *Gerontologist, 36*(4), 441–447.

Marek, K., Rantz, M., Fagin, C., & Krejci, J. (1996). OBRA '87: Has it resulted in positive change in nursing homes? *Journal of Gerontology Nursing, 22,* 32–40.

Maxwell, C., Zimmerman, D., Karon, S., Sainfort, F., & Purnell, M. (1998). Estimating quality indicators for chronic care from the minimum data set 2.0: Risk adjustment and concerns. *Canadian Journal of Quality in Health Care, 14*(3), 4–13.

Medicaid state operations manual (1989). Washington, DC: US Department of Health and Human Services, Health Care Financing Administration.

Moore, T., & White, A. (1998). *Drug utilization and MDS-based outcomes for elderly nursing homes residents.* Briefing Paper. Abt Associates, Cambridge, MA.

Mor, V., Branco, K., Fleishman, J., Hawes, C., Phillips, C., Morris, J., & Fries, B. (1995). The structure of social engagement among nursing home residents. *Journal of Gerontology: Psychological Sciences, 50*(1), 1–8.

Mor, V., Intrator, O., Fries, B., Phillips, C., Teno, J., Hiris, J., Hawes, C., & Morris, J. (1997). Changes in hospitalization associated with introducing the resident assessment instrument. *Journal of the American Geriatrics Society, 45*(8), 1002–1010.

Mor, V., Intrator, O., & Laliberte, L. (1993). Factors affecting conversion rates to medicaid among new admissions to nursing homes. *Health Services Research, 28*(1), 1–25.

Mor, V., Morris, J, Lipsitz, L., & Fogel, F. (1997). The Q-Metrics system for long-term care outcomes management. *Nutrition, 13,* 242–244.

Mor, V., Morris, J., Lipsitz, L., & Fogel, B. (1998). Benchmarking quality in nursing homes: The Q-Metrics system. *Canadian Journal of Quality in Health Care, 14*(2), 12–17.

Morris, J., Hawes, C., Murphy, K., & Nonemaker, S. (1995). *Long term care resident assessment instrument user's manual: Version 2.0.* Baltimore: Heath Care Financing Administration.

Morris, J. N., Fries, B. E., Mehr, D. R., Hawes, C., Phillips, C., Mor, V., & Lipsitz, L. A. (1994). MDS Cognitive Performance Scale. *Journal of Gerontology: Medical Science, 49*(4), M174–M182.

Morris, J. N., Hawes, C., Fries, B. E., Phillips, C. D., Mor, V., Katz, S., Murphy, K., Drugovich, M. L., & Friedlob, A. S. (1990). Designing the national resident assessment instrument for nursing homes. *Gerontologist, 30*(3), 293–307.

Morris, J. N., Nonemaker, S., Murphy, K., Hawes, C., Fries, B. E., Mor, V., & Phillips. C. (1997). A commitment to change: Revision of HCFA's RAI. *Journal of the American Geriatrics Society, 45*(8), 1011–1016.

Mosley, C. (1996). Nursing home ownership and quality of care. *Journal of Applied Gerontology, 13*(4), 386–397.

Mukamel, D. B. (1997). Risk-adjusted outcome measures and quality of care in nursing homes. *Medical Care, 35*(4), 367–385.

Mukamel, D. B., & Bower, C. A. (1998). The influence of risk adjustment methods on conclusions about quality of care in nursing homes based on outcome measures. *Gerontologist, 38*(6), 695–703.

Murtaugh, C. M., & Freiman, M. P. (1995). Nursing home residents at risk of hospitalization and the characteristics of their hospital stays. *Gerontologist, 35*(1), 35–43.

Nursing Home Law Letter, May 16, 1995.

Nyman, J. (1989). Improving the quality of nursing home outcomes. Are adequacy or incentive oriented policies more effective? *Medical Care, 26*(12), 1158–1171.

Nyman, J., Levey, S., & Rohrer, J. E. (1987). RUGs and equity of access to nursing home care. *Medical Care, 25*(5), 361–372.

O'Brien, J., Saxberg, B., & Smith, H. (1983). For-profit or not-for-profit nursing homes: Does it matter? *Gerontologist, 23*(4), 341–348.

Oborne, C. A., Batty, G. M., Maskrey, V., Swift, C. G., & Jackson, S. H. (1997). Development of prescribing indicators for elderly medical inpatients. *British Journal of Clinical Pharmacology, 43*(1), 91–97.

Office of Inspector General (1997). *Prescription drug use in nursing homes. Report 1.* Department of Health and Human Services, Washington, DC.

Office of Inspector General (1997). *Prescription drug use in nursing homes. Report 2.* Department of Health and Human Services, Washington, DC.

Office of Inspector General (1997). *Prescription drug use in nursing homes. Report 3.* Department of Health and Human Services, Washington, DC.

Ooi, W. L., Morris, J., Brandeis, G., Hossain, M., & Lipsitz, L. (In press). Do facility characteristics affect outcomes in nursing homes? *Journal of Aging and Health.*

Owens, N. J., Sherburne, N. J., Silliman, R. A., & Fretwell, M. D. (1990). The senior care study: The optimal use of medications in acutely ill older patients. *Journal of the American Geriatric Society, 38,* 1082–1087.

Phillips, C., Morris, J. N., Hawes, C., Fries, B. E., Mor, V., Nennstiel, M., & Iannacchione, V. (1997). Association of the Resident Assessment Instrument (RAI) with changes in function, cognition and psychosocial status. *Journal of the American Geriatrics Association, 45*(8), 986–993.

Phillips, C., Zimmerman, D., Bernabei, R., & Jonsson, P. (In press). Using the Resident Assessment Instrument for quality enhancement in nursing homes. *Age and Aging Special Issue.*

Porell, F., & Caro, F. G. (1998). Facility-level outcome performance measures for nursing homes. *Gerontologist, 38*(6), 665–683.

Ramsey, J. D., Sainfort, F., & Zimmerman, D. (1995). An empirical test of the structure, process and outcome quality paradigm using resident-based, nursing facility assessment data. *American Journal of Medical Quality, 10*(2), 63–75.

Ray, W. A., Federspiel, C. F., & Schaffner, W. (1980). Antipsychotic drug use in nursing homes: Epidemiologic evidence suggesting misuse. *American Journal of Public Health, 70,* 485–491.

Riportella-Mueller, & Slesinger, D. P. (1982). The relationship of ownership and size to quality of care in Wisconsin nursing homes. *Gerontologist, 22*(4), 429–434.

Rovner, B. W., Edelman, B. A., Cox, M. P., & Shmuely, Y. (1992). The impact of antipsychotic drug regulations on psychotropic prescribing practices in nursing homes. *American Journal of Psychiatry, 149,* 1390–1392.

Rubenstein, L. Z., Wieland, D., & Bernabei, R. (1995). *Geriatric assessment technology: The state of the art.* Editrice Kurtis: Milano.

Rudder, C., & Phillips, C. (1998). Citations and sanctions in the nursing home enforcement system in New York state: Their use and effects. *Generations: Journal of the American Society on Aging, 21*(4), 21–24.

Schmader, K., Hanlon, J. T., Weinberger, M., Landsman, P. B., Samsa, G. P., Lewis, I., Uttech, K., Cohen, H. J., & Feussner, J. R. (1994). Appropriateness of medication prescribing in ambulatory elderly patients. *Journal of the American Geriatrics Society, 42*(12), 1241–1247.

Shapiro, E., & Tate, R. (1995). Monitoring the outcomes of quality of care in nursing homes using administrative data. *Canadian Journal on Aging, 14*(4), 755–768.

Shaughnessy, P. W., & Kramer, A. M. (1990). The increased needs of patients in nursing homes and patients receiving home health care. *New England Journal of Medicine, 332,* 21–27.

Shorr, R. I., Fought, R. L., & Ray, W. A. (1994). Changes in antipsychotic drug use in nursing homes during implementation of the OBRA-87 regulations. *Journal of the American Medical Association, 271,* 358–362.

Snowden, M., & Ray-Byrne, P. (1998). Mental illness and nursing home reform: OBRA-87 ten years later: Omnibus Budget Reconciliation Act. *Psychiatry, 49*(2), 229–233.

Soumerai, S. B., McLaughlin, T. J., Spiegelman, D., Hertzmark, E., Thibault, G., & Goldman, L. (1997). Adverse outcomes of underuse of β-blockers in elderly survivors of acute myocardial infarction. *Journal of the American Medical Association, 277,* 115–121.

Spector, W. (1991). Cognitive impairment and disruptive behaviors among community-based elderly persons: Implications for targeting long-term care. *Gerontologist, 31*(1), 51–59.

State moves to close two nursing homes. (1998, July 25). *Miami Herald,* article 324.

Stuck, A. E., Aronow, H. U., Steiner, A., Alessi, C. A., Bula, C. J., Gold, M. N., Yuhas, K. E., Nisenbaum, R., Rubenstein, L. Z., & Beck, J. C. (1995). A trial of annual in-home comprehensive geriatric assessments for elderly people living in the community. *New England Journal of Medicine, 333*(18), 1184–1189.

Teno, J., Bird, C., & Mor, V. (2000). *Prevalence and management of pain in US nursing homes.* Report to the Robert Wood Johnson Foundation.

Teno, J., Branco, K. J., Mor, V., Phillips, C. D., Hawes, C., Morris, J., & Fries, B. E. (1997). Changes in advance care planning in nursing homes before and after the Patient Self-Determination Act: Report of a 10-state survey. *Journal of the American Geriatrics Society, 45*(8), 939–944.

Vladeck, B. C. (1995). From the health care financing administration. *Journal of the American Medical Association, 273*(19), 1483.

Weisskopf, M. (1998). The good provider. *Generations: Journal of the American Society on Aging, 21*(4), 5–9.

Wilcox, S. M., Himmelstein, D. R., & Woodhandler, S. (1994). Inappropriate drug prescribing for community dwelling elderly. *Journal of the American Medical Association, 272,* 292–296.

Wollstadt, L. J., & Porter, C. S. (1992). Nursing home antipsychotic drug use changes after OBRA'87. *Clinical Research, 40,* 575A.

Zimmerman, D., Karon, S., Arling, G., Ryther, C., Collins, T., Ross, R., & Sainfort, F. (1995). The development and testing of nursing home quality indicators. *Health Care Financing Review, 16*(4), 107–128.

Zinn, J., Brannon, D., & Mor, V. (1995). Organizing for quality in nursing home settings: A contingency approach. *Quality Management and Health Care, 3*(4), 37–46.

Zinn, J., & Mor, V. (1994). Nursing home special care units: Distribution by type, state and facility characteristics. *Gerontologist, 34*(3), 371–377.

Zinn, J., & Mor, V. (1998). Organizational structure and the delivery of primary care to older Americans. *Health Services Research, 33*(2), 354–380.

PART II

Quality of Care: Life in Long-Term Care Settings

4

Quality Long-Term Care: Perspectives From the Users of Home Care[1]

Neena L. Chappell

T he decade of the 1990s has been marked by discussion of fundamental health care reform throughout the industrialized world. Much of
the rhetoric has included the notion of client participation in care
decisions. The vision of a more comprehensive and appropriate health care
system includes the belief that better quality of care will be received if
clients themselves have a say in that care. As Lawton expresses it in chapter 7, quality of life rather than quality of care should be the focus. Quality
of life necessarily includes issues of autonomy and self-determination. Yet
historically, clients are not asked their view of health, nor what care they
believe they should receive. As Noelker and Harel note in their opening
chapter, home care today evolved from a time when publicly funded care
was met with moral disapproval and characterized by paternalism that
required passive and submissive recipients. As acceptance grows for
long-term care in the home for seniors, the area of client autonomy is critical, heightened by the fact that home care by definition means that services are coming into a personal and private place—one's home.

This chapter examines the issue of client participation and empowerment in home care in British Columbia, Canada. It begins with a discussion of universal Medicare in Canada and the vision of health reform that

[1] Funding for the data reported herein was provided by the Capital Regional District and
NHRDP, Health Canada to M.J. Penning, N.L. Chappell, P.E. Stephenson, H.A. Tuokko and
L. Rosenblood, Centre on Aging, University of Victoria.

has been widely accepted throughout the country. It then turns to the literature on empowerment in service delivery, notably home care, for seniors. It presents Canadian data from recipients of home care services on their views of the home care that they receive and how they would like to participate within decision making. The reactions of service providers and policy makers to the findings from extensive structured interviews and a more in-depth focus group with recipients of services are discussed. The chapter concludes with a discussion of the future of client empowerment given the current situation.

UNIVERSAL MEDICARE IN CANADA

Unlike the United States, Canada has universal Medicare. Canadians accept the argument that the risks of sickness and invalidity in old age are relatively easy to establish, relatively constant, and not subject to cyclical fluctuations or sudden emergencies; that the universal risks be underwritten by the community as a whole; that one should not become impoverished because of illness. In 1957, the Hospital Insurance and Diagnostic Services Act ensured hospital care including outpatient clinics, medical, and nursing schools for the entire country. As hospitals became the place where physicians practiced, physician insurance followed in 1966, with the Medical Care Act (implemented in 1968). By 1972, all provinces and territories had joined the federal government's cost-shared comprehensive medical insurance program. Initially, this was on a fifty-fifty basis but in 1977, was changed to a system of cash or block grants from the federal to the provincial governments. Starting in 1986, the federal government began withdrawing its funding from the provinces but this ended in the first budget speech of 1999, in which they started providing funds once again to the provinces for health care.

Canada's health care system, like that in many industrial countries around the world, is therefore, oriented toward physician care largely provided in acute care hospitals. This focus was intentional; medicine was believed to hold the answers to a healthy population and physicians held the necessary knowledge in order to cure us. It should be noted that while Canada has universal health care, it does not have socialized medicine. Physicians operate mainly as private entrepreneurs with guaranteed incomes that, until recently, were largely unlimited. In addition, Canada has never and still does not have universal or national programs for community-based, nonmedical forms of care. While there was substantial growth in home health services in the 1970s, they have not been added to Medicare. There is no comprehensive coverage for non-hospital, non-physician related services. Health care is a provincial responsibility. Virtually all provinces provide some home care (in British Columbia it is referred to as home support) services, but the specific services that are available, the ones that are charged a user fee, and the ones that are based on the ability to pay, vary from province to province and indeed from jurisdiction to jurisdiction within provinces.

The 1990s in Canada, as in other industrialized countries, marked a fundamental change in how the health care system was viewed. Until this time, the century had been characterized by building the welfare state. However, the 1990s saw a major shift, fueled largely because of continual cost increases in health care, that led to an acceptance of cumulative evidence that argued a biomedical focus on illness was too narrow. A broadened definition of health, together with a social determinant of health model, became accepted. In addition, the organization of the delivery of health care also came under attack. Until recently, countries, including Canada, had been more concerned with equity, extending equal financial protection and access to health services to most or all of the population, than with questioning the adequacy of the care being provided. There had been no overall mechanism to evaluate interventions, to assess delivery efficiency or effectiveness, or to ensure cost accountability (Chappell, 1998a).

For the first time since Medicare achieved prominence in health care in the industrialized world (about 100 years ago), the buyers of care, both public and private, began questioning the quality of that care. The critical questions became: How much of current medical intervention is warranted? Would some of the dollars currently spent on medical care be better spent (i.e., have a greater effect on health) on other things such as home care or housing or air quality? How do we ensure that medical intervention is beneficial rather than simply causing no harm? The 1990s marked an acceptance of the critiques of the health care system that claimed it was inefficient, lacking comprehensiveness, and in many instances, inappropriate. Much of the criticism is not new. The 1990s reflected an official acceptance of these arguments and an apparent willingness to act upon them—this is new. It is equally important to note that most critics of Medicare embrace some of its features. In Canada, universal access and public funding are overwhelmingly desired by the general population of Canadians within a Canadian health care system. An EKOS (1998) public opinion poll finds that Canadians want their health care system protected and want home care added to it.

With a political willingness to examine change in the health care system came a multitude of commissions, task forces, and committees, both federal and provincial, that examined health reform. Remarkable consensus emerged on a vision of a new health care system for Canada. In the early part of the 1990s, Mhatre and Deber (1992) reviewed available reports from provincial and federal working groups constituted to examine the health care system. They found remarkable similarity on the direction that health reform should take. It is to be noted that subsequent working groups have arrived at the same conclusions. The characteristics of the new health care system should include:

- Broadening the definition of health to include social and psychological aspects, in addition to the biomedical aspects of health.
- Shifting the emphasis from curing illness to promoting health and preventing disease.
- Switching the focus to community-based, rather than institutional-based, care.
- Providing more opportunities for individuals to participate with service providers in making decisions on health choices and policies.
- Decentralization of the provincial systems to some form of regional authorities.
- Improved human resources planning, with particular emphasis on alternative methods for remuneration of physicians other than fee-for-service.
- Enhanced efficiency in the management of services through the establishment of councils coordinating bodies and secretariats.
- Increasing funds for health services research, especially in the areas of utilization, technology assessment, program/system evaluation, and information systems.

There is widespread acceptance that there needs to be a redistribution of emphasis and dollars from medical and institutional care to a broader base of community health care services with its promise of a more appropriate system of care for less than, or at least no more than, the dollars expended on the current medical care system. The report of the National Forum on Health (1997), chaired by the Prime Minister, concluded from its consultations and discussion groups that Canadians unmistakably support the basic principles on which Medicare was built. They also value equity, compassion, collective responsibility, individual responsibility, respect for others, efficiency, and effectiveness. The report also recommends that home care be added to Canada's universal health care system.

By the close of the 1990s, there is clear evidence that federal and provincial ministries of health want to restructure the health care system in Canada. In rhetoric, there is an unmistakable acceptance of a broadened definition of health and efforts to ensure collaboration with multiple sectors, including the private sector, different levels of government, the informal sector, and volunteer agencies. There has also been unmistakable rhetoric embracing community care and informal caregivers. There are efforts to at least cap acute and institutional care. There is structural decentralization as provinces move to regionalization and there are increased research dollars for health services research (see Segall & Chappell, 2000, for an elaboration).

However, there has been less visible action in terms of shifting the emphasis from curing illness to promoting health and preventing disease; switching the focus to community-based care; providing more opportunities for individuals to participate with service providers in making decisions in health choices and policies; improving human resource planning and, in particular, alternative methods of remuneration of physicians; and enhancing efficiency in the management of services.

Interest in this chapter focuses on one of the areas of health reform, namely, autonomy for clients in community care. Autonomy generally refers to mastery, a sense of control, decision making in one's life, and freedom from the control and influence of others (for a recent review, see Chappell, 1998b). It is multidimensional, including, for example, autonomy of judgment as opposed to conformity; autonomy of action and the capacity to act in accordance with self-made decisions; and autonomy of decision as free will, meaning one can decide among a number of alternatives within constraints imposed by other factors (Fuchs et al., 1998). We turn next to a discussion of home care within the context of health reform in Canada.

HOME CARE

This chapter examines the focus on providing more opportunities for individuals to participate with service providers in making decisions specifically in community-based care. The rhetoric for citizen participation and empowerment in health care choices is a new rhetoric. Until recently, the health care system has not believed it was necessary or that it should pay particular attention to the wishes of the recipients of care, nor to their participation in the decision-making process regarding what, how much, and when they receive care. Rather, care recipients may express "want," but health professionals determine "need" in the context of an assessment that is assumed to provide an objective measure (Dill, 1993). Assessors also have competing pressures from families and other professionals to ensure safety through placement, from the system to contain costs, and from legal practices to ensure protection (Clemens, Wetle, Feltes, Crabtree, & Dubitzky, 1994).

There are three general service delivery models for home care. One is the brokerage model in which case the managers purport to play the role of impartial manager responsible for determining needs and arranging, coordinating, and monitoring services contracted from provider agencies (Ontario Ministry of Health, 1992; Zawadski & Eng, 1988). This approach is currently in use in Ontario. In two other provinces, New Brunswick and Quebec, an integrated team model is used. In this instance, case management is facilitated by a professional provider team where one has leadership responsibility. In British Columbia, Alberta, and Manitoba some select clients have a consumer managed model in which either clients or informal caregivers, provided that they are assessed as appropriate for self-managed care, receive information (and, in some instances, financial assistance) and they themselves select and coordinate the resources they need. Evaluation is limited although findings suggest that each approach may work in different circumstances for different clients and, therefore, there are some calls for a flexible client-driven approach (Rose, 1992). The consumer-managed model at the present time is implemented least often.

The area of client empowerment has received little attention within the flurry of health reform. As Mansour (1994) points out, despite a preoccupation with reforming the health care system and the argument that citizens should have a say in health concerns, there is a striking lack of consultation with citizens even about what they mean by the term "health." Research suggests that people have different definitions of what health includes: for example, a general sense of well-being, the absence of disease, and performance or functional ability. Others distinguish holistic, physical, and mental health (Morse, 1987), or between functional adapted and self-actualization aspects of health (Stuifbergen, Becker, Sands, & Ingalsbe, 1990).

Home care, known as the Home Support Program in the Capital Regional District (greater Victoria) in British Columbia where data reported here were collected, is part of that province's universal, province-wide health care system. In British Columbia, the provincial government provides policy guidelines and funding to the regions. The regions are responsible for budget allocations, and in the Capital Regional District, where the research was conducted, the region dispenses payments to a host of for-profit and not-for-profit home support agencies that are responsible for hiring the workers and delivering the care. However, assessment and eligibility take place at the regional level, not at the agency level. Furthermore, while assessment is provided without charge to any potential recipient, once deemed eligible for services, the services are available on an ability to pay basis.

Estimates concerning the use of home care prior to health reform ranged from 10–15% of older adults in general (Chappell, 1989; Doty, 1986) and from 25–36% of frail elderly in particular (Soldo, Agree, & Wolf, 1989). In the United States, average annual rates of growth for home care services have been estimated at around 20–25% (Applebaum & Philips, 1990). There were 208 agencies providing home care in the United States in 1969; there were approximately 8,000 in 1985. (In the 1990s, however, there have been declines.) In British Columbia, there were 77 agencies providing care in 1978 to 11,714 clients. There were 121 agencies and an estimated 25,500 clients by 1985 (Kane & Kane, 1985). In the Capital Regional District, the number of agencies remained the same at 15 between 1988 and 1993, but the number of clients increased 44.4% (from 4,269 to 6,166). However, the number of clients declined to 3,430 in 1995. In the Capital Regional District a policy against adding new long-term institutional beds and an expansion of home-based services was operative from 1991 to 1994.

Eustis and Fischer (1991) list several factors contributing to the growth of home care, including the increasing number of older adults with chronic health problems needing long-term care; patients increasingly being discharged from the hospital more quickly than in the past; substitution of limited home care for long-term care in institutions; and technological advances that allow treatment in the home.

Even during the expansion of home care services, there was little research on the quality of care delivered and even less on quality from the user's point-of-view. Furthermore, several factors are operative that suggest maintaining quality may be difficult. For example, recent changes in the construction of new long-term institutional beds and hospital discharge practices result in more frail and vulnerable clientele unable and unwilling to criticize services. Other factors include the fact that the majority of services (70–80%) are provided by care professionals such as homemakers, who frequently have low wages, inadequate supervision, inadequate training, and high absenteeism and turnover rates (60–70%); fiscal constraints; inadequate or inappropriate legislation; a lack of appropriate models defining quality of home care; and conflicting priorities and policies, such as cost containment, together with provision of high-quality care (Applebaum & Philips, 1990).

Although there is little research on the quality of home care, especially from the client's point of view, there are several calls for greater client participation in the literature. The few empirical studies available suggest little progress has been made in this direction.

CALLS FOR EMPOWERMENT

The literature contains many calls, under various names, for greater participation by clients, including a client-centered approach, client-focused approach, client-driven approach (Rose, 1996). All argue for involving clients as "the experts" in identifying their needs and goals and working with them in the decision-making process. However, as this author notes, case management is fraught with varying degrees of professional paternalism. Or, as Clemens et al. (1994) state, the contradiction between client-centered theory together with directive practice is evident in case management. Kapp (1997) argues that there are several reasons for the paternalistic approach to caring for seniors, including fear of lawsuits resulting from overprotective policies, obsession with formal structures and regulations, care providers' wish to maintain control over prevention of risks, and professionals' emphasis on the needs of the patient.

Research examining the participatory extent of older clients in home care is not abundant. Nevertheless, that which exists confirms that seniors and their informal caregivers have marginal roles in decisions concerning their receipt of health care services, including community services (Holstein, Bjorn, Holst, Due, & Almind, 1993; Lloyd, 1991). Professional staff make the decisions. Furthermore, studies of care relations between dependent elders and home care workers suggest that both are aware of the imbalance in the relationship, accounted for at least partially by the elders' undeniable need to rely on them (Aronson, 1991a, 1991b; Cox, 1993; Lustbader, 1991). When the informal caregiver is also involved in the decision-making process, the informal caregiver tends to have some say but less than the professional, and the elder emerges as still without much input (Hasselkus, 1994). An assumption of frailty and dependency is made by the professional provider about the elderly person (Becker & Kaufman, 1988; Keller, Leventhal, Prohaska, & Leventhal, 1989) that extends to a lack of consideration of the senior's wishes.

Even less research is available on seniors' interest in increasing their empowerment in the receipt of home care services. However, Glickman, Stocker, and Caro (1997) found that, despite widespread satisfaction (92%) with their home care worker and expressions of continuing need for the involvement of a case manager, approximately one quarter of clients indicated they would be willing to take on more responsibility for the supervision and direction of their own care. One third said they would accept less case manager involvement, although it was not necessarily their preference. Doty, Kasper, and Litvak (1996) also report high satisfaction with attendant services, with less than 10% not being very satisfied or at all satisfied. They report that consumer choice and satisfaction were maximized when a public program encouraged clients to hire their own attendants directly and hire whomever they wished. Furthermore, when given the choice, consumers favored persons already known to them (family members, neighbors, friends), resulting in what they call an integration of their formal and informal support systems. The states using these models argue that they curb costs and produce greater satisfaction, independence, and empowerment among clients.

Kane, Illston, Eustis, and Kane (1991) report that for home care consumers, their advocates, providers of care, and regulators, compatibility between worker and client is of utmost importance. All groups also note the importance of skills. Edebalk (1995) studied home care users and notes that first and foremost they want continuity of care in terms of both function and workers. Also of importance are the relationship and competence. Eustis and Fischer (1991) argue that informality is the key feature of home care.

Scala, Mayberry, and Kunkel (1996) found that case managers and assessors identified only 16.5% of clients as appropriate for consumer-directed care. Those identified as appropriate were more likely to be female, have fewer impairments, receive fewer services, have lower incomes, and to live alone. The case managers and assessors suggested that those who are appropriate for consumer directed care are likely to have stable health, a good support system, an understanding of the service system, and a willingness to make contacts if or when problems arise. In a Canadian study, Micco, Hamilton, Martin, and McEwan (1995) surveyed case managers to find that they generally believed that clients' well-being and quality of care would suffer if clients assumed sole responsibility for management and scheduling of their care, that it would increase the risk of abuse to both client and support worker, and it would increase job demands for case managers.

It would appear, then, that many clients may be interested in greater participation in the services they receive, although there is little evidence that health care providers are equally enthusiastic. Indeed, health care workers may not embrace the new vision of empowerment for clientele. One of the reasons appears to be a greater concern by health care providers for safety over self-determination for clients. Hennessy's (1989) study of On Lock argues that as client risk grows, service providers view autonomy with decreased importance. If there was low risk, the client's wish would be honored provided it could also be met for a reasonable cost. Clemens and colleagues (1994) argue that case managers express commitment to the principle of client self-determination or freedom but frequently act against autonomy in order to maximize safety. Similarly, Degenholtz, Kane, and Kivnick (1997) report from their research that elders seemed primarily focused on maintaining continuity of self amidst change while family and professionals seemed focused on caring for their safety. Among their sample of consumers of community long-term care, 49% preferred to have the freedom to come and go while 41% preferred to accept some restrictions to be safe. In another state, 62% of clients preferred to come and go while 26% preferred restrictions to be safe.

SOME CANADIAN DATA

We were interested in knowing how recipients of home support services felt about the amount of say that they had in the receipt of services and the areas in which they wanted more participation. A random sample of 567 recipients were interviewed face to face for an average of 2½ hours, of whom 59 (10.4%) were under the age of 65 (Penning & Chappell, 1996). In addition, 36 proxy interviews were included for those who were too ill or cognitively impaired and could not participate in the study directly. All interviews were conducted in English between July and December of 1995, usually in the client's home. The refusal rate was a low 13.4%. As expected, most of the users were female (78%), and the average age was 77. None of the clients were employed; most lived alone (69%). Most (62%) were Canadian born. Almost all (N = 563 or 99.3%) had contact with at least one family member, friend, or neighbor, and almost three-quarters said they had at least one person whom they could rely on for emotional support. Clients had a significant number of chronic illnesses, with all being limited to some extent in their ability to undertake instrumental activities of daily living, especially with regard to housework, yard work, shopping, and walking a city block. Most clients were also limited in basic activities of daily living, such as going up and down stairs and bathing. Approximately one-fifth appeared to be cognitively impaired, using a modified version of the Mini-Mental State Examination (Tombaugh, McDowell, Krisjansson, & Hubley, 1996).

The results from the survey were discussed with service providers, and a focus group of recipients was brought together in order to pursue details of how they would like to increase their participation. These results were discussed in a day-long workshop with managers and providers to understand their perception of how much say clients have, should have, and obstacles to implementation (Centre on Aging, 1997).

WHAT HOME CARE CLIENTS THINK

First, a discussion of home care clients. Almost everyone was receiving household cleaning (94%), with personal care including help bathing, dressing, and grooming, following next at 51%, and meal preparation including grocery shopping, at 32%. Very few seniors received any other services, but those under 65 were also somewhat likely to be receiving help with mobility, toileting, lifts or transfers, and urinary drainage. Services had been received on average for 10 years. Just over one-quarter (28%) pay for some or all of the services they receive. Most home care users receiving household cleaning do so together with either/or both meal preparation help and/or help with bathing, dressing, and grooming. It should be noted that the receipt of home making services only is not eligible within the program.

Overwhelmingly, clients believed that the home care services they were receiving were important for enhancing their quality of life (98%), when asked directly. Similarly, almost everyone believed they were important for preventing hospitalization and long-term institutional care (89%). Three-quarters believed they were important for helping them improve so they could manage on their own, and virtually everyone (98%) believed they were important for helping them to manage and ensure their basic needs were met. When asked separately about the effectiveness of the services for each of these goals, similar percentages were received.

Most were satisfied with the services they received (97%), and most rated their workers highly in courteousness and competence. Using these same survey data, multivariate analyses were performed (Penning & Chappell, 1996; Penning & Allan, 1997) to examine the predictors of clients' perceptions of overall satisfaction with services in facilitating independence and quality of life, and another multivariate analysis of the predictors of clients' perceptions of overall effectiveness of the services they received. In both instances it is the quality of the worker in terms of interpersonal skills and competence that was the main predictor. Those who have more choice are also more satisfied. Greater skill and flexibility of the worker contribute to an assessment of effectiveness. The findings point to the primary importance of the personal relationship established between the front line care provider and the client, as well as the perceived competence of the care provider for clients' assessment of overall effectiveness of services and their satisfaction with them.

It is of note that age, gender, living alone, and access to informal support were all unrelated to satisfaction or perceived effectiveness, unlike some other studies (see, e.g., Rabiner, 1992; Rabiner, Mutran, & Stearns, 1995). Although client involvement in decision making and their assessment of the quality of the agency providing care were not significant predictors of either perceived effectiveness or satisfaction, both of these variables were significantly correlated with assessment of worker quality, a variable that is an important predictor of both effectiveness and satisfaction. Client involvement in decision making is significantly correlated with assessments of worker quality and with their assessments of the quality of the agency providing care. These bivariate correlations suggest that these other factors are important for client satisfaction and assessment of service effectiveness, in an indirect way, mediated by assessments of worker quality.

Most (87%) believed they should have a say in the care that they receive. However, half (49%) said it is rare to have a say in who (the worker) provides care; 40% in what services were provided; and 34% in when the services were received. That is, users of home care services express satisfaction with the services that they are receiving and the workers who enter their homes. At the same time, they want to have a say in what services they receive, the workers who assist them, and the times these services are delivered. It is important to note that a satisfaction survey alone would not have revealed the desire for more participation.

Individuals were asked about their concerns, to express any areas in which they thought there was room for improvement, recognizing that one can always improve service delivery. They had no difficulty suggesting ideas. They listed several areas, including the inability and unwillingness of workers to be flexible and provide assistance in areas outside of the care plan; lack of skill on the part of home support workers in teaching and having clients participate in self-care; lack of adequate supervision of workers; and lack of involvement by agencies of clients' families in care programs. The first two in particular are areas that could easily be seen as outside of the existing home support program, discussed further in the focus group (see below). Lack of supervision, however, speaks immediately to an area where the home support program has jurisdiction. Involvement of families is an area that could be enhanced. It is an area where home support programs traditionally have some involvement but could easily expand.

That is, users of home care services do express satisfaction with services. However, they also want more say. These two views are held simultaneously.

SUGGESTIONS FROM HOME CARE CLIENTS

Almost all clients believed that they should have a say in the care they receive, and fully 68% believed that having a choice with regard to services is very important. However, the survey itself provided little specific information on how clients could have a greater say. Therefore, five elderly participants of the survey who expressed a wish to have a greater say were asked to take part in a focus group to provide ideas on how to improve the system.

Some of the suggestions referred to ensuring appropriate information is passed on to clients. For example, when one individual called to express dissatisfaction with the result of a reassessment, she was instructed to write a letter to the minister of health (which she did). An appeal process is in place in the CRD, but this individual was not told about it. There was concern expressed that clients often did not know who to call for information or where to lodge a complaint. One suggestion was to establish an ombudsperson for clients so they would have a representative. This would have to be implemented so that neither client nor worker would feel intimidated. The clients would have to be assured of confidentiality; the ombudsperson could have the power to conduct random checks so that, whenever a particular worker was being investigated, they would not necessarily conclude there had been a complaint. Another suggestion was to have random phone calls made to various personnel who deal with clients to ask for information or to lodge a complaint to ensure that clients are being treated in a courteous manner and the correct information is being conveyed.

Many of the suggestions were for system changes. For example, an individual reported having called the CRD to disagree about a reassessment that had been done and requested another. The same assessor was sent. Common sense suggests that a different assessor be sent in such cases. Other complaints included the lack of continuity of the worker, particularly when personal care is involved.

The general area of attitudes demonstrating respect and dignity is critical. Clients complained that they sometimes felt they were being interrogated in the assessment or reassessment process. It was suggested that each client or potential client be encouraged to have a family member or friend with them during an assessment/reassessment. It was pointed out that once the assessment is done, an assessor goes away, writes a formal assessment, and on that basis the individual receives or does not receive services. Yet, the individual client is never shown a copy of the assessment or given an opportunity to argue that it should be modified. Clients felt that not all the assessors and workers believe that clients themselves know what is best for them. One suggestion to assist workers and assessors to relate to a client's situation is to have them role play.

There were suggestions for social support. It was suggested that opportunities be provided for clients with similar problems to share ideas and concerns. It was also suggested that groups of clients meet with CRD representatives to foster better relationships.

In addition, the CRD provided specific questions and asked that they be discussed as well. These questions are interesting, not only in terms of client responses, but also in terms of the lack of congruence of world views revealed between CRD managerial staff and clients. The CRD wanted the clients to be asked what things workers are unwilling to do and whether or not these were things that were just nice to have done or are related to their health. Clients felt strongly that they are not asking simply for nice things. They would like workers to post letters for them, not to constantly have to follow workers around to see that they are not missing anything, and to have things done without having to ask the worker. Heavy housework is an interesting example, because individuals frequently seek assistance from community support when they are unable to do their own heavy housework, such as moving heavy furniture, removing drapes to be cleaned, and so on, and they are assessed partially on their ability to do these activities of daily living. Yet, workers are forbidden from doing heavy housework because of union rules! The obvious contradiction needs to be resolved.

The CRD also wanted to know examples of self-care that clients would be interested in learning. Clients had no difficulty providing examples, including the following: how to get about after an operation; how to make dressing easier without giving up style; how to use a wheelchair to get about; self-care areas generally. Clients were also asked how they thought there could be better supervision/training of workers. They had several suggestions, including: training in housecleaning; training in personal care; learning how to accept constructive criticism without taking it out on the client; having the assessor examine the job being done when they come to do the assessment; teaching workers how to empathize with the client.

Clients were asked what difference not having a choice makes. Clients responded that, if they don't have a choice, they feel very frustrated and angry. They do not know that the other person knows what they want or what is best for them. When they are not asked their perception of their needs and wants and what it is that is most difficult for them to do, the worker frequently ends up doing the things that the client is capable of doing herself. Clients gave examples of workers dusting nicknacks that clients are perfectly capable of doing themselves. Clients were also asked the type of family involvement they would like to see. The particular individuals in the support group did not necessarily want their families more involved but thought this would be important, especially for quieter clients, and suggested that they be available during assessments and reassessments. Clients also expressed concern about their financial situation and about health reform that had been taking place in British Columbia.

It should, of course, be pointed out that the suggestions mentioned here come from only a few individuals and are not necessarily representative. However, good ideas do not have to come from a representative sample of the clientele. The focus group was intended to illustrate specifics for a general question as to how clients could have greater say and become at least a little empowered. One focus group demonstrated dramatically the wealth of commonsensical ideas readily available by asking clients themselves to share their knowledge and experiences. These data reveal the value of seeking client knowledge to improve the delivery of home support services within a philosophy of client empowerment.

SERVICE PROVIDERS

Information from the survey of clients and the focus group was then presented to a day-long workshop with service providers, who were asked to discuss the issues of empowerment of clients, feasibility, barriers, and suggestions. The providers attending the workshop included management level. They were asked whether service deliverers at both the policy and practice levels believe in client empowerment (Centre on Aging, 1997). Much of the discussion focused on the many obstacles to change within the system, including the fact that it is quicker to give care than to promote independence; workers are not rewarded for focusing on independence; there is no focus on the emotional; there are insufficient dollars for community care; the political uncertainty results in confusion that is not conducive to service delivery; established policies, including where the assessment happens (for example, having it in the hospital is very stressful); seniority rules in the union for home care workers and other aspects of the collective agreement; and the pervasiveness of the medical model.

In discussing how to overcome these obstacles they also had many suggestions, including: one client file instead of numerous assessments; client input as the assessment unfolds; family sharing in the care plan; corporate funding to gain additional resources; client access to assessment information; the availability of an ombudsperson; changing and raising the image of home care workers to attract more workers; broadening the care plan, including a general discussion at the beginning of the assessment of what independence means to the client; providing easily accessible 24-hour information and learning about the culture and religion of the client.

The workshop with care providers demonstrated a world in which they work that is filled with constraints and obstacles to providing empowerment for clients. This is directly contrary to the expressed wishes of clients themselves and to the vision of health reform. This is not entirely surprising. The little research that is currently available on providers' views of client empowerment suggests that this notion will take a long time to become accepted. The research by Micco et al. (1995) is but one example wherein they report that case managers generally believed that independent provider care would not significantly improve clients' well-being and quality of care and that it would pose risks of abuse to both the client and support attendant and would result in greater job demands for case managers. Providers clearly have a differing world view than clients and also work in a bureaucracy with a history of paternalism that must be dealt with if client empowerment is to have a chance of becoming a reality.

Furthermore, change is taking place in health care in the province of British Columbia where these data derived, suggesting that increased demands for intensive post-acute care within home care are leading to a decline in long-term chronic care rather than the reverse. For example, Penning, Chappell, Stephenson, Rosenblood, and Tuokko (1998) examined the expenditures on home care services for the 8-year period, 1988–89 to 1995–96, and report gradual declines in the proportion of the health care budget going to medical and hospital services and increases in the proportion to community and other health services, including continuing care. However, within continuing care, the proportion of the budget allocated to home care services, that is, non-nursing services only, while increased in the earlier years, declined more recently. Similar evidence was revealed in relation to the number of clients served and the number of hours of service provided to home care clients. Both increased from 1989 to 1994, but then declined.

The intensity of services, though, increased. Fewer people received services, but those receiving services received more hours. The types of clients served also changed. Those at the lowest level of care (personal care) declined significantly. However, those in intermediate and extended care increased. These data suggest some reduction rather than expansion of community-based home care services and a redirection of services away from clients at the lower level of care who tend to require nonmedical and supportive services, such as housekeeping, laundry, and so on, and towards more intensive and medically focused needs, such as those higher levels of care. These trends suggest a medicalization of community care during recent health reform.

Current health reform appears to be imposing structural change that may be exasperating both the recognition of client empowerment and attempts to ensure that clients have a greater say. This is especially the case for seniors, who typically require less intensive, chronic care within the community. Increased demand for more post-acute care within an already constrained home care system leaves little maneuverability to enhance client participation.

DIFFERING WORLDS

The past decade has been filled with rhetoric, throughout the industrialized world, about fundamental reform of the health care system. This chapter has focused on one aspect of the new vision, namely, client participation in care decisions as a fundamental requirement for quality of care and quality of life, beginning with a brief discussion of universal medicare in Canada, the country from which these data come. Medicare in Canada is focused around physicians and acute care hospital treatment, where those who work in the system have been presumed to know best. This bias is evident in the literature on empowerment and service delivery, where there is much rhetoric calling for client empowerment but less evidence that it is occurring.

Data are presented from British Columbia, Canada, from recipients of home support services. While they express satisfaction with these services, there is no question that they would also like greater participation and say in the receipt of services, how those services are delivered, who delivers them, and when they are delivered. The primary importance of the personal relationship between the front-line care provider and the client, and the perceived competence of the care provider for the client's assessment of overall effectiveness, and their satisfaction with services, was revealed. In the face-to-face interviews, clients had no difficulty discussing their situation with home care providers and making suggestions for improvements (such as a greater flexibility on the part of the workers, teaching clients more self care, etc.). Similarly, a focus group of home care clients revealed the feasibility and the value of clients' participation. They easily made worthwhile suggestions from their experience of needing and receiving home care (such as an ombudsperson for clients, ensuring a different assessor is used when a reassessment is requested by the client, etc.).

A day-long workshop with home care providers and managers revealed a major concern with the many obstacles to system change and thinking that is pervaded with constraints and obstacles to providing empowerment to clients (such as not being rewarded for focusing on the emotional or on independence, insufficient dollars, etc.). These constraints are real and imposed by the system and, indeed, some of the structural changes that are taking effect within health reform (such as increased demand for intensive post-acute care from the home care budget, which is adding much strain to this system) are working against client empowerment. Yet, client empowerment has been accepted as a necessary component for quality of care to achieve quality of life.

Despite a decade emphasizing health reform that includes the notion of greater client participation and empowerment, these data suggest there is still a long way to go. An assumption of excess dependency (Baltes, 1988) appears to still be operative; however, there seems to be little question that seniors themselves want increased participation. Unfortunately, at the present time, clients and providers share different world views within a system that allows for little flexibility. The rhetoric of client empowerment shows little evidence of becoming reality until this changes.

REFERENCES

Applebaum, R., & Philips, P. (1990). Assuring the quality of in-home care: The "other" challenge for long-term. *Gerontologist, 30*(4), 444–450.

Aronson, J. (1991a). Dutiful daughters and undemanding mothers: Constraining images of giving and receiving care in middle and later life. In C. Baines, P. Evans, & S. Neysmith (Eds.), *Women's caring: Feminist perspectives on social welfare* (pp. 138–168). Toronto, ON: McClelland & Stewart.

Aronson, J. (1991b). Women's perspectives on informal care of the elderly: Public ideology and personal experiences giving and receiving care. *Ageing and Society, 10*, 61–84.

92 Quality of Care

Baltes, M. (1988). The etiology and maintenance of dependency in the elderly. *Behavior Therapy, 19,* 301–319.

Becker, G., & Kaufman, S. (1988). Old age, rehabilitation and research: A review of the issues. *Gerontologist, 28,* 459–468.

Centre on Aging (1997). *Home support services, client decision-making and independence: A collaborative workshop.* Summary Report. Seniors Independence Research Program, University of Victoria, BC.

Chappell, N. L. (1989). *Formal programs for informal caregivers to elders.* Report prepared for the Policy, Communications and Information Branch, Health and Welfare Canada.

Chappell, N. L. (1998a). Maintaining and enhancing independence and well-being in old age. In *Determinants of health, adults and seniors: Vol. 2* (pp. 89–137). Canada Health Action: Building on the Legacy, Papers commissioned by the National Forum on Health.

Chappell, N. L. (1998b). *Conceptual aspects of independence: What are the policy, programming, practice and research implications?* Final report. Systematic Literature Review and Synthesis National Consensus Process: Creating Evidence-Based Consensus on Health, Social and Economic Issues Related to Seniors' Independence. Centre on Aging, University of Victoria, BC.

Clemens, E., Wetle, T., Feltes, M., Crabtree, B., & Dubitzky, D. (1994). Contradictions in case management: Client-centered theory and directive practice with frail elderly. *Journal of Aging and Health, 6*(1), 70–88.

Cox, E. O. (1993). *Elderly care-receivers' perceptions of the care process: A multi-cultural view.* Denver, CO: University of Denver, 92 pp.

Degenholtz, H., Kane, A., & Kivnick, Q. (1997). Care-related preferences and values of elderly community-based LTC consumer: Can case managers learn what's important to clients? *Gerontologist, 37*(6), 767–776.

Dill, A. (1993). Defining needs, defining systems: A critical analysis. *Gerontologist, 33*(4), 453–460.

Doty, P. (1986). Family care of the elderly: The role of public policy. *Milbank Memorial Fund Quarterly, 64,* 34–75.

Doty P., Kasper, J., & Litvak, S. (1996). Consumer-directed models of personal care: Lessons from Medicaid. *Milbank Quarterly, 74*(3), 377–409.

Edebalk, P. G. (1995). How elderly people rank-order the quality characteristics of home services. *Aging and Society, 15*(1), 83–102.

EKOS (1998). EKOS Research Associates, Inc. Ottawa, private communication.

Eustis, N. N., & Fischer, L. R. (1991). Relationships between home care clients and their workers: Implications for quality of care. *Gerontologist, 31,* 447–456.

Fuchs, E., d'Epinay, C. L., Michel, J. P., Scherrer, K., Stettler, M., & Bickel, J. F. (1998). *The idea of autonomy: An interdisciplinary reformulation.* Presented at the XIV World Congress of Sociology.

Glickman, L. L., Stocker, K. B., & Caro, F. G. (1997). Self-direction in home care for older people: A consumer's perspective. *Home Health Care Services Quarterly, 16*(1–2), 4–54.

Hasselkus, B. R. (1994). From hospital to home: Family professional relationships in geriatric rehabilitation. *Gerontology and Geriatrics Education, 15*(1), 91–100.

Hennessy, C. (1989). Autonomy and risk: The role of client wishes in community-based long-term care. *Gerontologist, 29*(5), 633–638.

Holstein, B. E., Holst, E., Due, P., & Almind, G. (1993). Formal and informal care for the elderly: Lessons from Denmark. In A. Evers & G. van der Zanden (Eds.), *Better care for dependent people living at home: Meeting the new agenda in services for the elderly* (pp. 275–297). Netherlands Institute of Gerontology, European Center for Social Welfare Policy and Research, Bunnik, Netherlands.

Kane, R. L., & Kane, R. A. (1985). *A will and a way.* New York: Columbia University Press.

Kane, R. A., Illston, L. H., Eustis, N. N., & Kane, R. L. (1991). *Quality of home care: Concept and measurement.* Minneapolis: University of Minnesota, School of Public Health.

Kapp, M. B. (1997). Who is responsible for this? Assigning rights and consequences in elder care. *Journal of Aging and Social Policy, 9*(2), 51–65.

Keller, M., Leventhal, H., Prohaska, T., & Leventhal, E. (1989). Beliefs about aging and illness in a community sample. *Research in Nursing and Health, 12*, 247–255.

Lloyd, P. (1991). Empowerment of elderly people. *Journal of Aging Studies, 5*(2), 125–135.

Lustbader, W. (1991). *Counting on kindness: The dilemmas of dependency.* New York: Free Press.

Mansour, A. A. (1994). The conceptualization of health among residents of Saskatoon. *Journal of Community Health, 19*(3), 165–179.

Mhatre, S. L. & Deber, R. B. (1992). From equal access to health care to equitable access to health: A review of Canadian provincial health commissions and reports. *International Journal of Health Services, 22*(4), 645–668.

Micco, A., Hamilton, A. C., Martin, M. J., & McEwan, K. L. (1995). Case manager attitudes toward client-directed care. *Journal of Case Management, 4*(3), 95–101.

Morse, J. M. (1987). The meaning of health in an inner city community. *Nursing Papers, 19*, 27–41.

National Forum on Health (1997). *Canada health action: Building on the legacy.* Volume I: The final report of the National Forum on Health and Volume II: Synthesis reports and issues papers. Ottawa, Ontario.

Ontario Ministry of Health (1992). *Debriefing note of the Ontario Ministry of Health and the Ontario Home Care Programs Association Meeting.* Toronto: Queen's Park, December 21, 1992.

Penning, M. J., & Allan, D. (1997). Symposium: Issues of independence and autonomy in chronic illness: Self, informal and formal care. Presentation: Patterns of self, informal and formal care: Implications for independence. *Gerontologist, 37*, Special Issue II.

Penning, M. J., & Chappell, N. L. (1996). *Home support services in the Capital Regional District: Client survey.* Final report of the Centre on Aging for the Capital Regional District, Department of Health.

Penning, M. J., Chappell, N. L., Stephenson, P. H., Rosenblood, L., & Tuokko, H. A. (1998). *Independence among older adults with disabilities. The role of formal care services, informal caregiving and self-care.* Final Report. University of Victoria, Centre on Aging.

Rabiner, D. J. (1992). The relationship between program participation, use of formal in-home care and satisfaction with care in an elderly population. *Gerontologist, 32,* 805–812.

Rabiner, D. J., Mutran, E., & Stearns, S. C. (1995). The effect of channeling on home care utilization and satisfaction with care. *Gerontologist, 35,* 186–195.

Rose, S. M. (Ed.) (1992). *Case management and social work practice.* New York: Longman.

Rose, T. (1996). In search of a humanistic approach to long-term care case management. *Aging, Health and Society: News and Views.* Guest Editorial, 1(2), McMaster University.

Scala, M. A., Mayberry, P. S., & Kunkel, S. R. (1996). Consumer-directed home care: Client profiles and service challenges. *Journal of Case Management, 5*(3), 91–98.

Segall, A., & Chappell, N. L. (in press). *Sociology of health and health care in Canada.* Toronto, Ontario: Prentice-Hall.

Soldo, B. J., Agree, E. M., & Wolf, D. A. (1989). The balance between formal and informal care. In M. Ory & K. Bond (Eds.), *Aging and health care: Social science and policy perspectives.* New York: Routledge.

Stuifbergen, A. K., Becker, H., Sands, D., & Ingalsbe, K. (1990). Perceptions of health among adults with disabilities. *Health Values, 14,* 18–26.

Tombaugh, T., McDowell, I., Krisjansson, B., & Hubley, A. (1996). Mini-Mental State Examination (MMSE) and the Modified MMSE (3MS): A psychometric comparison and normative data. *Psychological Assessment, 8,* 48–59.

Zawadski, R. T., & Eng, C. (1988). Case management in capitated long-term care. *Health Care Financing Review, Annual Supplement,* 75–81.

5

Quality in Small Residential Care Settings

J. Kevin Eckert
Leslie A. Morgan

Only recently have researchers begun to carefully examine the range of long-term care options and alternatives within the middle ground between institutional nursing and home care. As noted by Rubinstein (1995), research on the middle range includes such alternatives as sheltered housing (Sherwood, Gutkin, Sherwood, & Mor, 1981), domiciliary care (Sherwood, Morris, & Sherwood, 1986), intermediate care housing (Brody, 1975), adult foster care (McCoin 1983; Sherman & Newman, 1988), assisted living (Kane, Wilson, & Clemmer, 1993), small congregate homes (Murray, 1988), and other planned housing (Mollica & Ryther, 1987). The term board and care is often applied generically to describe many of the above-mentioned residential care arrangements (Conley, 1989). These nonmedical, community-based residences provide shelter (room) and meals (board) for unrelated adults requiring daily living assistance and services that typically include 24-hour supervision, housekeeping, laundry, personal care, and recreation. They can range from large to small size and from an institutional to intimate environment (Mor, Sherwood, & Gutkin, 1986), with confusing terminology and problems distinguishing such homes from other places offering care without medical treatment (Stone & Newcomer, 1986).

This chapter focuses on the quality of life, quality of care, and resident satisfaction in the small residential care settings sometimes referred to as small board and care homes, adult foster care homes, or small domiciliary homes, among others. Small residential care homes represent one alternative filling the gap between home and nursing home for dependent adults who require assistance in activities of daily living but do not require skilled nursing care (Morgan, Eckert & Lyon, 1995). They differ from institutional settings (i.e., nursing homes) in that their primary purpose is to provide nonmedical personal care (McCoy & Conley 1990, p. 148). Although board and care homes may vary in size from one to more than 100 residents, what constitutes small generally includes homes ranging from one to 15 residents. For example, Hawes et al. (1995), in their multistate study of the effects of regulation on board and care quality, came to define the size strata as small (2–10 beds), medium (11–50 beds), and large (51 or more beds). They note that many earlier studies and several state licensing laws define small as up to five or six beds. In California for example, small includes homes from 1–14 beds (Newcomer, Breuer, & Zhang, 1993). For practical purposes, we will draw from research literature that includes homes ranging from 1 to as many as 15 residents.

CONTRASTING BOARD AND CARE AND ASSISTED LIVING

Traditional board and care homes are currently being compared with a new phenomenon known as assisted living. In reviewing studies of the board and care industry, both size and coresidence of the operator differentiates between the small, familial type homes we focus on in this chapter and the more institutional, "staffed" homes that resemble larger forms of care, such as congregate homes, nursing homes, and what has come to be called "assisted living." Studies of small board and care homes (Eckert, Namazi, & Kahana, 1987; Sherman & Newman, 1988) have found them to be much like typical family settings in single-family homes. The majority of operators were middle-aged women, many of whom had limited education, as is characteristic of women providing direct care to dependent adults in other settings (Abel & Nelson, 1990).

Assisted living housing can be defined as a model of residential long-term care based on the concept of outfitting a residential environment with professionally delivered personal care services in a way that delays or avoids institutionalization and keeps older frail individuals independent as long as possible (Regnier, Hamilton, & Yatabe, 1991). In theory and design, as a housing type between congregate housing and skilled nursing care, it serves the needs of persons with less severe mental and physical problems (Morgan et al., 1995). Mollica (1998), in an examination of policies in 14 states, notes that, while there is no common definition of assisted living for regulators to use, state rules generally include a reference to a philosophy that emphasizes consumer or resident independence, autonomy, dignity, privacy, and decision making. The label assisted living has been used to differentiate this type of housing from conventional board and care housing and the negative connotations that some people associate with it (Kane et al., 1993). While board and care homes tend to be small and informal community-based settings, assisted living facilities tend to be larger, ranging from 25 to more than 100 persons (Golant, 1992).

Facilities built with the express purpose of providing assisted living appear to attract a population with different demographic characteristics than those living in traditional board and care. Hawes and associates (1995) found that the racial mix of facilities was more inclusive of minority elders in smaller homes. Morgan et al. (1995), in a two-state study of small board and care homes, found that board and care residents were more likely to be African American than were populations living in the community or in nursing homes. In a very recent study of assisted living/residential care, Zimmerman, Sloane, and Eckert (in press) found that a key demographic difference between residents of small board and care homes and those living in new purpose-built assisted living was the latters' likely economic advantage—a not surprising finding, since such facilities are often expensive and "private pay."

The most observable difference between these two types of housing/care options is related to the physical environment. Ideally, assisted living settings have private living quarters, such as efficiency apartments, with doors that can be locked for privacy. The small residential care homes, in contrast, while often offering private rooms, may not have doors that can be locked or separate kitchen and bathing facilities (Morgan et al., 1995). Hawes and her colleagues (1995), after studying homes of varying sizes in 10 states, concluded that board and care homes fit in the niche between residential settings with few services and nursing homes.

The Benefits of Small Homes

Smaller size homes have been characterized as unique in that they may provide an environment more conducive to the development of close personal relationships, individualized care, or a family-like atmosphere (Morgan et al., 1995; Sherman & Newman, 1988). They have also been the focus of heated public debate focusing on abuses described as widespread among small residential care homes, especially those that are unregulated (U.S. House, 1989).

In contrast with this negative view, some believe that a highly desirable social environment can be created in these smaller homes, in which residents are treated as family members, sharing in the normal life activities of the household (Sherman & Newman, 1977; Silverstone, 1978). In reference to the smaller foster family arrangement, Silverstone (1978) suggests that these environments can offer older adults in need of care relatively permanent primary group relations, wherein their needs for individualized attention, including the need for affection, can be met as they arise. In addition, the foster family potentially offers closer links to the community of which they are a part and independence from conforming tendencies of institutional populations. Smaller homes are more likely to have live-in staff and reflect the "mom and pop" model of operation, while larger homes are staffed from the outside and are more likely to be regulated by the state and run by business interests (Dittmar, 1989). Whether smaller homes can respond to their residents in a more individualized fashion (e.g., taking food preferences into account and responding on an as needed basis for personal care) than larger facilities remains a focal point for this debate.

DEFINING QUALITY IN SMALL RESIDENTIAL HOMES

Definitional and Measurement Issues in Quality: Three Related Concepts

Traditional approaches to measuring quality of life, quality of care, and resident satisfaction are evident in studies of small residential care settings, including the conflation of these concepts in thinking and writing about the issues. Nonetheless, the implicit assumption in much of the research is that quality of care (measured in varied ways, most often reflecting regulatory or medicalized views) results in quality of life and resident satisfaction. By far the dominant work on this setting focuses on the regulatory/institutional point of view, examining regulation and reimbursement in multistage, national, or single state studies (Dittmar, Smith, Bell, Jones, & Manzanares, 1983; Hawes, Wildfire, Lux, & Clemmer, 1993; Hawes et al., 1995; Reichstein & Bergofsky, 1983). As in other settings, the dominant approach to measuring quality utilizes Donabedian's structure/process/outcome model developed for health care settings (Donabedian, 1966). In this approach, structure (traits and resources of the physical and organizational setting) and process (activities taking place between those providing and receiving care) remain much easier to evaluate than do meaningful outcomes for residents (Gibbs & Sinclair, 1992). Outcomes remain the "gold standard" for quality of care in residential care settings, but remain elusive when it comes to measurement, since health changes are slow to appear and often reflect degenerative processes (Porell & Caro, 1998).

Rubinstein (in press) has expanded this discussion by addressing the interface between quality of care, consumer choice and satisfaction, and quality of life. He notes that satisfaction as a construct should be embedded in cultural and ideological contexts linked to the person, rather than remaining an abstraction. He argues strongly for a "person centered" view of the quality of life or of satisfaction. Instead, resident satisfaction and quality of life are most often reflective of professional definitions of these concepts, reflecting points of view that differ from those residents might use to give meaning to their lives.

Rubinstein also acknowledges the frequent confusion of the resident as person or as patient. This mirrors the confusion of quality of life with health-related quality of care in settings such as nursing homes, which are essentially medical institutions rather than homes for residents (Johnson & Grant, 1985). The extent to which we medicalize and professionalize care settings contributes to a disjunction in perspectives and expectations about quality (Rubinstein, in press). In small residential care settings, in contrast to larger settings, many of these institutional and medical aspects are less evident, resulting in greater focus on home and person in evaluating quality or satisfaction.

In the studies described in the remainder of this chapter, seldom do researchers discuss an overall concept of quality or distinguish between quality of care and quality of life. Instead, specific measurement elements serving as indicators of an underlying concept of quality—often not designated as quality of care versus quality of life—are measured and reported. Table 5.1 lists some of the indicators of quality of care and quality of life used in studies of small residential care settings discussed in this chapter. Conclusions regarding overall quality are frequently left to the reader's interpretation of results, which may be problematic since findings on varied indicators are sometimes mixed. In small residential care settings, however, the range of measured indicators has been somewhat different than that in more formal and medical long-term care settings, providing an interesting contrast in terms of what is considered essential in these settings. Issues such as the quality and quantity of interactions among residents, sharing of meals with care providers, and homelikeness of the environment are often utilized in small settings in addition to select indicators used in larger, more institutionalized settings.

Whose Point of View?

In small residential care facilities, elements of what constitute quality may vary depending on *who you ask* and *how you ask*. Researchers defining quality of life, resident satisfaction, or quality of care in small residential care settings have operated on multiple levels, attempting to assess several of the points of view on quality. Most commonly represented is an institutional/regulatory point of view, wherein aspects of quality that most frequently appear in regulations (i.e., lighting, hall width, staffing ratios, and other measures) are defined as indicators of quality of care,

TABLE 5.1 Perspectives on Quality

Perspectives	Quality of Care		Quality of Life
	Structure	*Process*	
Regulator/policy makers	• Size • Auspices • Licensure	• Service availability • Staffing adequacy • Turnover	
Providers	• Amount of space • Types of space • Homelikeness	• Shared social activities • Backup support • Family likeness	
Families	• Safety • Transportation • Private space	• Turnover • Individualized care plans • Staffing	
Residents			• Privacy • Personal • Caring for self • Caring for others

and assumed to correlate with quality of life and resident satisfaction (see Table 5.1). Some of the confusion of quality of life (QOL) with quality of care (QOC) and resident satisfaction arises from these varying points of view (Cohn & Sugar, 1991). Seldom, however, is the empirical question addressed directly as to whether researchers' choices among these sets of indicators of quality are good ones (i.e., whether meeting standards in a facility such as adequacy of lighting has the desired or expected outcomes) and whether the quality indicators important to regulators are also those important to residents, care providers, or relatives (for an exception see Cohn & Sugar, 1991). In a study that included residents, family, and staff from both board and care and nursing homes, qualitative analysis showed that resident responses focused much more on issues of morale, while family and staff comments revolved around issues of the care provided (Cohn & Sugar, 1991). Therefore in addressing the issue of quality in smaller settings, we organize our presentation according to the dominant point of view on quality that is underlying the research. Not all of the multiple points of view on quality have been addressed adequately in research on the small homes examined in this chapter. In addition to the institutional/regulatory point of view on quality are those of front line care providers, residents' kin and significant others, and the residents themselves. Note that we utilize the term care providers, since smaller homes lack the hierarchical distinctions in staff typical of larger, institutional facilities in that the owner/operator may also be the primary provider of personal care, housekeeping, and meals. In larger settings the distinctions between floor staff and administrators are much more meaningful.

When researchers move away from the regulator/institutional definition of quality, they enter a less known territory, where the first step of research must be to define what constitutes quality by selecting a point (or points) of view. Although there may be overlap among the perspectives of these interested groups, it remains an empirical question as to how many elements they share in defining what constitutes quality of life or care. Regulators, for example, may value safety over autonomy when it comes to the issue of risking falls, taking medication, or locking doors, while residents may have the opposite views on some of these items. Staff may consider interpersonal relationships more important than do regulators, and kin may think that staff qualifications are more important than do the residents. One small, qualitative study in a nursing home, for example, found that quality of life from a resident's point of view, solicited in open-ended questions, did not reflect the physical environment or social activities that the researchers had expected to play a role (Aller & Van Ess Coeling, 1995). The initial question that must be posed, therefore, is *whose definition of quality* is of interest? The second question then becomes whether we actually know what elements of quality are important to the group in question?

Figures 5.1 and 5.2 display two possible views of the conceptual domains of quality for the constituent groups in small residential care settings. In the background of the figures are the overlapping conceptual domains of quality of care, quality of life, and resident satisfaction. Each of these domains contains an array of indicators, which may be selected by researchers to serve as indicators for one or more of these latent concepts. We suggest that the various actors sample a subset of this conceptual and measurement domain in constructing their definitions of what constitutes quality. The unanswered question is the degree to which these conceptual definitions actually overlap (i.e., the degree of consensus as to quality from varied points of view) among perspectives.

In Figure 5.1, the quality domains of the four groups show considerable overlap, suggesting that a relatively large number of possible indicators of quality are shared among the four groups. Definitions of regulators are oriented more toward the quality of care, while those of family and residents are slanted toward resident satisfaction or quality of life as concepts. Figure 5.2, however, suggests relatively little and uneven overlap in the elements which constitute quality for the various groups involved in small homes. Whether these or some other configuration of the elements of quality empirically reflects various groups' definitions remains unknown for small homes and probably for most care settings. In any case, when research is conducted, the point of view of whichever group or groups is being considered is filtered through the point of view of researchers before an operational definition of what constitutes quality is put into the field. Thus, the measurement of quality in small settings generally reflects two points of view at minimum—those of the targeted group or groups and of researchers—in defining what constitutes quality.

Fewer researchers to date have collected data on insiders' perspectives (i.e., residents, care providers, or families and friends) on quality in small residential care settings. Studies utilizing the various insiders' points of view shed light on the everyday, human experience of life in small homes and begin to address the lived experiences of people working, visiting, or residing in these settings. Paying attention to these other points of view illustrates in important ways how quality is expressed in smaller settings and how they differ from larger, more formally structured and medically based settings.

QUALITY IN SMALL HOMES: VARIED PERSPECTIVES

Regulatory and Policy-Oriented Studies of Quality in Board and Care

To address the questions and concerns of regulators and policy makers, several single and multistate studies of board and care quality have been

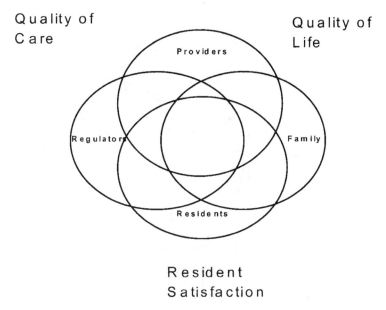

Quality of
Care

Quality of
Life

Resident
Satisfaction

FIGURE 5.1   Maximum overlapping of quality domains.

conducted (Hawes et al., 1995; Newcomer et al., 1993; Reschovsky & Ruchlin, 1993). Little of this research focuses exclusively on small residential care facilities, but instead attempts to provide uniform and comprehensive information about board and care facilities generally, to inform state and/or federal level policy debate. Studies address questions important to state and federal agencies and organizations such as: 1) Who is served by residential care? 2) What are the physical features and staffing capabilities? 3) What are the effects of regulation on structural, process, and resident-level quality measures? The impetus is to assist policy making and administrators' attempts to enhance quality and ensure maximum safety (i.e., minimize risks) for those being cared for in such homes (Hawes et al., 1993). Measures used often derive from those used in nursing homes, which may not be equally relevant in smaller settings. Additionally, regulatory and policy-oriented studies reflect few indicators of quality of life in favor of quality of care (e.g., safety and physical aspects of the environment), avoiding especially quality of life issues that are difficult to quantify such as quality of resident/staff interaction (Baggett, 1989; Dobkin, 1989; Stone & Newcomer, 1986).

As noted above, the dominant model for evaluating quality in small care settings focuses on structural and process features of the environment, including space and privacy, size, the physical environment, and

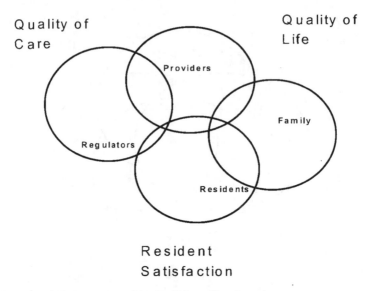

Resident
Satisfaction

FIGURE 5.2   Minimum overlapping of quality domains.

fire and other safety provisions—which derive from a quality of care
approach (Reschovsky & Ruchlin, 1993). In several of these studies selective indicators of quality have been related to facility size. Reschovsky
and Ruchlin (1993) analyzed data on 205 board and care homes serving
the poor elderly in seven states to examine elements of quality that contribute to the safety and quality of life of residents. Seven indexes of quality bridging conceptual domains and points of view (including resident
oversight, fire safety, other safety, space and privacy, supplemental services, resident and staff interactions, and overall facility environment)
were examined in relationship to structural, financial, and regulatory
variables. Their findings highlight several quality-related aspects of small
homes from a regulatory/policy perspective. For example, better staffing
levels were associated with lower-quality interactions within homes, challenging commonly held notions that higher staff/resident ratios enhance
quality in all respects (Reschovsky & Ruchlin, 1993). Also surprising was
the finding that dimensions of care important to the quality of life of residents (e.g., resident/staff interaction) had no clear relation to the cost of
operating a home. Moreover, nonprofit organizations that operate board
and care homes performed better along quality of life dimensions of care.

In terms of space and privacy, residents in small homes studied in
Maryland and Ohio frequently shared bedrooms, but the majority of
Maryland residents have private rooms (Morgan et al., 1995). This stands
in contrast to assertions that privacy is the domain of assisted living and

to the experience in larger homes, where sharing is the norm (Reschovsky & Ruchlin, 1993). Rooms in the smallest "mom and pop" foster care homes typically were not lockable by residents, again differentiating them from the aspiration of some for assisted living environments (Morgan et al., 1995). Ratings by interviewers suggest that the quality and condition of space in most small homes studied in Maryland was good to excellent (Morgan et al., 1995).

Another element central to the regulator point of view is the availability of services for residents. Small homes provide more care and services than congregate apartments and boarding homes, but fewer skilled and rehabilitative services, less routine monitoring, assessment and care planning, and less nursing and restorative care than nursing homes (Hawes et al., 1995). Small homes in Ohio and Maryland provide a wide range of services including meals and snacks, laundry, transportation, assistance with medication, and personal care. Other services, including those required to meet medical needs, were typically arranged outside the home, with assistance of kin or the care provider (Morgan et al., 1995). The range of services, as expected, expanded with more residents.

Other studies have focused on the adequacy of staffing. In a single state study of Residential Care Facilities for the Elderly (RCFEs) in California, Newcomer and associates (1993) studied facilities ranging from 1 to over 100 beds. Findings on quality of care related to the two smaller strata (1–6 beds and 7–14, respectively) showed differences based on the size of facilities. For example, residents in smaller facilities were more likely than those in larger facilities to report an unmet need for assistance with functional activities or social/recreational activities. Hawes and her associates (1995) reported that, in homes where the resident population is more impaired, facility staffing and training are more important.

Staff roles also differ in small homes. Although the tenure of home operators was longer in smaller homes, their duties encompassed most of the major activities of the Residential Care Facilities for the Elderly (RCFE), such as housekeeping, cooking, maintenance, medication supervision, and personal care (Newcomer et al., 1993). These findings raised questions regarding the adequacy of relief or backup for the owner/operators in the smallest homes, a point to which we return later.

Echoing some concerns found in the study of RCFEs in California (Newcomer et al., 1993), Hawes and her associates (1995) reported important staffing differences based on facility size. For example, they found that operators of small board and care homes were less likely to be well-educated than those in larger homes, with 43% of operators of small facilities having a high school education or less, compared to 20% or more in large facilities. Staff turnover was rapid in many homes. Over one-third of staff (35%) had worked in their current facility for less than 1 year. Smaller homes fared somewhat better, with about half of the staff at the same home from 1 to 5 years, compared to 40% of staff in large facilities. Staff in small facilities also had a wider range of responsibilities, while the responsibilities in larger homes were more defined and prescribed (Hawes et al., 1995).

Another element of quality reflecting primarily the regulatory point of view is the effect of licensure on quality in small residential care settings. Hawes and her colleagues (1995), in a 10-state study of board and care which sought to determine whether the extent of state regulations was associated with the quality of care in licensed and unlicensed board and care homes, found that more extensive regulations are associated with having more experienced operators and stringent staff training require-ments. They caution, however, that this does not necessarily mean that more extensive regulations improve overall quality of care. Regardless of size, licensed homes were more likely to report providing personal care services. "The homes were usually a family business, although not neces-sarily a family home" (Hawes et al., 1995, pp. 3–8).

Perhaps the most striking finding in these single and multistate, empir-ically based studies of board and care homes was their failure to substan-tiate claims of abuse or neglect—the "snake pit" image—portrayed through the popular media and hearings arranged by congressional committees (U.S. House, 1989). Instead, studies revealed that the board and care industry fills an important niche in the long-term care continuum across the economic spectrum. Both process and structure features associated with quality of care were present in most facilities regardless of regulation or licensure. These studies suggest that the concerns and policy issues requiring the most attention are those associated with providing adequate reimbursement levels for care and wages and benefits for care workers (Hawes et al., 1995; Newcomer et al., 1993).

QUALITY FROM THE CARE
PROVIDERS' PERSPECTIVE

In studies of quality in larger residential facilities, data from the perspec-tives of those directly providing services are seldom included. While many studies describe the characteristics of care providers (e.g., demographic traits, educational/training, and experience), these reflect the quality def-initions from the regulatory/institutional perspectives. In small residen-tial care facilities, where the staff is limited in size and typically the owner/operator is involved personally with delivery of care, a different type of inquiry may occur. By being closer to the residents, these "direct care operators," as Hawes and associates (1995) call them are both more aware of day-to-day quality issues in the provision of care and potentially more subject to social desirability in their responses regarding quality issues. Responses to inquiries regarding quality are perhaps more valid than those of an administrator in a large facility, but may be colored by the care provider's involvement in all aspects of the care, which make them less comparable to administrative/regulatory responses.

For example, issues of the quality of personal and shared spaces in small homes is shaped by the "family home" model, where public spaces may be shared by the care provider and her kin as well as the residents (Hawes et al., 1995; Morgan et al., 1995). Interviews with operators of small homes suggest that the amount and types of space are issues that they view as important to the ability to provide care, but for most providers was not necessarily problematic. Operators of small homes in Maryland frequently acknowledged the need to expand or improve the physical environment for providing care, most often mentioning the need for more space, improvements to bathrooms, or external areas such as porches and decks (Morgan et al., 1995). Most did not see their physical environments as an impediment to good quality care.

Within the family home model, when residents share living space and meals with care providers and often their kin (Morgan et al., 1995), important value questions arise. One example is the value of privacy versus that of social interaction in such homelike settings. Recent studies regarding assisted living show a strong consumer preference for private rooms (Jenkins, 1997), sharing an aspirational goal of those at the policy and regulatory level for assisted living. On the other hand, a quality living experience in small homes is also expected to involve sharing in social activities, according to the provider perspective. In one recent study in assisted living, for example, staff members saw more advantages of shared spaces in the environment than did residents (Kane, Baker, Salmon, & Veazie, 1998).

The quality of interpersonal relationships with providers and among residents appear to be central to provider definitions of quality. Operators emphasized the quality of the interpersonal bonds and the ability to customize care for their residents as positive aspects of quality in small residential care settings (Morgan et al., 1995). Issues of "homelikeness" of the environment and "family likeness" of the social relationships resonate with the providers' views of what is central to quality in small residential care homes. Providers in two-thirds of small homes studied in Maryland described their small residential care homes as like a real "home" and described relations between themselves and residents as "just like family" (Morgan et al., 1995). In open-ended questions, providers volunteered reasons that the environment was like a home, including sharing activities, showing love and affection, and quality caring. These and other comments suggested that the homelike and family-like nature of small homes, including the opportunity to develop strong one-to-one relationships with residents that continued over years and to personalize care, were central issues in their definitions of quality.

Perhaps most important in light of the concerns raised by other researchers (Hawes et al., 1995; Newcomer et al., 1993) was the finding that operators of small board and care homes were not isolated caregivers. Through careful interviews with 103 operators about their social networks, it was found that operators had both formal and informal supports to sustain them. The formal supports included professionals, programs, and others who provided assistance within and outside the home. The informal supports included families, friends, and neighbors of the operators and, to a lesser extent, the families and friends of the residents (Morgan et al., 1995). These represented a mixed support system benefiting the operator and residents on an as-needed and flexible basis. This is not to say that operators did not voice concerns about financial resources, service availability, and health care coverage for clients, but it did offer a counterpoint to concerns voiced in the literature regarding burden on the solo care provider (Dittmar & Smith, 1983; Hawes et al., 1995; Newman, 1989; Newcomer et al., 1993).

"For the operators and residents of these small board-and-care homes, definitions of quality go far beyond the easily quantifiable dimensions of the physical environment, staffing, and services. The familial and home-like characteristics of the environment were the core themes defining quality of life and quality of care. The operators and residents alike viewed the homes as family homes, unlike nursing homes in almost every respect." (Morgan et al., 1995, p. 180)

Quality From the Perspective of Residents' Families

Little is known about how families perceive quality in board and care facilities. As noted above, policy makers, providers, and researchers largely frame the debate about quality in board and care. Greene, Hawes, Wood, and Woodsong (1998) have attempted to fill this void by conducting focus groups with family members of people with dementia who live in or had recently been discharged from an assisted living facility. Their goal was to gain insight into how family members' perceptions, experiences, and attitudes about quality in assisted living facilities as a means to define quality from a consumer's perspective. Although evidence suggests that family members' views may differ from those of the care recipient (DiBernardis & Gitlin, 1979), they are often the most appropriate informant about quality issues for people unable to provide direct information about their care (Greene et al., 1998). While their findings are not limited to small facilities, inclusion of participants from Oregon's foster care system suggests that participants' represented family members with experiences in both large and small facilities.

Family members' comments about quality clustered into four major topic areas: facility staffing, services, environmental features, and general operational policies and practices (Greene et al., 1998). Family members felt strongly about the key role played by staff, especially type and level, training, knowledge (especially as related to dementia care), attitude, communication, turnover, and continuity. Several of their comments regarding staff seem especially favorable to small homes; for example, the family's desire for all staff to care about the welfare of residents, not simply perform discrete tasks without apparent concern for the general well-being of residents. Low turnover of staff and continuity were other important indicators of quality. As other studies suggest (Newcomer et al., 1993), staff turnover may be lower in smaller residential care facilities. Conversely, training for direct care staff in how to deal with Alzheimer's disease or other dementias may favor larger, more formal facilities (Morgan et al., 1995). Family members also felt strongly that services should be targeted to the needs, preferences, and strengths of the resident. Emphasis here was placed on individualized plans of care that support their family member's remaining skills and self-esteem. In addition, transportation for social outings and health care appointments was important for many family members.

Family members' main concerns about the physical environment were that it was safe and pleasant, with access to outside areas (Greene et al., 1998). In another study of relatives of those in assisted living facilities, privacy was a valued component of quality in the physical environment and an important issue in moving to a residential care environment (Kane et al., 1998). Also important in the focus group study was personal space that was homelike and clean, allowing for personal belongings. Family members particularly disliked environments with multiple floors and long halls (Greene et al., 1998). Again, several of these family preferences seem to favor small residential settings rather than larger, institutional settings. Finally, family members expressed a desire for separate units for people with Alzheimer's disease and other forms of dementia and multiple levels of care within the same facility or multiple level campus (Greene et al., 1998). These preferences in particular are relevant to the newly emerging, purpose-built, chain-affiliated assisted living industry.

Quality as Viewed by Home Residents

Consideration of quality for residents should focus on the quality of life and satisfaction with residential care. Again for this group, it remains unclear as to whether we actually know the range of elements that are important to assessment of quality in small care settings, and whether they are broadly shared across types of settings, socioeconomic strata, racial/ethnic groups, and residents of both sexes.

Studies of what constitutes quality of life and/or satisfaction are few among residents of long-term care facilities generally. Where they do exist, they interview cognitively intact residents who can be asked open-ended questions about what quality of life means to them and/or administered surveys about a limited range of quality indicators, including social interactions, resident satisfaction, and homelikeness. In a study of foster care residents, Kane and her colleagues (1998) reported that 70% found privacy an important consideration. Keeping control of personal space was connected in focus group discussions to being able to maintain possessions, controlling what and who is in that space, privacy of social relations, and keeping a personal timetable for daily events (Kane et al., 1998). In another study (Kane et al., 1993), residents of assisted living and nursing homes were compared on what factors they perceived as important in a care setting. Highly rated items for those residing in assisted living included: private rooms and baths, a safe place to live, access to medical care, good food, personal care staff, one's own refrigerator/stove, location/neighborhood, homelike atmosphere, among others. Abt Associates (1996) as part of an evaluation of a nursing home survey process, conducted a qualitative study to examine how nursing home residents viewed quality of life. Residents identified four themes: dignity, self-esteem, interpersonal relationships, and meaningful activity.

Aller and Van Ess Coeling (1995) interviewed eight cognitively intact residents of a 150-bed, long-term care facility to find out what contributed to their quality of life. Residents identified three themes of particular importance: the ability to communicate with other residents and staff within the facility, the ability to care for oneself, and the ability to care for and help others who were in more need than themselves. While their findings support the association between the desire for social interaction and quality of life found in other studies, two new factors—the importance of caring for oneself, and the importance of helping others—were mentioned by residents. These exploratory findings suggest that residents' views of what constitutes quality of life and personal satisfaction may be quite different from those of non-residents. Adding to this view, Cohn and Sugar (1991), in a study comparing the residents, staff, nurses' aides, and families' perceptions of quality of life across a range of long-term care facilities, found that various groups within homes differ when it comes to defining quality of life. Residents' perceptions of quality primarily focused on morale and attitude, while the other groups defined it in terms of care. They noted that each group tended to define quality of life in terms of their respective roles and domains over which they had responsibility. They conclude that differing perceptions about issues of autonomy and social contacts between staff and residents may lead to policies and actions that do not enhance residents' quality of life.

Namazi, Eckert, and Lyon (1987) studied quality of life among elderly residents of small board and care homes in terms of satisfaction with four domains of life: health, cost of care, hominess of the environment, and overall satisfaction with life. Four groups of independent variables were identified to influence quality of life: operators' practices and policies, operators' personal characteristics, residents' perceptions of the environment, and residents' own personal characteristics. Path analysis showed that all four groups of independent variables influenced the residents' quality of life. The greatest influences, however, were from the categories of residents' perceptions of the environment in which the social environment component had the strongest direct effect on their quality of life. Rechovsky and Ruchlin (1993) found an inverse relationship between facility size and the quality of interaction (based on subjective assessments by interviewers of staff interactions with residents), with very small homes (four to six residents) significantly outperforming larger homes with respect to resident/staff interaction. The importance of the social environment, especially as it is expressed through social interactions among residents and their caregivers, is a recurrent theme in studies of quality of life from the viewpoint of residents of long-term care. Within the domain of small residential care, the style of human relationships and manner of life that is often described as homelike or familylike is a distinguishing characteristic. It is assumed that an environment that is comfortable and "like home" is more desirable than one reflecting a more institutional atmosphere, but this assumption has not specifically been tested across the range of community-based residential care settings and health and non-related health quality of life outcomes.

Going beyond the traditional measures of the structure and process of care, Morgan and associates (1995) suggest that the social context of care provided in small board and care homes is central to the quality of life for residents and operators alike. Both the supports received by these groups and the nature of their bonds with one another can enhance or detract from the care given. "Both operators and the residents appear to emphasize board-and-care as a home or place of residence. They discuss the social relationships and caregiving aspects of day-to-day life in a home. From their viewpoint, caring is enmeshed in the domestic domain of family and friends, rather than in the formal relationships and arrangements typical of organizations such as nursing homes" (Morgan et al., 1995, p. 22).

QUALITY ISSUES IN SMALL RESIDENTIAL CARE HOMES

Although researchers agree that quality in board and care is largely subjective and difficult to define, they have, nonetheless, primarily approached it from the conceptual standpoint used to assess quality in health and other long-term care setting. The dimensions typically applied to small board and care homes reflect the traditional components of the structure, process, and outcomes of care model (Donabedian, 1966). Because the outcomes for residents in board and care (and other long-term care settings for that matter) are not readily available or agreed upon, there is an emphasis on comparing or describing settings based on measures of structure and process with no clear indication of how these components measurably affect residents' quality of care and quality or satisfaction with life. Assessments of quality in small board and care settings is further confused by research conducted to address regulatory or policy questions rather than quality from the residents' perspective or that of the primary caregiver(s).

Small board and care homes exist in the marginal worlds between family and nursing home, residential and service environment (Morgan et al., 1995) thereby raising questions about the adequacy of assessing quality using models developed for health and institutional long-term care settings. Is it meaningful to compare quality (by any definition) across settings that vary dramatically in size, purpose, and social organization? Is it meaningful or valid to apply the same metric for measuring aspects of the physical and social environments in settings that institute a "family" model of care with those instituting an "institutional" or "hotel" model of care?

Regulatory standards designed to ensure quality and safety in larger facilities may not be valid indicators of quality in smaller homes (e.g., staff to resident ratios). As other researchers have noted (Reschovsky & Ruchlin, 1993), smaller homes (those with 25 or fewer residents) are outperformed by larger homes on most objective measures of structure and process. However, smaller homes outperform larger homes when the subjective assessments of residents and their caregivers are taken into consideration. Within small homes, perhaps the most meaningful differences in perspectives on quality are between residents and non-residents. For example, residents and live-in operators and/or care providers may share similar perspectives on what constitutes quality, focusing more on interpersonal relationships directly related to satisfaction and quality of life than such things as services, decor, amenities, and scheduled activities. They are living life together rather than acting the roles of deliverer and consumer of services.

Indications are that one size (either in regulations or types of settings available) does not fit all. Regulations should take into consideration the

fundamental differences between small and large homes. Uniform legislation that enforces comprehensive standards for facilities of all sizes is sure
to work against smaller facilities, especially those that serve low-income
residents. Such homes are not able to take advantage of economies of
scale and are at best marginally profitable (Newcomer & Grant, 1989;
Chen, 1989; Morgan et al., 1995). Additionally, local zoning ordinances
may preclude their development due to limitations on the number of
unrelated people that may reside in residential neighborhood dwellings.

Currently, there exists a rich diversity in supportive living environments for frail adults. Settings vary in cost, size, style, and level of care
provided. Such diversity offers people a range of alternatives within the
limits set by such factors as income level and assets, state laws, and regulations governing residential care, and admission criteria. Findings from
the Denver Research Institute study undertaken between 1979 and 1983,
found that many poor, elderly persons were in need of community-based,
non-nursing, residential care (Dittmar et al., 1983). Dittmar (1989) notes
that the need for this type of service has not disappeared, but, in fact, has
increased as a result of population pressures from "above" and "below."
Pressures from above come from persons who, in the past, may have qual-
ified for nursing home care but, because of nursing home reform and
increased accountability for Medicaid and Medicare dollars, are no longer
eligible for such care. Pressures from below come from the rapid growth
in the number of elderly in need of personal care and oversight services
provided by board and care services. Homes built to meet this demand
favor for-profit ownership in larger facilities without the homey atmosphere of small "mom and pop" operations (Reschovsky & Ruchlin, 1993).
The problem, however, is that the supply of small board and care homes
that have traditionally served low income, publicly supported people is
decreasing as a result of gentrification, overly restrictive regulations, and
more attractive job opportunities for those who provide these services.
The challenge remains how to judge and reconcile the quality of personal
care services and quality of life that these facilities provide in light of the
valuable role they play in delivering housing and care to low income adults.

REFERENCES

Abel, E. K., & Nelson, M. K. (1990). Circles of care: An introductory essay. In E. K.
    Abel and M. K. Nelson (Eds.), *Circles of care: Work and identity in women's lives.*
    Albany: SUNY Press.
Abt Associates (1996). *Evaluation of the LTC survey process.* Cambridge, MA: Abt
    Associates. Report to the Health Care Financing Administrator.
Aller, L. J., & Van Ess Coeling, H. (1995). Quality of life: Its meaning to the long-
    term care resident. *Journal of Gerontological Nursing, 21,* 20–25.

Baggett, S. A. (1989). *Residential care for the elderly: Critical issues in public policy.* New York: Greenwood Press.

Brody, E. (1975). Intermediate housing for the elderly: Satisfaction of those who moved in and those who did not. *Gerontologist, 15,* 350–356.

Chen, A. (1989). The cost of operations in board and care homes. In M. Moon, G. Gaberlavage, & S. J. Newman (Eds.), *Preserving independence, supporting needs: The role of board and care homes.* Washington, DC: AARP Public Policy Institute.

Cohn, J., & Sugar, J. A. (1991). Determinants of quality of life in institutions: Perceptions of frail older residents, staff, and families. In J. E. Birren, J. E. Luben, J. C. Rowe, & D. E. Deutschmann (Eds.), *The concept and measurement of quality of life in the frail elderly* (pp. 28–49). San Diego: Academic Press.

Conley, R. W. (1989). Federal policies in board and care. In M. Moon, G. Gaberlavage, & S. J. Newman (Eds.), *Preserving independence, supporting needs: The role of board care homes.* Washington, DC: Public Policy Institute, American Association of Retired Persons.

DiBernardis, J., & Gitlin, D. (1979). *Identifying and assessing quality care in long term care facilities in Montana.* Report to the Department of Social and Rehabilitative Services, State of Montana. Center of Gerontology, Montana State University at Bozeman.

Dittmar, N. (1989). Facility and resident characteristics of board and care homes for the elderly. In M. Moon, G. Gaberlavage, & S. J. Newman (Eds.), *Preserving independence, supporting needs: The role of board and care homes.* Washington, DC: AARP Public Policy Institute.

Dittmar, N. D., & Smith, G. (1983). *Evaluation of board and care homes: Summary of survey procedures and findings.* Report to the Assistant Secretary for Planning and Evaluation, U.S. Department of Health and Human Services, Denver Research Institute, University of Denver.

Dittmar, N. D., Smith, G. P., Bell, J. C., Jones, C. B., & Manzanares, D. L. (1983). *Board and care for elderly and mentally disabled populations: Final report.* Denver, CO: Denver Research Institute.

Dobkin, L. (1989). *The board and care system: A regulatory jungle.* Washington, DC: American Association of Retired Persons.

Donabedian, A. (1966). Evaluating the quality of medical care. *Milbank Memorial Fund Quarterly, 44,* 166–196.

Eckert, J. K., Namazi, K. H., & Kahana, E. (1987). Unlicensed board and care homes: An extra-familial living arrangement for the elderly. *Journal of Cross-Cultural Gerontology, 2,* 377–393.

Gibbs, I., & Sinclair, I. (1992). Residential care for elderly people: The correlates of quality. *Age and Aging, 12,* 463–482.

Golant, S. (1992). *Housing America's elderly: Many possibilities, few choices.* Newbury Park, CA: Sage.

Greene, A., Hawes, C., Wood, M., & Woodsong, C. (1998). How do family members define quality in assisted living facilities. *Generations, 21*(4), 34–36.

Hawes, C., Wildfire, J. B., Lux, J. L., & Clemmer, E. (1993). *The regulation of board and care homes: Results of a survey in the 50 states and the District of Columbia.* Washington, DC: AARP Public Policy Institute.

Hawes, C., Wildfire, J., Mor, V., Wilcox, V., Spom, D., Iannacchione, V., Lux, L.,

Green, R., Grune, A., & Phillips, C. D. (1995). *A description of board and care facilities, operators and residents.* Report to the Office of the Assistant Secretary for Planning and Evaluation, U.S. Department of Health and Human Services, Research Triangle Institute and Brown University.

Jenkins, R. (1997). *Assisted living and private rooms: What people say they want.* Washington, DC: AARP Public Policy Institute.

Johnson, C. L., & Grant, L. A. (1985). *The nursing home in American society.* Baltimore: Johns Hopkins University Press.

Kane, R. A., Baker, M. O., Salmon, J., & Veazie, W. (1998). *Consumer perspectives on private versus shared accommodations in assisted living settings.* Washington, DC: AARP Public Policy Institute.

Kane, R. A., Wilson, K. B., & Clemmer, E. (1993). *Assisted living in the United States: A new paradigm for residential care for frail older persons.* Washington, DC: American Association of Retired Persons.

McCoin, J. M. (1983). *Adult foster homes: Their managers and residents.* New York: Human Sciences.

McCoy, J., & Conley, R. (1990). Surveying board and care homes: Issues and data collection problems. *Gerontologist 30,* 147–153.

Mollica, R. L. (1998). Regulation of assisted living facilities: State policy trends. *Generations, 21*(4), 30–33.

Mollica, R., & Ryther, B. (1987). *Congregate housing.* Washington, DC: Council of State Housing Agencies/National Association of State Units on Aging.

Mor, V., Sherwood, S., & Gutkin, C. (1986). A national study of residential care for the aged. *Gerontologist 26*(4), 405–417.

Morgan, L. A., Eckert, J. K., & Lyon, S. M. (1995). *Small board-and-care homes: Residential care in transition.* Baltimore: Johns Hopkins University Press.

Murray, C. C. (1988). The small congregate home. In G. M. Guttman & N. K. Blackie (Eds.), *Housing the very old.* Burnaby, BC: Gerontological Research Center, Simon Fraser University.

Namazi, K. H., Eckert, J. K., & Lyon, S. M. (1987). *Determining the quality of life of elderly residents of board and care homes.* Unpublished manuscript, University of Maryland, Baltimore County.

Newcomer, R., Breuer, W., & Zhang, X. (1993). *Residents and the appropriateness of placement in residential care for the elderly.* University of California, San Francisco: Institute for Health and Aging.

Newcomer, R. W., & Grant, L. (1989). *Residential care facilities: Understanding their role and improving their effectiveness.* Unpublished manuscript.

Newman, S. (1989). The bounds of success: What is quality in board and care homes? In M. Moon, G. Gaberlavage, & S. J. Newman (Eds.), *Preserving independence, supporting needs: The role of board and care homes.* Washington, DC: AARP Public Policy Institute.

Porell, F. & Caro, F. G. (1998). Facility-level outcome performance measures for nursing homes. *Gerontologist, 38*(6), 665–683.

Regnier, V., Hamilton, J., & Yatabe, S. (1991). *Best practices in assisted living: Innovations in design, management, and finances.* Los Angeles: National Elder Care Institute on Housing and Supportive Services, Andrus Gerontology Center, University of Southern California.

Reichstein, K., & Bergofsky, L. (1983). Domiciliary care facilities for adults: An analysis of state regulations. *Research on Aging, 5*(1), 25–43.

Reschovsky, J. D., & Ruchlin, H. S. (1993). Quality of board care homes serving low-income elderly: Structural and public policy correlates. *Journal of Applied Gerontology, 2,* 224–245.

Rubinstein, R. L. (1995). Special community settings: Board and care homes and assisted living. In Z. Harel & R. Dunkle (Eds.), *Matching people to services in long-term care.* New York: Springer Publishing Co.

Rubinstein, R. L. (In press). Resident satisfaction, quality of life and "lived experience" as domains to be assessed in long term care. In J. Cohen-Mansfield (Ed.), *Consumer satisfaction in the nursing home.* New York: Springer Publishing Co.

Sherman, S. R., & Newman, E. S. (1977). Foster family care for the elderly in New York State. *Gerontologist, 17,* 513–519.

Sherman, S. R., & Newman, E. S. (1988). *Foster families for adults: A community alternative in long-term care.* New York: Columbia University Press.

Sherwood, S., Gutkin, C., Sherwood, C., & Mor, V. (1981). *Domiciliary care programs across the nation: Implementing an option in long term care.* Boston: Hebrew Rehabilitation Center for the Aged.

Sherwood, S. J., Morris, N., &. Sherwood, C. C. (1986). Supportive living arrangements and their consequences. In R. J. Newcomer, M. P. Lawton, & T. O. Byerts (Eds.), *Housing an aging society: Issues, alternatives, and policy.* New York: Van Nostrand Reinhold.

Silverstone, B. (1978). The social, physical, and legal implications for adult foster care: A contrast with other models. In N. K. Haygood & R. E. Dunkle (Eds.), *Perspective on adult foster care.* Cleveland: Case Western Reserve University.

Stone, R., & Newcomer, R. L. (1986). Board and care housing and the role of state governments. In R. J. Newcomer, M. P. Lawton, & T. O. Byerts (Eds.), *Housing an aging society: Issues, alternatives, and policy.* New York: Van Nostrand Reinhold.

U. S. House (1989). Select Committee on Aging. Subcommittee on Health and Long-Term Care. *Board and care homes in America: A national tragedy.* No. 101–711. Washington, DC: U.S. Government Printing Office.

Zimmerman, S. I., Sloane, P. D., & Eckert, J. K. (In press). *Assisted living: Residential care in transition.* Baltimore: Johns Hopkins University Press.

6

The State and Quality of Assisted Living[1]

Sheryl Itkin Zimmerman
Philip D. Sloane
J. Kevin Eckert

Non-nursing home residential care for the elderly was first recognized in the United States in the 1940s (Morgan, Eckert, & Lyon, 1995). It began with small "mom-and-pop" homes, but within the last decade, it has taken on a new appearance and more specific nomenclature, and has proliferated under a multitude of names (e.g., sheltered housing, domiciliary care, intermediate care housing, adult foster care, congregate care) which have converged under the rubric of "assisted living." At minimum, assisted living refers to a type of care that combines housing and supportive services in a homelike environment that maximizes individual functioning and autonomy. In the most restrictive sense, assisted living connotes a distinct philosophy of care. This chapter will overview the definition and philosophy of assisted living, and will present data from a current National Institute of Health study of residential

[1] The research presented in this chapter was supported by grants from the National Institute on Aging (RO1 AG13871 and RO1 AG13863). Contributors to this work include Drs. Leslie Morgan (University of Maryland, Baltimore County); Ann Gruber-Baldini, J. Richard Hebel and Jay Magaziner (University of Maryland, Baltimore); Sally Stearns, Joan Walsh, Judith Wildfire and Gary Koch (University of North Carolina, Chapel Hill); as well as Ms. Verita Custis Buie (University of Maryland, Baltimore) and Ms. C. Madeline Mitchell (University of North Carolina, Chapel Hill). The authors wish to acknowledge the cooperation of the facilities, residents and families participating in the Collaborative Studies of Long-Term Care.

care/assisted living, to describe the current residents and practice of assisted living across four states. It will conclude with considerations regarding the quality of assisted living and resident quality of life, using standard concepts of the structure and process of care, and how they relate to resident outcomes.

ASSISTED LIVING IN THE CONTEXT OF NON-NURSING HOME RESIDENTIAL CARE

The commonality of all non-nursing home residential care is that it is a nonmedical community-based living arrangement that is not licensed as a nursing home; houses two or more unrelated adults; provides shelter (room), food (board), and 24-hour supervision or protective oversight or personal care services in activities of daily living; and can respond to unscheduled needs for assistance (Kane & Wilson, 1993). Over the years, residential care settings have evolved from containing a mixed population, including many younger persons with mental retardation and psychiatric conditions, to serving a predominantly elderly population. In the decade between 1983 and 1993, residents became increasingly aged (38% vs. 64% were 75 years of age and older); cognitively impaired (30% vs. 40%); incontinent (7% vs. 23%); wheelchair dependent (3% vs. 15%); requiring assistance with bathing (27% vs. 45%); and taking medications (43% vs. 75%) (Hawes et al., 1995).

Definition

Whether or not "assisted living" constitutes a distinct form of residential care depends on the definitional specificity applied to the term. There are multiple and varying definitions of assisted living set forth by trade associations and organizations, researchers, and lay authors, and terms such as "board and care" and "residential care" are often used interchangeably with "assisted living." Virtually all definitions stress support for activities of daily living; limited medical care; 24-hour service availability; and an aging-in-place philosophy of care. Beyond this basic definition, however, there is wide variation in how the term is used, the specific services provided, and the appropriate target population. There is no consensus as to the details of care provision and the importance of the assisted living philosophy. Further confusing the matter is that there are two differing perspectives on the role of assisted living: the first is that it lies along the continuum from home care to nursing home care; the second is that it constitutes an approach and philosophy that can apply to all persons, regardless of their level-of-care need (Lewin-VHI, Inc., 1996). In fact, in some cases, assisted living facilities provide care for residents who meet the level-of-care criteria for nursing homes (General Accounting Office, 1999).

While not necessarily creating uniformity, regulations have helped define assisted living. Federal regulations do not exist for assisted living facilities, but an impetus for increased state regulatory oversight has been fueled by multiple sources: increasing public expenditures for the care of disabled elderly in community settings; concerns regarding the quality of care, based on media reports of inadequate care and safety risks; emphasis on strengthening federal oversight of nursing home quality which high-lighted the lack of systematic information about assisted living; and the increasing demand for assisted living due to demographic trends and shifts in morbidity (Chairman of the Subcommittee on Health and Long-Term Care of the Select Committee on Aging, 1989; General Accounting Office, 1989, 1992a, 1992b). By 1998, 22 states had licensing regulations using the term assisted living, and draft regulations were being developed by an additional nine states. The major issues addressed by regulations concern requirements for the living unit; admission and retention of residents; the level of services allowed; and administrator and staff training.

Some regulations, for example, require apartment settings; others allow shared rooms. Some require that health-related services be delivered by licensed home health agencies; others allow facilities to hire nursing professionals to provide care. Many states now license facilities as assisted living only if they feature single-occupancy apartment units with full bathrooms and kitchenettes (Lewin-VHI, Inc., 1996). Other states use the terms assisted living and board and care interchangeably, and still others describe assisted living as a specific model of care.

Philosophy

One area in which assisted living tends to differ from board and care is in overt statements of philosophy (Mollica, 1998). Assisted living settings often present goals such as providing personal and health-related services to allow persons to age in place in a homelike environment that maximizes autonomy, independence, privacy, and dignity. It emphasizes individuals' rights to make decisions about their own care and to take responsibility for certain risk that may result from those decisions; self-governance; protection of individual rights; and the exercise of autonomy within the parameters of service provision (Wilson, 1996). It is also intended to accommodate changing needs and preferences and to encourage family and community involvement in care. All of these areas are meant to increase the quality of life possible for assisted living residents.

Much of what assisted living strives to achieve has been explicated by the Assisted Living Quality Coalition. The Coalition was formed in 1996, and includes representatives of the Alzheimer's Association; American Association of Homes and Services for the Aging; American Association of Retired Person; American Health Care Association/National Center for Assisted Living; American Seniors Housing Association; and the Assisted Living Federation of America. The Coalition has set forth a detailed list of the philosophies of assisted living, which are meant to be reflected in the setting's mission statement, policies, and procedures (see Table 6.1). Many of the 17 philosophies reflect the quality of care that is to be provided and the quality of life that is to be achieved in assisted living.

The specificity of this philosophy not withstanding, there remains no one accepted definition of assisted living or guidelines for how to operationally distinguish it from other forms of non-nursing home residential care (Lewin-VHI, Inc., 1996). The term is used by facilities that do not necessarily subscribe to the philosophy, and it is not always used by facilities that do. Of interest is that, in a recent national study of assisted living facilities, only 72% identified themselves as "assisted living" facilities, and these facilities were similar to those that didn't in reference to size, services, staffing, admission and discharge criteria, and resident characteristics; differences were evidenced in respect to occupancy, length of time in business, number of apartment and private units, and monthly fees (Hawes, Rose, & Phillips, 1999). This variation is reminiscent of the lack of specificity attendant to the special care movement, which likewise developed in response to market forces, and without regulatory oversight or attention to quality indicators (Magaziner & Zimmerman, 1994).

THE SCOPE OF ASSISTED LIVING

The assisted living industry is witnessing a period of phenomenal growth. This growth is due to multiple factors. First, the need for housing has increased in accordance with the increase in the numbers of elderly in the population; also, more of these persons can afford to pay for housing than in earlier generations, resulting in demands for higher quality care. Furthermore, changes in health care delivery, such as the availability of home health nurses, aides, and therapists, make residential care feasible. Finally, rapidly escalating health care costs have led to innovative service delivery approaches, such as assisted living (Assisted Living Quality Coalition, 1998). In early 1998, it was estimated that there were 11,459 facilities nationwide, serving approximately 521,500 residents (Hawes et al., 1999). By 1999, estimates of residents served ranged from 800,000 to 1.5 million (General Accounting Office, 1999). Overall, the annual growth rate of assisted living has been between 15% and 20% (National Center for Assisted Living, 1998); as a top growth industry, it is predicted that within 10 years

TABLE 6.1   The Philosophy of Assisted Living

1. Offer cost-effective quality supportive services that are personalized for each individual and delivered in a safe residential environment.
2. Maximize the independence of each resident.
3. Treat each resident with dignity and respect.
4. Promote the individuality of each resident.
5. Protect each resident's right to privacy.
6. Provide each resident the choice of services and lifestyles and the right to negotiate risk associated with his or her choices.
7. Involve residents and include family and friends in service planning and implementation when requested by a competent resident or when appropriate for incompetent residents.
8. Provide opportunity for the resident to develop and maintain relationships in the broader community.
9. Minimize the need to move.
10. Involve residents in policy decisions affecting resident life.
11. Make full consumer disclosure before move in.
12. Ensure that potential consumers are fully informed both verbally and in writing regarding the setting's approach and capacity to serve individuals with cognitive and physical impairments.
13. Ensure that specialized programs (e.g., for residents with dementia) have a written statement of philosophy and mission reflecting how the setting can meet the specialized needs of the consumer.
14. Ensure that residents can receive health-related services provided as they would be within their own home.
15. Ensure that assisted living, while health care–related, focuses primarily on a supportive environment designed to maintain an individual's ability to function independently for as long as possible.
16. Ensure that assisted living, with its residential emphasis, avoids the visual and procedural characteristics of an "institutional" setting.
17. Ensure that assisted living, with its focus on the customer, lends itself to personalized services with an emphasis on the particular needs of the individual and his/her choice of lifestyle. The watchwords should be "creativity," "variety," and "innovation."

Source. Assisted Living Quality Coalition (1998). *Assisted living quality initiative. Building a structure that promotes quality.* Public Policy Institute, American Association of Retired Persons: Washington, DC.

it will serve more elderly than do nursing homes (Meyer, 1998; General Accounting Office, 1999).

Despite definitional, regulatory, and philosophical attempts, there remains no typical assisted living facility or resident; within regulatory parameters, facilities have flexibility to set admission and discharge criteria, and to determine the type of services they will provide. The two recent national studies have not helped clarify this matter. One project (Hawes et al.,

1999) established few criteria to differentiate assisted living from other residential care; it defined eligibility as having more than 10 beds, serving a primarily elderly population, and identifying itself as assisted living or offering basic services. The second study (National Investment Conference, 1998), while imposing more specific criteria (i.e., facilities had to have eight or more units, be freestanding or have dedicated staff, be built or renovated after 1982, and have at least 70% of the resident population age 60 years or older), did not require that assisted living facilities provide select services or serve a select clientele to merit the name assisted living. The next section of this chapter uses a definition that begins to more fully address the concept underlying this mode of residential care, and provides information about the residents and services of assisted living facilities.

THE VARIABILITY OF ASSISTED LIVING RESIDENTS AND SERVICES: THE COLLABORATIVE STUDIES OF LONG-TERM CARE

The Collaborative Studies of Long-Term Care (CS-LTC) is a program of study of residential long-term care across four states (Florida, Maryland, New Jersey, North Carolina), sponsored by the National Institutes of Health. These states have well-developed residential care industries, yet exhibit variability in reference to the degree to which assisted living has permeated the marketplace. Within each of these states, the CS-LTC sampled residential care facilities in four strata: facilities with fewer than 16 beds; facilities with 16 or more beds that reflect components of "assisted living" (defined below); facilities with 16 or more beds that are more "traditional" (do not meet the criteria of assisted living); and nursing homes. To arrive at a definition of assisted living, 66 facilities were identified in New Jersey and Maryland, one-half of which were known as "assisted living" facilities based on licensure status and expert knowledge of the investigators. A telephone survey was conducted, and data were analyzed to determine which combination of items yielded the highest sensitivity and specificity; these characteristics were used to identify assisted living facilities. To be considered assisted living (also known as "new-model" in other CS-LTC reports), a facility had to be built after January 1, 1987, and had to have at least one of the following criteria: two or more private pay rates, depending on resident need; 20% or more of residents requiring assistance in transfer; 25% or more of residents who are incontinent daily; or either an RN or an LPN on duty at all times. Admittedly, this definition does not capture all elements of the "pure" form of assisted living, but it is an empirical construction that begins to make headway in this area.

Forty facilities were randomly selected which met these criteria, 10 in each state of study. Data were collected between October 1997 and November 1998 on these facilities and on a random sample of approximately 20 residents from each (N=765). Data were collected related to the resident population and to the structure and process of care, and were based on observation and interviews with residents, administrators, and care providers; those used in this chapter are elaborated below. Resident cognition was assessed from information provided by caregivers, using the MDS Cognition Scale Score (MDS-COGS) (Hartmaier, Sloane, Guess, & Koch, 1994). In addition, care providers provided information regarding resident depression using the Cornell Scale (Alexopoulos, Abrams, Young, & Shamoian, 1988), and about resident behavior using the 14-item version of the Cohen-Mansfield Agitation Inventory (CMAI) (Cohen-Mansfield, 1986). Data related to environmental characteristics derived from expert observation using the Therapeutic Environment Screening Scale—Residential Care (TESS-RC). This measure is a refinement of the TESS-NH, which evolved from the TESS-2+ and the TESS (Sloane & Mathew, 1990); it is completed through a structured observation of the facility, and collects data on indicators believed to reflect goals of quality care. The original TESS was designed to capture elements of care important for chronic care populations, including safety, orientation, stimulation, continuity, cleanliness/maintenance, personal control, and social isolation (Lawton, Weisman, Sloan, & Calkins, 1997); to this list has been added items relevant to assisted living settings and reflecting valued care domains, such as the ability to lock doors and adjust the temperature of the room. Information related to the process of care was measured with a modification of the Policy and Program Information Form (POLIF), one of five instruments comprising the Multiphasic Environmental Assessment Procedure (Moos & Lemke, 1996). It includes measures that assess philosophical policies such as the extent to which facilities impose limitations on resident behaviors and the degree of control, choice, and privacy afforded to residents. POLIF domains have been expanded to capture the evolution of assisted living and presumed indicators of care; for example, questions about services are further differentiated as to whether they are provided on- or off-site, and more information is obtained regarding the provision of distinct medical services. Further information about these measures and the design of the CS-LTC can be found in the text *Assisted Living* (Zimmerman, Sloane, & Eckert, under contract) to be published by The Johns Hopkins University Press in 2000.

Residents

Slightly more than one-half of residents were 85 years of age and older (53%); 75% were female, and 95% were white. Three-quarters were widowed, and 14% were married. Forty percent had some education beyond high school; 33% completed high school but did not proceed further, and 27% did not complete high school. Forty-three percent had been resident in the facility for 1 year or less, and the remainder were equally distributed among those who had been living there for between 1 and 3 years and beyond 3 years. Almost 90% had a relative or friend who resided nearby; 83% had visited and 59% had spoken on the telephone with a family member in the prior 2 weeks. These figures indicate that the population residing in these assisted living facilities was rather select. The majority were females who had been born before 1915, three-quarters of whom had completed high school; thus, the assisted living market, as captured by the CS-LTC definition, includes a significant number of middle-to-upper income seniors. (Supporting this finding is that 45% of facilities would discharge a resident who required Medicaid, as shown later in Table 6.4).

Cognitive and functional limitations of these residents are displayed in Table 6.2. Using the MDS-COGS score, 48% of residents were cognitively intact, the remainder being split among those who were moderately or severely impaired. Residents were impaired in an average of two of eight activities of daily living; more than one-half were impaired in bathing, and one-third were impaired in dressing and hygiene. Sixty-two percent of residents used some mobility device. Therefore, it is clear that assisted living settings are serving an impaired population (although not necessarily exclusively so), which has implications for the level of care provided and the degree of resident autonomy that is feasible.

Consistent with cognitive limitations, between 13 and 18% of assisted living residents displayed behavioral problems, including cursing/verbal aggression; complaining; pacing/aimless wandering; constant requests for attention; repetitive sentences; and general restlessness/repetitious mannerisms. In total, 39% of residents sampled displayed one or more of these types of behaviors. Depressive symptoms also were common, including anxiety/worry (36% of residents); annoyance/irritability (28%); sad expression/tearfulness (26%); and slow movements/speech/reactions (20%).

Structure of Care

Physical criteria to define assisted living include continuity with the past (e.g., homelikeness of the setting); privacy (e.g., private units; door locks); completeness (e.g., full bathroom and kitchenette); and the provision of stimulation (Regnier, 1992, 1994). Other considerations, such as safety and orientation, are also important, considering the number of residents with cognitive impairment. Table 6.3 provides data for each of these domains, indicating the percent of facilities or the mean percent of resident rooms that embody each feature. Up to eight examples are provided within each

TABLE 6.2   Cognitive and Functional Impairment of Assisted Living Residents in the Collaborative Studies of Long-Term Care (N = 765)

	Percent
Cognitive status[a]	
• Intact	48%
• Moderately impaired	25%
• Severely impaired	27%
Function (limited assist to total dependence)	
• Bathing	59%
• Dressing	34%
• Personal hygiene	33%
• Toilet use	25%
• Bed mobility	10%
• Transfer	18%
• Locomotion on unit	14%
• Eating	7%

[a] Based on MDS-COGS score, with 0–1 indicating intact, 2–4 indicating moderately impaired, and 5 or greater indicating severely impaired.

category, two of each as observed in 0–25% of facilities (or mean percent of rooms); 26–50% of facilities or rooms; 51–75%; and 76–100%, respectively. It is first apparent that no fewer than 26% of facilities were deficient in the observable indicators of safety. This finding is not unexpected, as it constitutes the area most typically addressed in state regulations. Between one-quarter and one-half of rooms had bath handrails and safe bath floors, evidenced by a lack of slippery or uneven surfaces. Almost 60% of exits were secured with a lock, alarm, or continuous staff monitoring, and 63% of facilities had extensive handrails along the hallways. More common were the average percent of bathrooms that had emergency call buttons and bedrooms that had safe floors.

In reference to orientation, a variety of design strategies may aid orientation, but assisted living facilities did not appear to excel in this area. No more than 50% of any facilities or rooms contained the orientation devices under study. Fewer than 5% had no hallways or had toilets that were visible from the bed, thereby minimizing the utility of the natural orientation afforded by visual access.

Providing stimulation without stress requires both the limitation of noxious stimuli and provision of positive stimuli. Data indicate that 17% of assisted living facilities had odors of bodily excretion that were detectable in some public areas, and that noises and tactile stimulation were less than ideal in as many as 30% of facilities; television and radio

TABLE 6.3 The Structure of Assisted Living: Percent of Facilities or Mean Percent of Rooms Displaying Select Environmental Features among the Collaborative Studies of Long-Term Care Facilities (N = 40)

	Percent of facilities or mean percent of rooms displaying feature			
	0–25%	26–50%	51–75%	76–100%
Safety features	None	Bath handrails (38%) Safe bath floors (50%)	Secured exits (59%) Hallway handrails (63%)	Bath call buttons (85%) Safe room floors (87%)
Orientation cues	No hallways (3%) Toilet visible from bed (2%)	Open room door (33%) Personal object (38%)	None	None
Stimulation	Odors in public areas (17%) Loudspeaker/intercom (25%)	Minimal tactile stim. (30%) General noises (30%)	Visual stimulation (55%) Even lighting (64%)	Television/radio (78%) Attractive locale (85%)
Privacy and completeness	≥ 3 residents/room (1%) Shared bath (17%)	Own kitchenette (37%)	Private rooms (73%)	Ability to lock door (76%) Temp. control (82%)
Continuity with past	Somewhat homelike (15%)	Moderately homelike (28%)	Very homelike (58%)	Personal mementos (91%)

Note. None indicates that no selected items were endorsed within this category.

noises were evident in almost 80% of facilities. The majority of the neighborhoods in which these facilities were located were rated as attractive or very attractive, however.

In the domain of privacy and completeness, both highly touted as a philosophical foundation of assisted living, facilities seemed to fare well. Only 1% of rooms had three or more residents; on average, 73% of resident rooms were private. Approximately 80% of rooms could be locked (from inside or outside), and most were equipped with controls to adjust the temperature.

Continuity with the past is considered important so that residence in assisted living is not seen as an abrupt departure from prior experience. Homelikeness had become a hallmark of continuity with the past, and is equated with patterned or visually textured fabric and wood on furniture; use of multiple furniture styles in the same room; furniture arrangement in small clusters (with chairs at right angles to each other); paper or border prints on walls; non-vinyl, non-terrazzo floor treatments; and lamps and/or incandescent lighting fixtures. In this study, 58% of facilities were considered very homelike, and none were considered not at all homelike. Evidence of some institutional flavor is apparent, though, as a significant minority were only somewhat or moderately homelike.

Process of Care

Similar to the structure of care, the process of care embodies multiple concepts. Facilities differ in the extent to which they allow, tolerate, or discourage certain resident behaviors (before insisting that residents be discharged) and admit or discharge certain residents; in their degree of policy clarity and resident choice, control, and privacy; and in the types of services they provide. Table 6.4 provides data in these areas, presented in accordance with the framework developed for the structure of care. Different from those data, however, which were collected by trained observation, these data derive from administrator report.

It appears that assisted living facilities are quite accepting of inappropriate behavior. While only 13% and 21%, respectively, would retain residents who steal or attempt suicide, more than one-quarter accept drunkenness or unreported absence, and more than one-half allow residents to wander and refuse medications. Also evident on Table 6.4, there are no resident characteristics for which only a minimal percent of facilities would allow admission; however, only 33% and 46% of facilities, respectively, admit residents who are bed-bound and exhibit problem behavior. Mental retardation, mental illness, and select medical needs do not prohibit admission in the majority of facilities. In a related manner, no criteria resulted in a majority of facilities indicating a need for discharge. Fewer than 50% of

TABLE 6.4 The Process of Assisted Living: Percent of Facilities Endorsing Select Components of Care Provision among the Collaborative Studies of Long-Term Care Facilities (N = 40)

	Percent of facilities endorsing			
	0–25%	26–50%	51–75%	76–100%
Requirements for residents				
Allow/tolerate/ discourage residents who:	Steal (13%) Attempt suicide (21%)	Exhibit drunkenness (26%) Exit without notice (44%)	Wander at night (59%) Refuse medications (72%)	Refuse activities (100%)
Admission policies				
Admit residents who:	None	Bed-bound (33%) Problem behavior (46%)	Mentally retarded (60%) Mentally ill (68%)	Need special diet (85%) Need daily bandage (93%)
Discharge policies				
Discharge residents who:	Unable to walk (10%) Confused/disoriented (13%)	Unable to feed self (33%) Medicaid recipient (45%)	None	None
Policy clarity				
Have policy:	Weekly staff meeting (24%)	None	Posted rules (72%) Resident orientation (74%)	Newsletter (77%) Resident handbook (85%)
Resident choice				
Have policy or allow/tolerate:	None	Dinner ≥ 1-hour range (26%) No set time to awaken (41%)	Drink alcohol in room (69%) Do some laundry (72%)	Select seat at meals (80%) Fish/bird in room (84%)

TABLE 6.4 (*Continued*)

	Percent of facilities endorsing			
	0–25%	26–50%	51–75%	76–100%
Resident control Involve residents in:	Discharging residents (18%) Planning entertainment (23%)	Dealing with hazards (31%) Setting rules (33%)	Deciding public décor (54%) Working in facility (59%)	Residents' council (85%) Moving rooms (87%)
Resident privacy Have policy/provide:	None	Individual mailboxes (46%)	Locks on all bath doors (64%) ≥ 50% private bath (72%)	≥ 50% private room (77%) < 3 residents/room (96%)
Health service/daily living activities Provide:	On-site defibrillator (15%) On-site adult day care (18%)	On-site medical clinic (28%)	Case management (64%) On-site physician (70%)	Weekly nursing (85%) On-site therapy (90%)
Social/recreational activities Provide:	Self-help groups (18%)	Classes, lectures (26%) Reality orientation (41%)	Arts, crafts (62%) Clubs, drama, singing (64%)	Outdoor activities (87%) Exercise (95%)

Note: None indicates that no selected items were endorsed within this category.

facilities reported policies that delineated resident characteristics that would impel discharge. (Note: The need for extensive medical care was not a variable under study.)

Facilities tended to communicate their policies in writing, either through posted rules (72%), newsletters (77%), or handbooks (85%); the majority (77%) also had a policy regarding procedures for resident orientation. In the next category, a minimum of 26% of facilities allowed resident choice in all activities under study, which ranged from flexibility in the time to eat (26%) and awaken (41%) to the ability to select seats at meals (80%) and keep pets (84%). Assisted living facilities also granted resident control in determining if and when to discharge other residents (18% of facilities); deciding the décor of the public areas of the facility (54%), and determining if and where to move resident rooms (87%). Policies on resident privacy favored locks on bathroom doors (64% of facilities), private baths (72%), and fewer than three residents per room (96%); these latter items were supported by observed data, as was shown in Table 6.3. Finally, service provision was varied, with 18% having on-site adult day care and self-help groups; 26–28% having classes and an on-site medical clinic; 64% providing case management/social work services and clubs/drama/singing groups; and 90% or more providing on-site physical therapy and exercise programs.

THE STATE OF ASSISTED LIVING

Despite the growing interest in and expansion of settings calling themselves assisted living, little is known about their actual role and performance and the degree to which they represent a viable option for frail and disabled elders. Increasingly, assisted living is a term that is seen as most correctly applied to residential settings that meet regulatory requirements and/or subscribe to the philosophy of assisted living. However, as demonstrated by the CS-LTC data, there is no uniformity in reference to the degree to which these facilities support principles of assisted living. Some physical characteristics of the settings appear institutional. Residents are not uniformly involved in policy decisions. Policies are not exquisitely clear or maximally flexible. State regulations limit services that might otherwise be received in private homes. Furthermore, some philosophies are inherently difficult to implement; for example, maximizing independent function may be unlikely when many residents have disabilities and are receiving care in a group setting. Given varying disabilities, and the fact that localities must be responsive to the needs of their population, a common definition of assisted living is not likely to be feasible (Mollica, 1998), nor necessarily desirable.

Quality of Care and Quality of Life

Unfortunately, nowhere in the evolution of the assisted living movement has there been an evaluative consideration of the cost-effectiveness and quality of care, or empirical evaluation of resident quality of life, as embodied in the principles of assisted living. It is only now, after assisted living has taken form, that industry leaders are attending to internal quality evaluation and improvement, and proposing rewards for high quality outcomes (Assisted Living Quality Coalition, 1998). Indeed, considering that the most recent General Accounting Office report (1999) found problems related to incorrect, incomplete, and misleading information provision; inadequate care; insufficient staffing; and medication errors, the necessity for such oversight is warranted.

Examination of quality typically uses Donabedian's framework (Donabedian, 1966), and incorporates three dimensions: (a) structure: the facility's capacity to provide care (i.e., the care setting, including the adequacy of the physical plant and equipment and the qualifications and training of staff); (b) process: the manner in which care is delivered (i.e., the application of care, such as the provision of organized activity programs); and (c) outcomes: the measure of change in the residents' status, such as new medical morbidities, functional change, or the use of acute care. In this paradigm, the human and material resources and actual care are measured and related to resident outcomes. Resident outcomes constitute the parameters that define quality of life.

Unfortunately, the study of the quality of assisted living and the quality of resident life is in its infancy. Some limitations about what is known relate to study design. Most notably, investigators have not always studied outcomes directly; instead, they have examined relationships between structure and process, and *assumed* that homes with select features provide better care which in turn results in better outcomes (Kurowski & Shaughnessy, 1983; Morgan et al., 1995; Newman, 1989; Reschovsky & Ruchlin, 1993; Segal & Hwang, 1994). Another difficulty with quality assessments in assisted living is that the few examinations conducted to date have been cross-sectional in design, determining quality by examining associations between resident well-being (or unmet need) and care provision. Data gathered in this manner suggest that less than one-half of residents have their needs met through assisted living (Mor, Sherwood, & Gutkin, 1986); that larger facilities and process components of care are related to well-being (Namazi, Eckert, Kahana, & Lyon, 1989; Timko & Moos, 1989; Weihl, 1981); and that cost savings can be achieved by substituting assisted living for nursing home care (Leon, Cheng, & Neumann, 1998). These studies are limited in that the relationship of need to service provision and outcomes is undetermined; resident report excluded those who were too cognitively impaired to respond for themselves (perhaps the most vulnerable segment of the population); the samples were not random; and the accuracy of respondent recall was not evaluated.

A second explanation for the lack of knowledge regarding quality relates to the fact that this is a new field of investigation. The CS-LTC is the broadest outcome study of assisted living, but it cannot answer all existing questions. What the CS-LTC can do is to elucidate the relationship of resident mortality, morbidity, health care utilization, and change in health and functional status, to components of the structure and process of care. The CS-LTC also can examine whether and how facilities that meet certain definitional and philosophical standards of assisted living differ from others in reference to resident outcomes and resulting quality of life. However, what the CS-LTC cannot do is flesh out all the indicators of quality care, or investigate them against all quality of life outcomes. In some cases, objective dimensions of care have been captured, but subjective components of care have not; for example, homelikeness that has been defined for research purposes may not be in agreement with the definition applied by an individual resident or by residents in aggregate. Thus, findings related to homelikeness may not capture the areas that are most salient in residents' lives. Other indicators have not been measured at all, such as familylikeness, which fosters primary group relations; because relationships have not been well-studied, they will be excluded from consideration as a possible indicator of quality care. Similarly, it is difficult to comprehensively study outcomes; areas such as maintaining meaning in life, or having a sense of hopefulness about life, which are likely to be at least as important to a resident as the number of infections she has had, have not been examined in the CS-LTC. Finally, it is important to recognize that not only will what constitutes quality differ across individuals, but it will also differ within individuals over time, as they change and their health and functional status worsen and their needs for assistance increase (Zimmerman et al., 1997).

These caveats notwithstanding, the cry for accountability is being heard nationwide, and it is promoting the need to focus on resident outcomes and quality of life. Guidelines established by the six leading LTC organizations that constitute the Assisted Living Quality Coalition contend that performance outcomes must constitute the indicator of quality, as opposed to compliance with minimum standards that serve as the focus of regulatory monitoring (Assisted Living Quality Coalition, 1998). Recognizing that research is lacking to develop and validate quality indicators, and that definitional complexities confound the very essence of the setting under study, there is much to be learned about the quality of assisted living and resident quality of life. In the end, the challenge is to evaluate and improve assisted living care, regardless of the attached label and inherent challenges.

REFERENCES

Alexopoulos, G. S., Abrams, R. C., Young, R. C., & Shamoian, C. A. (1988). Cornell scale for depression in dementia. *Biology Psychiatry, 23*, 271–284.

Assisted Living Quality Coalition (1998). *Assisted living quality initiative. Building a structure that promotes quality.* Public Policy Institute, American Association of Retired Persons: Washington, DC.

Chairman of the Subcommittee on Health and Long-Term Care of the Select Committee on Aging (1989). *Board and care homes in America: A national tragedy.* U.S. Government Printing Office, Committee Publication No. 101–711, Washington, DC: U.S. House of Representatives, One Hundred First Congress, First Session.

Cohen-Mansfield, J. (1986). Agitated behaviors in the elderly. II. Preliminary results in the cognitively deteriorated. *Journal of the American Geriatrics Society, 34*, 722–727.

Donabedian, A. (1966). Evaluating the quality of medical care. *Milbank Memorial Fund Quarterly, 44*, 166–196.

General Accounting Office, United States Congress (1989). *Insufficient assurances that residents' needs are identified and met.* Report to Congressional Requesters. Washington, D.C.: U.S. Government Printing Office.

General Accounting Office, United States Congress (1992a). *Board and care homes: Elderly at risk from mishandled medications.* Report to House Subcommittee on Health and Long-Term Care. Washington, D.C.: U.S. Government Printing Office.

General Accounting Office, United States Congress (1992b). *Drug use and misuse in America's board and care homes: Failure in public policy.* Report to House Select Committee on Aging. Washington, D.C.: U.S. Government Printing Office.

General Accounting Office, United States Congress (1999). *Assisted living: Quality of care and consumer protection issues in four states.* Report to Congressional Requesters. Washington, D.C.: U.S. Government Printing Office.

Hartmaier, S., Sloane, P. D., Guess, H., & Koch, G. (1994). The MDS cognition scale: A valid instrument for identifying and staging nursing home residents with dementia using the minimum data set. *Journal of the American Geriatrics Society, 42*, 1173–1179.

Hawes, C., Mor, V., Wildfire, J., Iannacchione, V., Lux, L., & Green, R. (1995). *Executive summary: Analysis of the effect of regulation on the quality of care in board and care homes.* Research Triangle Institute and Brown University.

Hawes, C., Rose, M., & Phillips, C. D. (1999). *A national study of assisted living for the frail elderly. Executive summary: Results of a national survey of facilities.* Meyers Research Institute, Beachwood, OH.

Kane, R., & Wilson, K. B. (Eds.) (1993). *Assisted living in the United States: A new paradigm for residential care for frail older persons?* Public Policy Institute, American Association of Retired Persons: Washington, DC.

Kurowski, B. D., & Shaughnessy, P. W. (1983). The measurement and assurance of quality. In R. J. Vogel & H. C. Palmer (Eds.), *Long-term care perspectives from research and demonstrations.* Health Care Financing Administration (DHHS), 103–132.

Lawton, M. P., Weisman, G. D., Sloane, P., Calkins, M. (1997). Assessing environments for older people with chronic illness. In J. A. Teresi, M. P. Lawton, D. Homes, & M. Ory (Eds.), *Measurement in elderly chronic care populations.* New York: Springer Publishing Company.

Leon, J., Cheng, C. K., & Neumann, P. J. (1998). Alzheimer's disease care: Costs and potential savings. *Health Affairs, 17,* 206–216.

Lewin-VHI, Inc. (1996). *National study of assisted living for the frail elderly.* Literature review update. Contract No. HHS–1–94–0024.

Magaziner, J., & Zimmerman, S. I. (1994). Evaluating special care units: The importance of definitional clarity. *Alzheimer Disease and Associated Disorders, 8*(1), S54–S57.

Meyer, H. (1998). The bottom line on assisted living. *Hospital Health Network, 72*(14), 22–26.

Mollica, R. L. (1998). *State assisted living policy: 1998. http://aspe.os.dhhs.gov/daltcp/ Reports/98state.htm*

Moos, R. H., & Lemke, S. (Eds.) (1996). *Evaluating residential facilities: The multiphasic environmental assessment procedure.* Thousand Oaks, CA: Sage Publications, Inc.

Mor, V., Sherwood, S., & Gutkin, C. E. (1986). A national study of residential care for the aged. *Gerontologist, 26,* 405–417.

Morgan, L. A., Eckert, J. K., & Lyon, S. M. (Eds.) (1995). *Small board-and-care homes: Residential care in transition.* Baltimore and London: The Johns Hopkins University Press.

Namazi, K. H., Eckert, J. K., Kahana, E., & Lyon, S. (1989). Psychological well-being of elderly board and care home residents. *Gerontologist, 29,* 511–516.

National Center for Assisted Living (1998). *Facts and trends: The assisted living source book.* Annapolis, MD.

National Investment Conference for the Senior Living and Long Term Care Industries (1998). *National survey of assisted living residents: Who is the customer?*

Newman S. (1989). The bounds of success: What is quality in board and care homes? In M. Moon, G. Gaberlavage, & S. J. Newman (Eds.), *Preserving independence, supporting needs: The role of board and care homes.* Public Policy Institute, American Association of Retired Persons: Washington, DC.

Regnier, V. (1992). Assisted living: Promoting independence choice and autonomy. *National Eldercare Institute on Housing and Supportive Services, 1*(1), 4–5.

Regnier, V. (1994). *Assisted living housing for the elderly. Design innovation from the United States and Europe.* New York: Van Nostrand Reinhold.

Reschovsky, J., & Ruchlin, H. (1993). Quality of board and care homes serving low income elderly: Structural and public policy correlates. *Journal of Applied Gerontology, 12,* 225–245.

Segal, S. P., & Hwang, S. D. (1994). Licensure of sheltered-care facilities: Does it assure quality? *Social Work, 39,* 124–131.

Sloane, P. D., & Mathew, L. J. (1990). The therapeutic environment screening scale. *American Journal of Alzheimer's Care, 5,* 22–26.

Timko, C., & Moos, R. H. (1989). Choice, control, and adaptation among elderly residents of sheltered care settings. *Journal of Applied Social Psychology, 19,* 636–655.

Weihl, H. (1981). On the relationship between the size of residential institutions and the well-being of residents. *Gerontologist, 21,* 247–250.

Wilson, K. B. (1996). *Assisted living. Reconceptualizing regulation to meet consumers' needs and preferences.* Public Policy Institute, American Association of Retired Persons: Washington, DC.

Zimmerman, S. I., Sloane, P. D., & Eckert, J. K. (in press). *Assisted living.* Baltimore and London: The Johns Hopkins University Press.

Zimmerman, S. I., Sloane, P. D., Gruber-Baldini, A., Calkins, M., Leon, J., Magaziner, J., & Hebel, J. R. (1997). The philosophy of special care in Alzheimer's special care units. *Journal of Mental Health and Aging, 3,* 169–181.

7

Quality of Care and Quality of Life in Dementia Care Units

M. Powell Lawton

T his chapter reviews information regarding the number and characteristics of special care units (SCUs) for cognitively impaired elders.
How SCUs differ empirically from nonSCUs is essential to the
major topic of defining quality care in the SCU, including the few studies
where their differential impact has been reported. The issue of impact is
the heart of this book's editors' conceptual model: performance and outcome are the elastic features of long-term care to which care policies and
practices are most fruitfully directed. After the review of research findings
dealing explicitly with SCUs, the chapter will suggest that process and
outcome are not so easily distinguished and that quality of life (QOL) is a
more fitting umbrella goal than quality of care for people in nursing homes.
Further, QOL will be seen as more generic to the nursing home milieu
than to dementia-specific settings, although there are exceptions. Discussion
of seven perspectives on QOL will constitute the final section.

DEFINITION OF SPECIAL CARE

Criteria defining the features of the SCU have not been agreed on by all.
Frequently noted criteria are (a) a geographically distinct area that is (b)
secured or locked, with (c) special environmental features suited to people with dementia, (d) special activities and programs tailored to people
with dementia, (e) specialized staff training, and (f) special admission and
discharge criteria. Despite the relative conceptual clarity of these criteria,
some have proved difficult to operationalize and objectify. As a result,

much research, including the large national surveys to be described, have used the facility's self-definition of whether they provided an SCU as the criterion.

The repetition over time of several surveys of SCUs has provided an interesting view of the growth in the SCU phenomenon. In 1987, 7.6% of nursing homes in the national Medical Expenditure Survey (NEMES, Leon, Potter, & Cunningham, 1990) reported having a special care unit or program for residents with dementia. Special surveys of SCUs in 1991 (Leon, 1994) and 1995–96 (Leon, Cheng, & Alvarez, 1997) found that percentage to have grown to almost 10% and 19%, respectively. The reason for the difference between this latter estimate and the lower estimate of 13% from the National Medical Expenditure Panel Survey (NMEPS) of 1996 (Friedman & Brown, 1999), the successor to the NEMES may relate primarily to definitions and the sampling-frame base. Both surveys estimated that SCUs (about 60% of them) were more likely to be found in for-profit facilities. They also were found in larger facilities. The average SCU had existed for about 6 years in 1996, 23% of them were purpose-designed, and their average size was 34 beds.

CHARACTERISTICS AND DISTINGUISHING FEATURES OF SCUS

The first SCUs to be reported tended to feature special environmental characteristics designed to support positive behaviors or counteract pathological behaviors such as disorientation, memory loss, deindividuation, or social withdrawal (Lawton, Fulcomer, & Kleban, 1984; Liebowitz, Lawton, & Goldman, 1979; Zarit, Zarit, & Rosenberg-Thompson, 1990; Zeisel, Hyde, & Levkoff, 1994). These efforts generated an impressive body of design knowledge (Calkins, 1988; Cohen & Day, 1993; Cohen & Weisman, 1991). More recently have come a variety of dementia-specific or dementia-relevant programs, such as reduced stimulation (Cleary, Clamon, Price, & Shullaw, 1988; Hall & Buckwalter, 1990), selective reinforcement of independent behavior (Baltes, Neumann, & Zank, 1994), stimulation-retreat (Lawton, Van Haitsma, Klapper, Kleban, & Katz, 1998), certified nursing assistant (CNA) training to deliver one-to-one interventions (Van Haitsma, Lawton, Kleban, Klapper, & Corn, 1997), and behaviorally oriented programs targeting specific problem behaviors (Burgio, Scilly, Hoar, Washington, & Tunstall, 1993).

As might be imagined, the claims made for the positive effects of the SCU have been many. An early warning and challenge to professionals was issued by Ohta and Ohta (1988) regarding the need of this care type to have its efficacy proven. Exhaustive review of the state of the art in the

SCU and other programs for residential care of dementia came from the U.S. Congress Office for Technology Assessment report (1992) which concluded that a differentially positive impact for the SCU was as yet unproven. Despite the many reasons for caution advanced in these and other writings, marketing of the SCU in nursing homes and its extension to assisted living has mushroomed to a present very high level.

Research has been unable to keep pace with such growth despite efforts like the formation of a Workgroup for Research and Evaluation of Special Care Units (WRESCU) as an interest group of the Gerontological Society of America and a major cooperative study supported by the National Institute on Aging (Ory, 1994). In reviewing research evidence regarding SCU efficacy, a first question concerns simple differences and similarities between SCUs and nonSCUs. The second and more important question is whether outcomes are different for SCUs and nonSCUs. And, of course, the outcome focus leads to the major topic of quality.

DIFFERENCES BETWEEN SCUS AND NONSCUS

The distinctive characteristics of SCUs noted earlier help define the SCU but are not necessarily present in all SCUs, except for the physically separate criterion, which is assumed to be the single necessary feature (note that Leon et al., 1997 also counted dementia-specific *programs* in addition to units, which would have added another 3% of all nursing homes to the original 19%). In fact, no empirical studies have come to light that systematically count the presence or absence of each of the SCU defining characteristics. As a whole, the literature on differences between SCUs and nonSCUs deals with a very broad set of facility, staffing, program, and resident characteristics. A comprehensive survey of the earlier literature on SCUs (U.S. Congress Office of Technology Assessment, 1992, pp. 92–103) suggests that on an absolute percentage basis, descriptions of SCUs report a majority with special environmental features (especially exit alarm systems), extra staffing, special staff training regarding dementia, and activity programs.

When SCUs were compared with nonSCUs, differences have not always been evident. Mathew, Sloane, Kilby, and Flood (1988) found more private rooms and a higher-quality total environmental score in SCUs than in nonSCUs, but SCUs actually were judged less homelike and were less likely to have personal possessions in view. In a large sample of facilities in Minnesota, Grant, Kane, and Stark (1995) found a greater prevalence of favorable design features in SCUs, and less "stimulation" and "complexity" were reported by nurses in SCUs. Resident characteristics, aside from the greater prevalence of dementia in SCUs, do not display a consistent pattern across all studies. SCU residents do seem to be more mobile, more continent, and less physically ill (Mehr & Fries, 1995; Sloane & Mathew, 1991; Teresi, Holmes, Ramirez, & King, 1998), but not more behaviorally disturbed (Sloane & Mathew, 1991). SCU residents are also more impaired in cognitively related, self-care abilities such as eating and dressing (Holmes et al., 1990).

A number of staffing characteristics have been compared. Several studies have documented greater staffing richness (Grant, Kane, Pothoff, & Ryden, 1996; Holmes, Teresi, Ramirez, & Goldman, 1997; Sloane & Mathew, 1991), although in a New York state sample, the ratio of social workers, activity, and other specialty staff was greater in nonSCUs (Holmes et al., 1997). On the other hand, Mehr and Fries (1995) found that fewer nursing staff hours and fewer total staff hours were reported in SCUs in a large national data set. The complexity of such data is illustrated by the lack of a difference once Mehr and Fries (1995) adjusted for case mix. The particular types of dysfunction presently found in residents of SCUs may be judged as requiring less staff than some of the more physically disabled and possibly acutely ill people who live in nonSCUs. Although Grant and colleagues (1996) found that staff training in SCUs had greater breadth, few differences were found between the two unit types in prevalence of specific types of training. In a New York state sample (Teresi et al., 1998), certified nursing assistants (CNAs) working in SCUs received fewer hours of training than those assigned to nonSCUs. The latter study also failed to show differences between SCUs and nonSCUs on three indicators of staff morale (Ramirez, Teresi, Holmes, & Fairchild, 1998). Less total staff turnover was found among professional nurses in SCUs but not among CNAs (Sloane & Mathew, 1991), while Grant et al., (1996) found no turnover differences associated with unit type. Stable assignment of a CNA to a resident (i.e., less-frequent rotation of assignment) was more frequent in SCUs (Teresi et al., 1998). All of the above findings of SCU differences, often observed in only one of the several studies, must be interpreted in the context of the much more prevalent lack of differences when the total number of comparisons is taken into account.

In the domain of activities, Sloane and Mathew (1991) found that among several types of activities, only reminiscence groups were more prevalent in SCUs. Nonetheless, residents were observed to have been out of their rooms more often and participating in activities in SCUs. Grant and Potthoff (1997) obtained staff informant judgments about types and levels of resident participation in different types of activities. They found that SCUs reported more activities tailored to the special characteristics of their residents and more residents reported as participating in structured group activities. Among a list of 30 activities, 13 were significantly more often reported in SCUs than in nonSCUs (Grant, Kane, & Stark, 1995).

Another quality indicator is prevalence of restraint use, which was less frequent among SCUs in the North Carolina sample (Sloane & Mathew, 1991) and also among SCUs in a large national sample (Mehr & Fries, 1995). In the latter study, however, SCU residents were almost twice as likely (42% versus 22% in nonSCUs) to be receiving psychoactive medication.

Finally, what might be thought of as a set of psychosocial milieu dimensions was derived and rated in 20 SCUs in Maryland (Zimmerman et al., 1997). Thirteen such dimensions yielded sufficient consensus to lead the authors to identify six core philosophies of special care: Promoting Safety and Security, Enhancing Connections to Others, Mitigating Disruptive Emotional and Physical Behaviors, Supporting Cognitive Functioning, and Regulating Stimulation. Their contrast with nonSCUs has not been reported. Grant (1996) used a set of milieu characteristics to contrast SCUs and nonSCUs. A total of 158 items were rated by one informant (primarily nurses) in each of 75 SCUs, 171 nonSCUs in facilities with SCUs, and 64 facilities without SCUs. The ratings yielded factors named Separation, Staff Assignment, Stability, Noxious Auditory Stimulation, Activity Complexity, Toleration versus Control of Deviance, and Homelike Environmental Continuity. SCUs were found to exhibit greater Separation and Stability and less Stimulation, Complexity, and Control than nonSCUs, each of these differences representing a preferred difference in favor of SCU quality.

RELATIVE IMPACTS OF SCUS AND NONSCUS

Cross-sectional comparisons of the types just reviewed may be influenced by admission standards and the case mix along many dimensions and thus do not speak to the issue of discerning whether the SCU has any effect on the resident. They document well the ecology of special care as it is now delivered but they cannot assess impact. A longitudinal randomized clinical trial is the only route to test impact. In the world of practice, randomized assignment to SCU and nonSCU is difficult. In addition, the SCU criteria are not always met. Indeed, there are only two studies using randomization in which one included the evaluation of a program (not a unit) by Rovner, Steele, Shumely, and Folstein (1996). The other evaluated a special-care program using randomization at the unit rather than individual level (i.e., the program was assigned randomly to one of two physically identical units specially designed for the care of dementia) (Lawton et al., 1998). Rovner et al. (1996) detected some improvement in behavioral disturbance but not on cognition or ADL. Similarly, Lawton and his colleagues (1998) found that cognition and ADL declined and negative behaviors and most affect states did not change in the SCU special program unit. However, several positive behaviors and positive affect increased at 6 months but not at 12 months. One possibility, in the absence of random patient assignment, is the longitudinal study of residents living in an SCU used their baseline level as the control measure but without comparison to an untreated group. Sloane, Lindeman, Phillips, Moritz, and Koch (1995, Table 1, p. 104) reviewed several such studies each with some scattered favorable effects, as did a later review by Bellelli and his colleagues (1998). The absence of any comparison group and the failure of the scattered positive findings to have been confirmed across several studies render the meaning of such findings at best ambiguous. A design in which SCUs and nonSCUs are compared longitudinally is superior, and obviously effective to the extent that baseline characteristics of the two groups are similar. Adequate-sized samples of this type were studied by Holmes and his colleagues (1990) in four SCUs; no differential benefit attributable to SCU residence was detected after 6 months. Volicer (1994) compared demented people segregated into one unit (with no other information on other defining characteristics of an SCU) with demented people scattered among nonSCU units in another hospital. As measured over 3 months, discomfort was less in the SCU, although mortality was also greater in the SCU (with no control for risk factors). Finally, the most complete study was done by Phillips, Sloane, Hawes, Koeh, Han, et al., (1997). In their three-state sample of 77,000 residents in 48 SCUs and 800 nonSCUs over a 12-month period, no differential effects attributable to residence in an SCU were seen in continence, weight loss, or five activities of daily living.

As a whole, the literature on SCU - nonSCU differences and effects does not support strongly the conclusion that benefits occur if special care is provided. In fact, the evidence is rather compelling that the course of basic abilities such as cognition and ADL is inexorably downhill (Lawton et al., 1998; Phillips et al., 1997). Effects on mortality are too scattered to allow any conclusion. The only other outcomes that fall clearly into the category of outcomes are psychological. The clearest such outcome is in a decrease in observed signs of distress among SCU residents in the study by Volicer and his colleagues (1994). Although a few other positive presumed correlates of SCU residence were reported, they were clearly in the process realm. More favorable design features (that may possibly relate to SCUs being newer), lower environmental stimulation and complexity, less use of restraints, and greater activity richness are among the positive process characteristics reported as more frequent in SCUs from more than one study. These environmental features have been defined consensually by experts to represent higher quality. Yet, to categorize them as process rather than outcome diminishes them in light of the call for outcome measurement as the only sure mark of quality (Kane, Bell, Reigler, Wilson, & Keeler, 1983). In the analogy with acute care, length of stay, mortality, and incidence of morbidity are the outcomes. Kane and her colleagues (1983) and the 1987 OBRA language clearly added resident well-being as an outcome appropriate for long term care. I argue that this definition requires still further enlargement.

QUALITY OF CARE, QUALITY OF LIFE, AND OUTCOMES

Above a threshold level of adequacy, concerning primarily physical health and sanitation, the critical definition of quality in the nursing home is more fittingly quality of life rather than quality of care. Further, quality of life is itself the outcome, not a means to more ultimate outcomes of health and longevity. Thus, I suggest that for long-term care in a nursing home and particularly for people with dementia, who will live the rest of their lives in residential care, there is a need to rearrange our concept of the outcomes of care. Specifically:

1. The term "quality of care" should be reserved to refer to the operations that contribute to cleanliness, meeting physical needs (elimination, eating, etc.), and treating, or counteracting, the threats to life associated with physical illness and their effects on the basic functions of cognition and function, as in the ADLs. An example is the development of a set of 12 indicators of quality of care that may be obtained from the Minimum Data Set of record: Accidents, Behavioral and Emotional Patterns, Medication Management, Cognition, Continence, Infection Control, Nutrition, Physical Function, Psychotropic Drug Use, "Quality of Life" (i.e., use of restraints and "little or no activity" on MDS), Sensory Functioning, and Skin Care (Zimmerman et al., 1995). Most of these indicators are in the basic-function category. Most can be risk-adjusted, that is, account taken of initial level. This latter characteristic is an advantage, because it implies that change from baseline may be reliably measured. Some of the indicators (e.g., change in depression, participation in activities) are clearly QOL rather than quality of care, but they are few in number and limited to what is already in the MDS.

2. Quality of life within a facility refers to the aspects of residential care associated with subjective states of the resident. A more formal definition might be, "The aggregate of positive and negative subjective states summed over time for all residents, plus the personal, social, and environmental features associated with residents' subjective status." Deviations from established standards of quality of care are likely to be associated with pain, subjective distress, and other negative

emotions. Deviations from usual subjective states may also be positive. Positive states may be consequences of a very broad range of characteristics of the residential milieu, going far beyond care operations.

3. Quality of life thus *is* the outcome toward which our efforts should strive. As the worst of care abuses become reduced through legislation, quality monitoring, and positive redefinition of the norms of care, mortality, and morbidity will recede in their comparative importance as outcomes, in favor of quality of life in its largest sense.

WHAT IS QUALITY OF LIFE IN THE NURSING HOME?

The foregoing statements clearly suggest that quality of life is something experienced by people, falling within the broad range from distress to elation. The emphasis on personal experience has led many to assume that quality of life can be *only* subjective. In our realm of long-term care, this assumption, partially embodied in OBRA 87, has led to a search for ways of assessing consumer satisfaction with many types of care (e.g., Zinn, Lavizzo-Morey, & Taylor, 1993). Is client satisfaction a sufficient complement to mortality and morbidity to form a complete set of quality outcomes capable of being measured and applied in quality control?

Subjective and Objective Quality of Life

The suggestion advanced here is that all definitions of quality of life that do not represent adequately *both* subjective and objective aspects of quality are deficient. Subjective quality of life is the idiosyncratic judgment of the experiencer; aggregated judgments of quality across many experiencers yield a distribution that can be characterized as representing the average perceived quality of the program.

Objective quality of life is a far more problematic concept, because the question "quality for whom?" is raised. Individual preferences and suitability vary greatly. Yet every designer, architect, planner, or service provider absolutely must make decisions based on their most-informed judgments about the number of users likely to benefit from a program. Although opportunity for individual choice must be included to the extent possible, every program includes some immutable and exclusionary elements. Best-informed judgments on how to design such elements obviously must rely on standards whose basis goes beyond any individual user's subjective judgment. In some instances, such objective standards are definable in clear physical terms: Physical cleanliness, absence of infection, full lighting in obstacle areas, and so on. More likely, social norms are likely to have defined characteristics of environments, staff behavior, or service delivery that are generally agreed upon as superior or inferior. For example, at the time of this writing, "homelike quality" is highly valued by professionals and has found its way into the HCFA-prescribed nursing home survey process. Homelike quality is defined idiosyncratically by each individual, but the survey process designers concluded that consensus regarding what is homelike was strong enough to warrant its use as a relatively objective facet of facility quality. Other examples of varying "objective" quality abound, such as frequency of activities, type and quantity of staff training, or prevalence of private versus shared rooms. Such a list of facility characteristics would resemble exactly what have been called process features, not outcomes. In Donabedian's (1966) and other later models of health organizations, process variables are antecedents of patient outcomes and thus explicitly defined as lying outside the outcome class. The reason is that the process characteristic may or may not result in a favorable outcome for everyone or people in the aggregate (for example, size or sponsorship of nursing home). Unless a characteristic results in a favorable (or unfavorable) outcome for all individuals, it cannot be characterized as an outcome.

The position taken here is that individuals experience favorable or unfavorable outcomes idiosyncratically but in the aggregate we can measure the proportions of individuals who experience such differential outcomes. Therefore, environmental characteristics which are defined objectively and which are empirically related to favorable individual outcomes should be thought of as facility-level quality of life outcomes because, in the aggregate, people exposed to them have a higher probability of subjective well-being or individual achievement. We have not hesitated to use small social-area characteristics such as average income, housing stock quality, or crime rate to represent quality of life for those that live there, so why not look to institutional characteristics as indicators of quality of life for residents?

The last thought related to the inclusion of both subjective and objective features in the definition of quality of life is that subjective quality in the aggregate is not necessarily the sole criterion against which objective qualities should be validated. As in the case of some bacterial infections, there may be some negative aspects of one's milieu about which people are unaware, or limitations in their ability to make quality judgments or foresee future consequences of present features of the milieu. Later in this chapter specific consequences of such limitations for assessing the quality of life of people with dementia will be discussed. Thus room must be left for expert opinion or quantitative standards (e.g., necessary wheelchair turning radius) to override individual judgment or, at the least, to be considered as factors in reconciling objective and subjective aspects of quality as outcome criteria.

Further Thoughts on Subjective Quality of Life

The previous section made brief reference to the equipotentiality of distress and elation as opposite aspects of quality of life. Research in general psychology (Bradburn, 1969; Diener & Emmons, 1984; Watson & Tellegen, 1985) as well as in gerontology has documented the partial independence of positive and negative affect states, prompting this author (Lawton, 1991) to conclude that in our zeal to treat psychological illness, we have downgraded the importance of half of all that should be included in our concepts of psychological well-being and mental health.

Research on dementia and research conducted in nursing homes has similarly selectively neglected the possibility of tracking positive states. Only relatively recently have we had such measures as the Pleasant Experiences Inventory for Alzheimer's Dementia (Logsdon & Teri, 1997), or self-response questionnaires for perceived quality of life by people with dementia (Brod, Stewart, Sands, & Walton, 1999; Logsdon, Gibbons, McCurry, & Teri, 1999). Lawton, Van Haitsma, and Klapper (1996) developed a nonverbal instrument for observing five affect states and reported the incidence and duration of such states among cognitively intact and impaired nursing residents. The conclusions from these types of research is that positive states occur at least as frequently as negative states among nursing home residents and that their occurrence is correlated with some eustressful and stressful contexts (Lawton, Van Haitsma, Perkinson, & Ruckdeschel, 1999).

This line of research should be followed in order to continue to map the relationships between context and affect; the more specific the details of the context and the concomitant affect the better. The burden is on the research community to build up such an inventory of validated relationships demonstrating that objective domains of asserted quality do in fact result in differential positive or negative outcomes. An example of a finding that begs for further investigation is that residents with dementia who interact more with others exhibited both more pleasure and more anger (Van Haitsma, et al., 1997). Can more careful study identify the specific interactions and the combinations of people and interaction type that were more associated with pleasure versus those resulting in anger? The guiding principle in the search for indicators of quality of life is actually two principles: What produces positive moments and what produces distressing moments?

Positive and negative states are not exact opposites or the sole complementary components of a quantum of quality of life. Everyday life also consists of affectively neutral time and we must allow for individual differences in preferences for high-affect versus low-affect quanta. Personal preference is thus another ingredient of quality of life whose understanding will assist in enhancing individual quality of life as well as quality of life in the aggregate. Knowing what proportion of clients assess an activity program positively but without caring much for the activity versus the proportion who both value the activity and assess it positively provides much better information on enhancing quality of life than does the simple percentage satisfied. OBRA's discussion of preferences has stimulated new research in this area. Such research is methodologically challenging, however, and we are still far from the point of being able to assess preferences systematically and organize the information in a way that is usable in providing direct services.

A CONCEPTUAL OVERVIEW OF ONE APPROACH TO ASSESSING QUALITY OF LIFE IN DEMENTIA CARE

This review of research comparing SCUs and nonSCUs revealed at best a scattering of such differences, an absence of upheld SCU effects, and doubt in this author's mind regarding the future potential in searching for SCU-specific outcomes in the QOL realm. The second section reviewed the much more general constructs of quality of care, quality of life, and outcomes, with little specific attention being given to dementia and none to SCUs. In this last section, a skeleton of a conceptualization of quality of life in the nursing home will be presented. Because more than half of long-term residents are cognitively impaired, any such framework must be designed to accommodate the needs of people with dementia as well as those with relatively intact function. The author's recent work has led to the conviction that a new framework for assessing quality of life in nursing homes is needed and that designing specifically for dementia represents a second-stage task, one that should follow on the satisfactory beginning of the more general task for assessing nursing homes in general.

Embarking on such a task demands immediate recognition of the major achievement of the Multiphasic Environmental Assessment Protocol (MEAP, Moos & Lemke, 1996) in providing a means for assessing residential environments for older people. Space is not available to describe this measure in the detail it deserves, or to state fully why a successor to it may be needed. Two reasons are evident, however. The first is that the nursing home environment has changed since the MEAP was designed. Full assessment of its characteristics does not seem possible when using an instrument that was designed to include a relatively broad range of facilities (i.e., independent housing and assisted living) for people of varying levels of competence. The second reason is that perceived quality of life and psychological well-being (i.e., the evaluated aspect of environment) were excluded by the MEAP's authors in favor of attributes that could be linked to observable phenomena, to the extent possible.

The present framework is one under development in ongoing research under the direction of Rosalie A. Kane and Robert L. Kane of the University of Minnesota, with contract funding from the Health Care Financing Administration (HCFA). The framework to be described here represents the early conceptions of this chapter's author (Kane, Kane, & Lawton, 1998). It is by no means fully incorporated into the assessment procedure that will ultimately be used and the examples are purely for illustration. The measures actually used in the HCFA research will undoubtedly differ substantially from those used as examples here. Responsibility for the weaknesses of the model to follow is the present author's.

Human Needs as a Way of Describing Quality of Life

The subjective-objective and pleasure-distress principles guide us in a general sense toward defining QOL. We need greater specificity than these abstractions, however. I have suggested that the next step is to look at the largest array of human needs and consider which ones are most relevant to QOC and QOL. The final list of most important needs has never been and will never be constructed because the value judgments of individuals are intrinsically a factor in deciding what is important. There have been several decades of thought on such topics, however. Many investigators' top-10 lists have been collated to arrive at the set shown in Table 7.1. In turn, it has been revised in the ongoing research. This list has three characteristics: (1) each need is a universal human need; (2) each can be served or frustrated in caregiving settings; and (3) each need may be represented by its fulfillment for each individual and by its capacity to be fulfilled by the facility. There are three methods for obtaining information on domain-specific quality of life and four foci for attention.

Methods for obtaining the information are direct observation, reports from others, and self-report of the client. *Foci for attention* are the physical environment of the program, the social environment of the program, the client, and the family. Combining the foci and the methods yields seven approaches to assessing quality. A Cadillac version of assessment would use all of them. In real life, each approach provides a valid portion of the truth about quality of life in a specified context, but each also has sources of error. In practice, a usable instrument should make it possible for portions of the total version to be used. Illustrations of the type of inquiries that might be used for several of the needs will be presented. Because there is as yet no formal QOL assessment instrument of this type, the items are merely examples.

TABLE 7.1 Facility Quality Indicators for 11 Needs

1. *Autonomy.* The extent to which resident initiative and choice are allowed or encouraged.

2. *Privacy.* The extent to which the structure, policies, and procedures allow physical, auditory, visual, and communicative privacy when wished.

3. *Dignity.* Sensitivity to residents' self-respect, values, modesty, and feelings, as expressed in staff behavior.

4. *Social interaction.* Person-to-person interchange, whether in dyadic or group form, including residents, staff, family, and others where the purpose is social.

5. *Meaningful activity.* Either obligatory (e.g., self-care) or discretionary behaviors where the task is the goal behavior more than any social goal, and the result is either self-affirmative competence or active pleasure in the doing or watching of the activity.

6. *Individuality.* The degree to which residents' personal preferences and markers of their backgrounds and present interests are evident in staff and resident behavior.

7. *Enjoyment versus aversive stimulation.* Expressions, verbal or nonverbal, of active pleasure in everyday life, whether in active care, activities, or nonactive times, including efforts of staff to express warmth or recognition, contrasted with pain and distress. Stimulation, novelty, sensory experience.

8. *Safety and security.* Evidence that the facility does all possible to produce the perception of safety and security and that residents feel able to move about freely and keep their possessions intact.

9. *Spiritual well-being.* Reports from staff and residents that concern for religion, prayer, meditation, and moral values is supported by the facility.

10. *Clarity of structure.* The rules and norms governing resident behavior are clearly stated and consistently applied without rigidity, use of punishment, or exclusive serving of staff and administrative needs. Space uses clearly designated, knowledge of appropriate behavior communicated through signs, visibility, clear signals. Orientational information present.

11. *Functional competence.* The extent to which the physical structure, policy, staff behavior, and the social milieu contribute to the improvement of, maintenance of, or slowed decline of skills important in everyday life (primarily ADL and IADL tasks).

The Seven Routes to Quality Of Life Assessment

1. *Observing the physical environment.* The physical environment is relatively stable and many of its components may be judged relatively objectively. The main problem is how to pick out from all that exists in "the environment out there" the limited number of features centrally relevant

to quality of life. Moos and Lemke's (1980) Physical and Architectural Features checklist includes environmental facets particularly relevant to residential settings. Focusing on the SCU environment, Sloane and Mathew (1990) constructed the Therapeutic Environment Screening Schedule (TESS) based on a research assistant's tour of the facility. A companion expert rating scale was built around 10 attributes selected from the literature to represent important personal needs that might be met by environmental design: Control, Orientation, Privacy, Function, Stimulation Quality, Stimulus Regulation, Continuity of Self, and Social Contact (Weisman, Lawton, Sloane, Calkins, & Norris-Baker, 1996). A number of these domains formed part of the thinking that led to the choice of need domains as served by environmental features.

An early version of our Physical Environmental Observation form (Table 7.2) began with the 11 needs and constructed a set of environmental indicators for each. Once having represented the domains by multiple indicators, the indicators may be arranged by places, rather than needs (e.g., resident rooms, dining room, lobby, etc.). One may thus construct a matrix of places (rows) and needs (columns) where each cell would be filled with one or more examples of environmental features that foster or impede the need fulfillment.

2. *Observing the psychosocial environment.* All programs are composed of a complex aggregation of goals, activities, rules, practices, and staff behaviors, which I refer to as the psychosocial environment, sometimes called the organizational environment. Characteristics such as these are the main ingredients of the Sheltered Care Environment Scale of the MEAP (Lemke & Moos, 1987). The potential scope of assessing this aspect of QOL is limitless and thus could consist of hundreds of observable behaviors or archival features. Many of these events are very rare. In order to bring this observation task within reach of the possible, a streamlined approach has been substituted for the more time-consuming practice of repeated formal observations of scores of specific times, events, or interactions. Instead, examples of indicators of positive or negative quality are provided to the observer in order to illustrate the concept, not to inventory all possible indicators. Table 7.3 shows illustrative indicators of this type. The psychosocial environment may then be rated on a Likert scale by a professional staff member (or outsider, if available) who meets the following criteria. The observer is: (a) already very familiar with the facility; (b) willing and able to study a set of 11 rating scales representing the resident needs; (c) in a position to observe informally for a period of 2 weeks before making the ratings; and (d) during these preparatory 2 weeks, take notes about anything observed that might be relevant to each need. The prepared list of indicators, plus all the new ones generated in the 2 weeks and judged relevant, would be used in producing each rating.

TABLE 7.2   Observational Indicators for the Physical Environment

1. Autonomy
   - Heat and air conditioning individually room controlled
   - Variation in lighting possible (minimum of overhead, over-bed, and one lamp or seat spotlight)
   - Is there a place where resident can purchase notions, necessities, cards, gifts, etc.?
   - Some bedroom doors observed closed (presumption of resident's choice)
   - Frequent observed use of restraints or mobility-limiting furniture (negative)
   - Room window curtains easily controlled by resident

2. Privacy
   - Proportion of all residents who live in single rooms
   - Proportion of all residents who have exclusive use of a toilet
   - Bathroom doors can be locked from within
   - Some seating in public places where one person can sit at a distance from others

3. Social interaction
   - Places to stop and sit in public halls and outdoor areas
   - Places to sit with views of high-traffic areas, enlarged area for seating near nursing station, nurses area, entrances, staff congregation areas)
   - Choices of one-, two- , and multiple-person seating in public areas

3. *Inquiring about the psychosocial environment.* Direct observation of activity such as that catalogued in the observed psychosocial environment takes much time; therefore, the way we assess the psychosocial environment must be streamlined. Some aspects of the psychosocial environment are nearly impossible to observe, however. For example, one would have to observe for many hours to be able to catalog the organized activities that take place in a week or to see whether residents are allowed to sleep late in each unit. The natural alternative is to obtain information from an informant, for example, the administrator or a staff professional (see the Policy and Program Information Form, Lemke & Moos, 1980), or from archival data such as attendance records or a staff training syllabus. The opportunity for reporting bias to be present from such sources is obvious. If we ask the director, for example, "How warm and friendly are the staff?" it would be superhuman for the answer not to be colored by some overall tendency to praise or criticize.

Such direct evaluations are best avoided in favor of information for which there is some objective basis. For questions such as those shown in Table 7.4, direct falsification and giving one's own program the benefit of the doubt can occur, but at least there is a fact lurking in the background against which any tendency to distort may be compared.

TABLE 7.3   Observational Indicators for the Psychosocial Environment

1. Autonomy:
   a. Staff encourages autonomous behavior and discourages dependent behavior.
   b. Residents observed in active community roles (at desk, as guide, etc).
   c. Staff observed offering residents a choice.
   d. Staff discourage occupancy of resident bedrooms (negative indicator).

RATE AT THE END OF YOUR TIME AT FACILITY

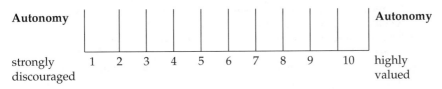

Autonomy

strongly discouraged   1   2   3   4   5   6   7   8   9   10   highly valued   Autonomy

2. Privacy:
   a. Staff knock before entering room.
   b. Staff discuss a resident in presence of others (negative indicator).
   c. Staff careless about privacy during personal care (door open, bathroom exposed, etc.).

RATE AT THE END OF YOUR TIME AT FACILITY

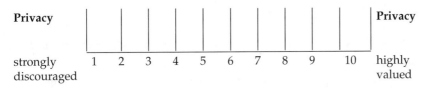

Privacy

strongly discouraged   1   2   3   4   5   6   7   8   9   10   highly valued   Privacy

3. Dignity:
   a. Address form (first name, Mr., Mrs.) used selectively.
   b. Staff use baby talk (negative indicator).
   c. Staff explains reason for request or command.
   d. Staff openly critical in nonsensitive way (negative indicator).
   e. Staff smile during interaction.

RATE AT THE END OF YOUR TIME AT FACILITY

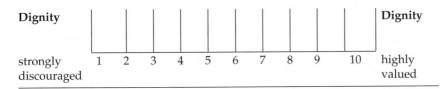

Dignity

strongly discouraged   1   2   3   4   5   6   7   8   9   10   highly valued   Dignity

TABLE 7.4 Informant-Based Indicators for the Psychosocial Environment

All of these indicators represent staff reports of objective facts/events, rather than asking for one informant's estimate of a way of thinking that characterizes the whole facility.

1. Autonomy
   • Can residents sleep late if they wish?
   • Can residents stay up if they wish?
   • Can residents get a drink or snack if they wish?
   • Do residents get meals at the same time or can they decide (within limits) when they want to get 1 or more meals each day?
   • Does the resident have a choice of 2 or more main dishes at 1 or more meals each day?
   • If a resident requests it, can he/she get a bath or shower at a requested time? (vs. only on schedule)
   • How many residents (or %) attended the last residents' council meeting?
   • If a resident wakes up at night, what does s/he usually do? (any response indicating resident choice)
   • Are there resident committees that meet regularly? Which ones? How many attended last meeting?

2. Privacy
   • Are residents allowed to be in their bedrooms with door closed whenever they wish?

3. Dignity
   • Is there an in-service training module about preserving resident dignity?

4. Social interaction
   • Have any groups from outside the NH come in to provide a program in the past month? Which?

---

4. *Asking professional caregivers about the resident.* Some of the problems of self-ratings may be counteracted by getting an "outside opinion" from care staff who have ongoing opportunities to watch the behavior of clients. In the nursing home setting, the Minimum Data Set (Morris et al., 1990) is designed to give staff the opportunity to rate the important facets of an individual's life: ADL function, cognition, social behavior, activity partic- ipation, and mental health, among others. (See Lawton et al., 1996 for psy- chometric analysis of these measures.) These indexes are available on all residents. They represent some, but not all of the 11 need domains. Such an MDS profile on a single individual is extremely useful for care plan- ning for that person, and the collection of profiles for all residents is use- ful for characterizing the nursing home as a whole. One great advantage

of the expert's rating is that all program participants can be rated on the scale, as contrasted with the self-report, which may be unusable on half or more of people with dementia. Many other scales may be used, limited primarily by the amount of time available to train raters and make ratings. Some that have been used in the NIA cooperative study of SCUs include the Cohen-Mansfield Agitation Inventory (Cohen-Mansfield, Marx, & Rosenthal, 1989), the Multidimensional Observation Scale for Elderly Subjects (MOSES, Holmes, Csapo, & Short, 1987) or the BEHAVE-AD (Reisberg et al., 1987), an inventory of behavioral symptoms.

Staff must be trained to make such ratings, however, and care must be taken to ensure that a professional rater has had adequate opportunity to know the resident and observe her or his behavior over a period long enough to make a valid rating possible. Many staff also must be taught to appreciate the value of structured ratings for assessing current state and progress over time. A barrier frequently is encountered when busy staff have the hasty reaction of feeling that the formal rating is interfering with their ability to work directly with the client. It is evident, however, that resident need fulfillment for some of the needs shown in Table 7.1 would be impossibly difficult for some staff rating some patients, to say nothing of the inordinate amount of valuable staff time required.

5. *Formal expert observation of the resident.* Because of these problems in obtaining ratings from staff observers, another source of data, direct observation by trained and relatively sophisticated researchers or staff, is desirable. Theoretically, a system for directly observing all behavior could be designed as in behavior maps or streams of behavior (Van Haitsma et al., 1997). But the expense of this type of observation time required is a barrier to extensive use of direct behavior observation. Limited categories of behavior, such as independent functional activity, social interaction, or wandering may be tallied, as illustrated in Table 7.5. Recent research has demonstrated that emotion may be measured in ways other than by self report. The Apparent Affect Rating Scale (included in Table 7.5 as a way of illustrating Enjoyment and Distress) yields observer ratings of Pleasure, Interest, Anger, Anxiety, and Sadness after 5 minutes of observation (Lawton et al., 1998). Several repeated ratings are needed for each client. It is possible for a trained observer to position herself in a room or a place with a view of ongoing activity for an hour and emerge with 5-minute affect ratings for 10 or more clients. This technique needs several hours of training and observed practice. Philadelphia Geriatric Center has produced a commercially distributed videotape that provides an introduction to what may be learned from recognizing resident feelings and a manual for instruction (Terra Nova Films, 1997). All residents' feeling states may be rated, whether they are cognitively impaired or not. In turn, these feelings give staff useful feedback about whether their programs, or their personal approaches to residents, are working.

TABLE 7.5   Observational Indicators: The Resident

1. Autonomy
   - Resident observed serving in functional roles (receptionist, working in store, helping set up meetings, etc.)

4. Social interaction
   - Occasions of observed conversation with other residents (tally)
   - Occasions of observed conversation with staff (tally)
   - Quality of interactions observed with staff and residents more positive than negative

5. Meaningful activity
   - Resident observed actively participating in organized activity program.
   - Resident observed watching, with directed attention (i.e., obvious eye focus, eye and head movements following activity of others) while not participating behaviorally.
   - Resident observed engaged in some other nonsocial, nonorganized, nongroup activity (tally number?).

7. Enjoyment/Distress
   PGC Apparent Affect Rating Scale (5-minute observation) 1 = Never to 5 = > 2 minutes

   PLEASURE
   Signs: Smile, laugh, stroking, touching "approach" manner, nodding, singing, arm or hand outreach, open-arm gesture.

   ANGER
   Signs: Clench teeth, grimace, shout, yell, curse, berate, push, physical aggression, or implied aggressive such as fist shaking, pursed lips, eyes narrowed, knit brow.

   ANXIETY/FEAR
   Signs: Furrowed brow, motoric restlessness, repeated or agitated motion, facial expression of fear or worry, withdrawal from other, tremor, tight facial muscles, calls repetitively, hand wringing, leg jiggling, eyes wide.

   DEPRESSION/SADNESS
   Signs: Cry, tears, moan, sigh, mouth turned down at corners, eyes/head turned down and face expressionless, wiping eyes.

   INTEREST
   Signs: Eyes following object, intent fixation on object or person, visual scanning, facial, motoric, or verbal feedback to other, eye contact maintained, body or vocal response to music, turn body or move toward person or object.

6. *Asking the resident.* The typical approach to assessing QOL is to ask the resident to rate satisfaction with a variety of facets of each domain, or the frequency with which various positive or negative events occur. There are many pressures that can make nursing home residents (in fact, people in general) overrate their satisfaction with anything. First, if they say they're satisfied, maybe they will actually feel better. Second, there is often a desire to please the interviewer. Third, cognitive impairment sometimes makes it difficult to discriminate among levels of judgment and it is simply easier to express a feeling of total satisfaction than to make more complex discriminations. Finally, the most potent source of positive bias is the huge differential in power perceived by the residents who are not only very old and sometimes frail but who feel at the mercy of their caregivers. It is often assumed that cognitively impaired people cannot voice their wishes or evaluate their current situation. This assumption has resulted in ignoring large numbers of mildly or moderately impaired residents, some of whom may be capable of making evaluation judgments. The limits for such judgments have not been established, however.

Some of the quality of life assessment instruments described earlier have framed questions very simply, provided easy response alternatives (e.g., yes versus no rather than a Likert scale), and have reduced the number of questions. A sample of such a version is shown in Table 7.6. Although there will always be a segment of any long-term care population who cannot respond knowledgeably to quality of life questions, the proportion who can do so is probably higher than typically thought. One possible alternative approach is to use a family member's judgment as a proxy for the quality of life assessments of cognitively impaired elders.

7. *Asking the family.* Many of the same evaluation and satisfaction questions asked of the resident may be asked of a family member. Every method has its problems. Asking the family has error associated with possible family biases and sources of defensiveness. Family members may also have some of the same cautiousness about expressing dissatisfaction that was noted for older clients. The major source of error is the family informant's simple lack of knowledge about what the elder does in the facility, together with any outsider's inability to see into the inside of another person in order to know the elder's feelings. It is thus very unlikely that family judgments can be used to represent the resident's. Thus it is essential to view the family perspective as an additional perspective that is part of the total picture but not a substitute for the resident's view.

THE PROSPECTS FOR IMPROVED QUALITY OF LIFE IN NURSING HOMES

The survey process by which the federal government attempts to monitor quality in nursing homes has had a difficult time in meeting its goal. It is

TABLE 7.6   Resident Interview

1. Autonomy
    1. Do you get as many showers or baths as you want at times when you want them?
    2. Do you decide when to go to bed?
    3. Do you decide what clothing to wear?
    4. Do the residents here have free choice in most things they do?
    5. If you don't like something here, who do you go to to try to change it? (positive response is any recourse)
    6. Do you have a choice about when to have your meals?

2. Privacy
    1. Do the people who work here knock on your door before entering your room and wait for your response before they enter?
    2. Can you find a place to be alone here when you wish?
    3. When you have a visitor, is there a place where you can visit in private? (IF YES) Where? _____ (positive response is any place named)

3. Dignity
    1. Do the people who work here take time to listen when you have something you want to talk about?
    2. Do the people who work here remember to do things you ask them to do, or get something you ask for?
    3. Do the people who work here handle you gently when they help you to move, dress, or bathe?
    4. Around here, staff talk down to residents.

much easier to specify the absence of threats to life, health, and sanitation than it is to specify the presence of the types of positive indicators of Quality of Life (QOL) which the preceding section has attempted to assemble. Nonetheless, the Health Care Financing Administration (HCFA), which monitors states' Medicare and Medicaid certification process, has moved over the last few decades toward better recognition of the importance of QOL indicators. In the year 2000, HCFA is sponsoring four major contracts designed to improve this process of improving both quality of care and quality of life. As this chapter is being written, President Clinton has just called for more funding to support national efforts to deal with the worst offenders in terms of unsafe and inhumane nursing home care. Thus, the outlook seems good for achieving this latter goal.

There is also the hope that these same initiatives may bring QOL into the range of the legally enforceable regulatory system. Potential indicators of the types shown in Tables 7.2 through 7.6 would presumably be successively sharpened in such a way as to be usable as criteria to be rated by the state surveyors as they perform their biennial or more frequent certification rounds. This goal may be somewhat more difficult to achieve. Mere inspection confirms that many of these indicators that seem consensually obvious markers of good or poor quality may still be much more subject to variation among observers than are some of the poor quality of care indicators. Unless QOL indicators can be specified so objectively that inter-rater agreement is easily obtained, the risk of error and the consequent risk to facility administrators, sponsors, and ultimately residents, is higher than desirable. Such unsettling questions may be addressed by ongoing research.

One possible scenario may be that punishing deficits may always be easier than rewarding assets. It may well be that incentives to create higher-than-average quality of life components in residential facilities are better reinforced by market forces than by regulation. Much of the current success of SCUs and of assisted living may be attributed to the recognition by sponsors that many of the amenities represented in the illustrative QOL assessments discussed earlier are highly appealing consumer items. If, as we hope, unutterably bad nursing facilities can be obliterated by the legal monitoring initiatives now in process, consumer choices may well be based on discriminating among the positive quality features.

The negative aspect of this scenario is that such choices are far more available to the economically privileged than to the poor. Thus, social policy efforts aimed at bringing better QOL into residential care generally should use models now established for the affluent to actively guide the design of facilities for the more deprived consumer. Possibly, even those for the poor may evolve eventually into a more consumer-driven course. Also, the threat of demise in a future era where the present boom turns into an oversupply of facilities might be a motivation to court even poor and disenfranchised consumers. In the meantime, a bootstrapping effort to identify the most objectively ratable QOL features and add them to the pool of those already included as survey indicators should add incrementally to the overall effort of improving quality.

CONCLUSION

The central point to be made is that quality of care constitutes one of many aspects of quality of life. Quality of life is the central goal of all programming. Quality of life is measured in terms of minutes of life during which one's affect state may be positive, neutral, or negative. If our focus is on the individual, only that person can tell us (either in words or nonverbally) the quality of a moment or of a longer span of time. If our focus is the quality of life for residents in general, then aspects of the care environment known to be statistically associated with the most favorable balance of positive and negative for the group of people receiving care must be thought of as elements of quality of life.

Alzheimer's disease does not stop all processes by which poor and good qualities are experienced. Although the goal of program and environmental design that meets the idiosyncratic needs of people with dementia is worthwhile, empirical support for differential design is still in short supply. The evidence in favor of high quality being embodied in the SCU is still notably absent. It is suggested that the hundreds of possible program and design variations need to be studied in a way that produces a firm enough body of knowledge that allows the design of an SCU with optimal features. Until that time, good quality of care and of life will be possible in areas designated as SCUs or those not so designated.

REFERENCES

Baltes, M. M., Neumann, E. M., & Zank, S. (1994). Maintenance and rehabilitation of independence in old age: An intervention program for staff. *Psychology and Aging, 9*, 179–188.

Bellelli, G., Frisoni, G. B., Bianchetti, A., Boffelli, S., Guerrini, G. B., Scotuzzi, A. M., Ranieri, P., Ritondale, G., Guglielmi, L., Fusari, A., Raggi, G. C., Gasparotti, A., Gheza, A., Nobili, G. L., & Trabucchi, M. (1998). Special care units for demented patients: A multicenter study. *Gerontologist, 38*, 456–462.

Bradburn, N. (1969). *The structure of psychological well-being.* Chicago: Aldine.

Brod, M., Stewart, A. L., Sands, L., Walton, P. (1999). Conceptualization and measurement of quality of life in dementia: The Dementia Quality of Life Instrument. *Gerontologist, 39*, 25–35.

Burgio, L. D., Scilly, K., Hoar, T., Washington, C., & Tunstall, A. (1993). Behavioral interventions for disruptive vocalizations in elderly nursing home residents with dementia. *Gerontologist, 33* (special issue), 110.

Calkins, M. P. (1988). *Design for dementia: Planning environments for the elderly and the confused.* Owings Mills MD: National Health Publishing.

Cleary, T. A., Clamon, C., Price, M., & Shullaw, G. (1988). A reduced stimulation unit: Effect on patients with Alzheimer's disease and related disorders. *Gerontologist, 28*, 511–514.

Cohen, U., & Day, K. (1993). *Contemporary environments for people with dementia.* Baltimore MD: Johns Hopkins University Press.

Cohen, U., & Weisman, G. (1991). *Holding on to home.* Baltimore MD: Johns Hopkins University Press.

Cohen-Mansfield, J., Marx, M. S., & Rosenthal, A. S. (1989). A description of agitation in a nursing home. *Journal of Gerontology: Medical Sciences, 44*, M77–M84.

Diener, E., & Emmons, R. (1984). The independence of positive and negative affect. *Journal of Personality and Social Psychology, 47*, 1105–1117.

Donabedian, A. (1966). Evaluating the quality of medical care. *Millbank Memorial Fund Quarterly, 44*, 166–206.

Friedman, M., & Brown, E. (1999). Special care units in nursing homes—selected characteristics 1996. Rockville, MD: Agency for Health Care Policy and Research. *MEPS Research Findings* No. 6.

Grant, L. A. (1996). Assessing environments in Alzheimer special care units. *Research on Aging, 18,* 275–291.

Grant, L. A., Kane, R. A., Potthoff, S. J., & Ryden, M. (1996). Staff training and turnover in Alzheimer special care units: Comparisons with nonspecial-care units. *Geriatric Nursing, 17,* 278–282.

Grant, L. A., Kane, R. A., & Stark, A. J. (1995). Beyond labels: Nursing home care for Alzheimer's disease in and out of special care units. *Journal of the American Geriatrics Society, 43,* 569–576.

Grant, L. A., & Potthoff, S. J. (1997). Separating the demented and cognitively intact: Implications for activity programs in nursing homes. *Journal of Mental Health and Aging, 3,* 183–193.

Hall, G. R., & Buckwalter, K. C. (1990). From almshouse to dedicated unit: Care of institutionalized elderly with behavioral problems. *Archives of Psychiatric Nursing, 4,* 3–11.

Holmes, E., Csapo, K. G., & Short, J. A. (1987). Standardization and validation of the Multidimensional Observation Scale for Elderly Subjects (MOSES). *Journal of Gerontology, 42,* 395–405.

Holmes, D., Teresi, J., Ramirez, M., & Goldman, D. (1997). The measurement and comparison of staff source inputs in special dementia care units and in traditional nursing home units using a barcode methodology. *Journal of Mental Health and Aging, 3,* 195–208.

Holmes, D., Teresi, J., Weiner, A., Monaco, C., Ronch, J., & Vickers, R. (1990). Impacts associated with special care units in long-term care facilities. *Gerontologist, 30,* 178–183.

Kane, R. L., Bell, R. M., Reigler, S. Z., Wilson, A., & Keeler, E. (1983). Predicting outcomes of nursing home patients. *Gerontologist, 23,* 200–206.

Kane, R. A., Kane, R. L., & Lawton, M. P. (1998). Measurement, indicators, and improvement of the quality of life in nursing homes. Contract HCFA 98-002PK, Health Care Finance Administration. Baltimore MD.

Lawton, M. P. (1991). A multidimensional view of quality of life in frail elders. In J. E. Birren, J. E. Lubben, J. C. Rowe, & D. E. Dutchman (Eds.), *The concept and measurement of quality of life* (pp. 3–27). New York: Academic Press.

Lawton, M. P., Casten, R., Parmelee, P. A., Wu, H., Van Haitsma, K., & Corn, J. (1996). *Psychometric characteristics of the Minimum Data Set II: Validity.* Philadelphia: Philadelphia Geriatric Center.

Lawton, M. P., Fulcomer, M. C., & Kleban, M. H. (1984). Architecture for the mentally impaired elderly: A post-occupancy evaluation. *Environment and Behavior, 16,* 730–757.

Lawton, M. P., Van Haitsma, K., & Klapper, J. (1996). Observed affect in nursing home residents with Alzheimer's disease. *Journal of Gerontology: Psychological Sciences, 51,* P3–P14.

Lawton, M. P., Van Haitsma, K., Klapper, J., Kleban, M. H., & Katz, I. R. (1998). A stimulation-retreat special care unit for elders with dementing illness. *International Psychogeriatrics, 10,* 379–395.

Lawton, M. P., Van Haitsma, K., Perkinson, M., & Ruckdeschel, K. (1999). Observed affect and quality of life in dementia; Further affirmations and problems. *Journal of Mental Health and Aging, 5,* 69–82.

Lemke, S., & Moos, R. H. (1980). Assessing the institutional policies of sheltered care settings. *Journal of Gerontology, 35,* 96–107.

Lemke, S., & Moos, R. H. (1987). Measuring the social climate of congregate residences for older people. The Sheltered Care Environment Scale. *Psychology and Aging, 2,* 20–29.

Leon, J. (1994). The 1990-1991 National Survey of Special Care Units in nursing homes. *Alzheimer's Disease and Related Disorders, 8*(Suppl. 1), S72–S86.

Leon, J., Cheng, C. K., & Alvarez, R. J. (1997). Trends in special care: Changes in SCU from 1991–1995 ('95/96 TSC). *Journal of Mental Health and Aging, 3,* 149–168.

Leon, J., Potter, D., & Cunningham, P. (1990). *Current and projected availability of special nursing home programs for Alzheimer's disease patients.* DHHS Pub. No. PHS 90–3463. Rockville, MD: Public Health Service.

Liebowitz, B., Lawton, M. P., & Goldman, A. (1979). Designing for confused elderly people: Lessons from the Weiss Institute. *American Institute of Architects Journal, 68,* 59–61.

Logsdon, R. G., Gibbons, L. E., McCurry, S. M., & Teri, L. (1999). Quality of life in Alzheimer's disease: Patient and caregiver reports. *Journal of Mental Health and Aging, 5,* 21–32.

Logsdon, R. G., & Teri, L. (1997). The Pleasant Events Schedule—AD: Psychometric properties and relationship to depression and cognition in Alzheimer's disease patients. *Gerontologist, 37,* 40–45.

Mathew, L., Sloan, P., Kilby, M., & Flood, R. (1988). What's different about a special care unit for dementia patients? *American Journal of Alzheimer's Care and Related Disorders Research, 3,* 16–23.

Mehr, D. R., & Fries, E. B. (1995). Resource use on Alzheimer's special care units. *Gerontologist, 35,* 179–184.

Moos, R. H., & Lemke, S. (1980). Assessing the physical and architectural features of sheltered care settings. *Journal of Gerontology, 35,* 571–583.

Moos, R. H., & Lemke, S. (1996). *Evaluating residential facilities: The Multiphasic Environmental Assessment Procedure.* Thousand Oaks CA: Sage.

Morris, J. N., Hawes, C., Fries, B. E., Phillips, C. D., Mor, V., Katz, S., Murphy, K., Drugovich, M. L., & Friedlob, A. S. (1990). Designing the national resident assessment instrument for nursing homes. *Gerontologist, 30,* 293–302.

Ohta, R. J., & Ohta, B. M. (1988). Special units for Alzheimer's disease patients. *Gerontologist, 28,* 803–808.

Ory, M. G. (1994). Dementia special care: The development of a national research initiative. *Alzheimer Disease and Associated Disorders, 8*(Suppl. 1), S389–S404.

Phillips, C. D., Sloane, P. D., Hawes, C., Koch, G., Han, J., Spry, K., Dunteman, G., & Williams, R. L. (1997). Effects of residence in Alzheimer disease special care units on functional outcomes. *Journal of the American Medical Association, 278,* 1340–1344.

Ramirez, M., Teresi, J. A., Holmes, D., & Fairchild, S. (1998). Ethnic and racial conflict in relation to staff burnout, demoralization, and job satisfaction in SCUs and nonSCUs. *Journal of Mental Health and Aging, 4,* 459–480.

Reisberg, B., Borenstein, J., Franssen, E., Salob, S., Steinberg, G., Schulman, E.,

Ferris, S., & Georgotis, A. (1987). BEHAVE-AD: A clinical rating scale for the assessment of pharmacologically remediable behavioral symptomatology in Alzheimer's disease. In H. Altman (Ed.), *Alzheimer's disease: Problems, prospects, and perspectives* (pp. 1–16). New York: Plenum Press.

Rovner, B. W., Steele, C. K., Shumely, Y., & Folstein, M. (1996). A randomized trial of dementia care in nursing homes. *Journal of the American Geriatrics Society, 44,* 7–13.

Sloane, P. D., Lindeman, D. A., Phillips, C., Moritz, D. J., & Koch, G. (1995). Evaluating Alzheimer's special care units: Reviewing the evidence and identifying potential sources of study bias. *Gerontologist, 35,* 103–111.

Sloane, P. D., & Mathew, L. J. (1990). The Therapeutic Environment Screening Scale. *American Journal of Alzheimer's and Related Disorders Care and Research, 5,* 22–26.

Sloane, P. D., & Mathew, L. J. (Eds.) (1991). *Dementia units in long term care.* Baltimore MD: Johns Hopkins University Press.

Teresi, J., Holmes, D., Ramirez, M., & King, J. (1998). Staffing patterns, staff support, and training in special care and nonspecial care units. *Journal of Mental Health and Aging, 4,* 443–458.

Terra Nova Films (1997). *Recognizing emotion in persons with dementia.* Training videotape. 9848 South Winchester Avenue, Chicago, Illinois 60643.

U.S. Congress Office of Technology Assessment (1992). *Special care units for people with Alzheimer's and other dementias.* OTA—H-543. Washington DC: U.S. Government Printing Office.

Van Haitsma, K., Lawton, M. P., Kleban, M. H., Klapper, J., & Corn, J. (1997). Methodological aspects of the study of streams of behavior in elders with dementing illness. *Alzheimer's Disease and Associated Disorders, 11,* 228–238.

Volicer, L., Collard, A., Hurley, A., Bishop, C., Kern, D., & Karon, S. (1994). Impact of special care unit for patients with advanced Alzheimer's disease on patients' discomfort and cost. *Journal of the American Geriatrics Society, 42,* 597–603.

Watson, D., & Tellegen, A. (1985). Toward a consensual structure of mood. *Psychological Bulletin, 98,* 219–235.

Weisman, J., Lawton, M. P., Sloane, P. S., Calkins, M., & Norris-Baker (1996). The *Professional Environmental Assessment Protocol.* Milwaukee WI: School of Architecture, University of Wisconsin at Milwaukee.

Zarit, S. H., Zarit, J. M., & Rosenberg-Thompson, S. (1990). A special treatment unit for Alzheimer's disease: Medical, behavioral, and environmental features. *Clinical Gerontologist, 9,* 47–64.

Zeisel, J., Hyde, J., & Levkoff, S. (1994). Best practices: An environment-behavior (E-B) model for Alzheimer special care units. *American Journal of Alzheimer's Disease, 9,* 4–21.

Zimmerman, D. R., Karon, S. L., Arling, G., Ryther-Clark, B., Collins, T., Ross, R., & Sainfort, F. (1995). Development and testing and nursing home quality indicators. *Health Care Financing Review, 16,* 107–126.

Zimmerman, S. I., Sloane, P. D., Gruber-Baldini, A., Calkins, M., Leon, J., Magaziner, J., & Hebel, J. R. (1997). The philosophy of special care in Alzheimer's special care units. *Journal of Mental Health and Aging, 3,* 169–181.

Zinn, J. S., Lavizzo-Morey, R., & Taylor, L. (1993). Measuring satisfaction with care in the nursing home setting. The Nursing Home Resident Satisfaction Scale. *Journal of Applied Gerontology, 12,* 452–465.

8

Measuring and Assuring Quality Care in Nursing Homes

Charles D. Phillips

THE COURSE OF THIS DISCUSSION

This chapter will provide the reader with an overview of some of the important issues currently being addressed in efforts to measure and assure quality in nursing homes in this country. The discussion begins with a brief discourse on those characteristics of nursing homes and their residents that make the pursuit of quality in nursing home care a particularly challenging enterprise. Next comes a related discussion of whether quality of care or quality of life is the most general term one can use in thinking about quality in nursing homes. The state's central role in monitoring and enhancing quality in nursing homes is then the topic of interest. The latter part of the chapter is devoted to discussion of a recent innovation in quality monitoring, the introduction of the Health Care Financing Administration's program of using quality indicators, and the search for some way of identifying better quality facilities using such indicators.

DIFFICULTIES IN DISCUSSING NURSING HOME QUALITY

Two fundamental challenges have haunted the analysis and discussion of quality in nursing home care. These derive from the peculiar nature of the institution itself and the characteristics of those served by the institution. A nursing home is a peculiar institution in that it is at once a health care facility and a person's residence. Nursing home residents live with a variety of health and functional challenges, the care for which must be a part of their everyday lives. But, unlike those receiving medical or nursing care in other settings, nursing home residents are not "patients." They are residents, or more appropriately, they are members of a community, with all the needs, desires, and strengths that status implies. A full evaluation of quality of care in nursing homes must deal with both of these realities. Such an evaluation must look at the quality of health care that residents receive and determine the degree to which residents function as members of a community, rather than simply as the "objects of care."

This characterization of nursing homes is not meant to imply that other health care providers, such as physicians or hospitals, are absolved from any responsibility for dealing with their "patients" as something other than a compilation of conditions. Instead, it constitutes recognition of the special challenges inherent in the provision of long-term care in an institutional setting. Nursing home residents are, unlike short-stay hospital patients and individuals receiving out-patient medical care, for their remaining life-course enmeshed in a setting that can operate as a "total institution," enveloping and invading the entire fabric of their lives (Goffman, 1961).

The second difficulty encountered in discussions of quality in nursing homes is rooted both in the diversity and in the nature of the individuals whom these institutions serve. As Robert Kane (1998) indicates, the modern nursing home serves at least five distinct subgroups of individuals, each of which has different care needs. These include:

- Residents recovering from an acute episode and likely to return to the community;
- Residents who are terminally ill;
- Residents with chronic problems in physical health who are cognitively intact;
- Residents with significant cognitive impairment; and
- Residents in permanent vegetative states.

Shorter-stay residents' basic needs revolve around their presenting conditions and the implementation of a rehabilitative regimen that gives them the greatest likelihood of a return to their pre-morbid status. Pain management, development of advance directives, and family involvement are crucial issues in caring for the terminally ill. Monitoring and management of chronic conditions and altering the trajectory of decline due to these conditions are important for all longer stay residents. Issues of personal control, independence, and autonomy are also major concerns for longer stay residents. Maintenance of function and dignity are crucial to care for those with cognitive impairment. For those residents in a persistent vegetative state, adherence to advance directives and special attention to the sequela of immobility are important. Even this abbreviated recitation of the most obvious differences among residents makes clear the diversity of the issues that arise in nursing home care and rest under the rubric of "quality."

RELATIONSHIP BETWEEN QUALITY OF CARE AND QUALITY OF LIFE

Talking about quality of service in the special environment of the nursing home thus becomes a difficult endeavor. The multidimensionality of the nursing home's mission and the diversity of the population receiving care has led some observers over the years to assume an interesting stance on defining quality. Their perspective is similar to that of U.S. Supreme Court Justice Potter Stewart who admitted the great difficulty in developing a meaningful definition of pornography, while remaining clear in his belief that "I know it when I see it." Such a stance concerning nursing homes correctly acknowledges the inherent complexity of thinking about and measuring quality in this setting. Unfortunately, the "I know it when I see it or smell it" school of measurement also constitutes a complete "dead-end" for those interested in improving, assuring, or even discussing quality.

However, many of the difficulties faced in thinking about quality in nursing homes become somewhat more manageable when one makes the distinction between "quality of care" and "quality of life" in nursing homes. One important advantage of this distinction is that it brings into clearer focus the dual role of nursing home as health care facility and personal residence. But, this distinction raises an initial issue that deserves attention.

Arguably, there is some ambiguity about the relationship between quality of life and quality of care. One may wish to argue that quality of care is simply a subset of quality of life issues, a subset that focuses on health care–related concerns. Conversely, one can consider quality of life a special subset of quality of care, one focusing on residents' psychosocial well-being. This issue is not trivial. In fact, the way in which it is resolved serves as the foundation for how one thinks about, measures, evaluates, assures, and regulates quality in nursing home care.

The key to the resolution of this issue is best found by reflecting on the nature of the setting under consideration and our aspirations for individuals in that setting. It is life in all its fullness that transpires in nursing homes, whether for short-stay or longer-stay residents. To think of the range of human interactions that do and should occur in nursing homes as simply "care," devalues both the actions of those identified as caregivers and strips those who would be seen as simply care recipients of much of their individuality and humanity. The most useful characterization of what goes on in a nursing home is simply "life." Caring is part of that life, an important part, but it is not the whole of it. Thus, in the nursing home, issues related to quality of care are most appropriately seen as a subset of quality of life concerns.

THE STATE'S ROLE IN MEASURING, ASSURING, AND ENHANCING QUALITY

But, whether it is quality of life or the more limited issue of quality of care that is of concern, much of the responsibility for assuring and enhancing quality in long-term care lies with governmental regulatory bodies. In few areas of health does one find the government so pervasive in its involvement in supporting the delivery of services and in its responsibility for the quality of services as one sees in nursing home care.

A variety of factors have brought this set of circumstances into existence. First, the government is the major payor for nursing home care. Of the $82.8 billion expended in 1997 on nursing home care, just over 62% of that sum derived from public sources of funds (Braden et al., 1998). As the major purchasers of nursing home services, the U.S. Health Care Financing Administration and the Medicaid agencies in each state are the major "consumers" of nursing home care in this country. As such they assume major responsibility for assuring the quality of the product for which they are paying.

Second, the majority of nursing home residents are members of vulnerable populations. Over 63% of nursing home residents are Medicaid recipients and constitute a vulnerable population because of their economic status. Almost 90% of residents are elderly, and a majority must deal with a variety of chronic health problems, which include high rates of cognitive impairment (Krauss & Altman, 1998). Thus, most nursing home residents have a series of disadvantages that make them members of one or more vulnerable populations. As such, governmental agencies have a special responsibility to protect the interests of these populations (President's Advisory Commission, 1998).

Third, the nursing home industry itself has, until recently, eschewed any responsibility for quality assurance or improvement in nursing homes. The modern nursing home industry has its roots in the explosion of for-profit corporate involvement in nursing home care resulting from the influx of public monies into the industry due to the implementation of the Medicaid and Medicare in the mid-1960s. These early health care entrepreneurs often saw nursing homes as little more than lucrative real estate ventures. The results of this approach generated sufficient bad press to create a climate ripe for some remedy, while the industry itself showed little interest in the process of professionalization that might have served as a surrogate for state regulatory action (Hawes & Phillips, 1986; Kane, 1998).

Each of the three factors noted above would, in isolation, justify strong governmental involvement in monitoring the nursing home industry. Given the presence of all three factors in one setting—large amounts of public funds, the presence of a vulnerable population, and the abdication of responsibility by providers, the entry of the state into the regulation of nursing homes was unavoidable and its continued presence is inevitable.

GOVERNMENTAL EFFORTS TO ENHANCE QUALITY

The early regulatory focus in nursing homes was little different from that in other service areas with which states were more familiar. At first rules focused very heavily on such issues as adherence to building codes, food preparation and storage, staff licensure requirements, and fire safety regulations. These regulations were later elaborated to include a number of elements of the process of care provided. Minimum standards were set by federal agencies; annual inspections were carried out by state agencies; citations for deficiencies could be issued for failure to meet those standards.

However, passage of the Nursing Home Reform Act as part of the Omnibus Budget Reconciliation Act of 1987 altered the entire regulatory scheme for nursing homes by redefining the standards, the process for determining compliance with the standards, and the enforcement system charged with monitoring and assuring compliance (Hawes, 1998). The new standards required that facilities provide care that would result in each resident achieving the "maximum practicable" level of functioning. They also included recognition of issues such as residents' psychosocial well-being and residents' rights. The inspection process was also changed. As Catherine Hawes (1998) notes: "The new inspection procedures . . . focused on process and outcome quality, incorporating interviews with residents, families, and ombudsmen about their daily experiences in the homes and requiring direct observation of residents and the care they were receiving" (Hawes, 1998, p. 6). Finally, a wider range of enforcement remedies, including civil monetary penalties, were also developed, though their use varied dramatically both across and within states (Rudder & Phillips, 1998).

THE FOCUS ON QUALITY OF CARE
RATHER THAN QUALITY OF LIFE

Unfortunately, nursing homes are arguably unique in the degree to which quality of life is an issue. Instead, quality of care has historically been, and remains, the primary focus of state-sponsored quality assurance and quality measurement in long-term care (Cella, Gabay, Teitelbaum, Walker, & Kramer, 1996). The recent changes in the enforcement process and recent HCFA initiatives have appropriately placed greater importance on quality of life issues. However, the quality of care focus has not been supplanted for a number of reasons.

First, nursing homes are still seen by many regulatory bodies as health care institutions, and this perception is reinforced by a wide range of serious problems in the provision of basic health services that persist in these settings. A recent Government Accounting Office study (1998) of a sample of residents who died in California found that more than half had received unacceptable care, including failure to properly treat pressure ulcers and provide attention to dramatic weight loss. Another study of 14 facilities in 11 states reported inadequate treatment in important health-related areas for residents in one-third of the facilities (Johnson & Kramer, 1998). Other studies of larger groups of facilities report continued problems in such fundamental areas of care as nutrition and pain management (Bernabei et al., 1998; Blaum, Fries, & Fiatarone, 1995; Hawes, 1998). Given these continuing problems in the provision of good health care in the industry and the resource constraints faced by state regulatory agencies, a real incentive exists for agencies to devote their energies to more health-related issues, rather than quality of life.

Second, the measurement of quality of life is a difficult enterprise. As Powell Lawton notes, one of the appeals of the term, quality of life, may be "its ability to mean anything to anybody—it is only an illusion that consensus [on the meaning of quality of life] exists" (Lawton, 1997, p. 45). Though some level of confusion and ambiguity does exist, the views of residents themselves tend to imply that quality of life is built around a number of quite broad dimensions. Residents have, in personal interviews (Cella et al., 1996), identified these dimensions as:

- Dignity—maintenance of independence and a positive self-image
- Privacy—adequacy of space and others' respect for personal space
- Interactions with staff—the quality and quantity of both personal and professional interactions
- Nursing facility—facility décor and physical features
- Nursing home operations—quantity and quality of staffing and services for residents
- Relationships—ongoing relationships with family/friends, other residents, and staff.

As one would hope, these dimensions do seem to capture in an almost exhaustive fashion those things that might fall under the rubric, "quality of life." However, they may constitute something of a measurement nightmare. Each dimension can be divided into an almost infinite set of specific indicators, which may or may not exhibit meaningful correlations. We lack valid, reliable, and administratively feasible measures of many of the aspects of quality of life, and we surely lack the means to aggregate some set of indicators into an overall measure of quality of life for a single individual, much less an entire facility.

In addition, many of the individuals in nursing homes, due to health conditions or problems in cognitive function, cannot be interviewed concerning their quality of life. Through direct, in-depth observation by trained observers some insight can be gained into some aspect of quality of life for these residents (Cella et al., 1996). But, how one creates a meaningful process that could be part of some state monitoring effort is a difficult issue. The idea that one can simply ask "interviewable" residents about such issues and that they can serve as "surrogate" respondents (Kane, 1998) seems more in the realm of wishful thinking than in the realm of possibility. Trained observers have, for example, noted distinct differences in the way that facility staff interact with "interviewable" and "noninterviewable" residents (Cella et al., 1996).

These factors have combined to make quality of life issues secondary to quality of care in the monitoring processes carried out under state authority. In the survey process,

- the traditional pre-eminence of issues around physical health and well-being,
- the continued problems with quality of care,
- the difficulty of measuring quality of life, as well as
- the unfamiliarity of such issues to those staff currently involved in state surveys push an appropriate focus on quality of life for nursing home residents well into the future.

QUALITY OF CARE AND HCFA'S QUALITY INDICATORS (QIS)

While the full integration of quality of life into the regulatory process has not occurred, innovation within that process has not stopped. A major innovation in the assessment and measurement of quality of care in nursing homes has grown out of the OBRA '87 reforms. One aspect of The Nursing Home Reform Act was the requirement that a uniform multidimensional assessment be performed periodically for all nursing home residents (Hawes et al., 1995; Hawes et al., 1997; Morris et al., 1990). This assessment tool, the Minimum Data Set (MDS), has been used by HCFA to develop a series of quality indicators that the developers believe can, ". . . provide a foundation for both external and internal QA and quality-improvement activities [in nursing facilities]" (Zimmerman et al., 1995).

The QIs are based on individual-level MDS data aggregated to the facility-level. The QIs include a number of prevalence and incidence measures covering 12 areas of resident status:

- accidents,
- behavioral and emotional problems,
- clinical management,
- cognitive patterns,
- elimination and continence,
- infection control,
- nutrition and eating,
- physical functioning,
- psychotropic drug use,
- quality of life,
- sensory function and communication, and
- skin care.

Some of the measures under these more general categories deal with the process of care, while others focus on resident outcomes. Some of the indicators are prevalence measures, and others measure the incidence of some event. These indicators are to be used by the states in the nursing home inspection or survey process. The QIs will be used to identify areas of concern in a facility (e.g., psychotropic drug use). They may also be used to identify specific residents who might be included in the sample of residents (e.g., individuals with significant weight loss), whose care will be more intensively reviewed by the surveyors (Zimmerman et al., 1995).

One wants differences on the QIs to reflect differences solely in the patterns of care in facilities, not differences in the characteristics of their residents. For example, there are a variety of resident characteristics outside the control of the facility that affect a resident's likelihood of developing a pressure ulcer (Berlowitz et al., 1996). So, the most useful quality indicator will be "case-mix adjusted" to reduce the possibility that differences among facilities derive from differing resident populations than from differing skin care (Zimmerman et al., 1995). The adjustment strategy chosen for HCFA's QIs was the development of risk groups with separate QIs for each group. For example, individuals with difficulty in transferring, impaired bed mobility, diabetes, desensitized skin, and a variety of other conditions are much more likely, in any facility, to develop a pressure ulcer. So, these individuals constitute a "high-risk" group, for whom a separate pressure ulcer prevalence rate is calculated. All other residents are considered "low-risk," and they have their own prevalence rate for pressure ulcers (Arling, Karon, Sainfort, Zimmerman, & Ross, 1997). As important as case-mix adjustment is recognized to be (Mukamel, 1997; Porell & Caro, 1998), only a few of the HCFA QIs are now risk-adjusted.

States and vendors use various combinations of the QIs in feedback reports to providers and as part of their oversight of facilities involved in the Medicare and Medicaid programs. These reports are usually developed on a quarterly basis. A common format used in these reports appears in Table 8.1. Regulators and facilities are provided information on:

- the number of individuals in the facility with a specific condition (the number in the numerator),
- the total number of individuals who could have presented with or developed that condition (i.e., the number in the denominator),
- the facility prevalence or incidence rate (i.e., numerator divided by the denominator), the prevalence or incidence rate for some comparison group (e.g., usually all other facilities in the state), and
- how the rate for the facility compares with that for the comparison group (e.g., usually a percentile ranking).

In our illustration in Table 8.1, the 15 out of 100 residents (15%) fell in this facility, while the average across all facilities in the state for the same period was 20%. This places the facility in the 25th percentile, meaning that 75% of the facilities in the state had higher fall rates and 24% of the facilities had lower fall rates. Table 8.1 also presents an illustration of the reporting format using one of the risk-adjusted QIs, pressure ulcer prevalence. As the illustration indicates, the reported information for the risk-adjusted indicators duplicates that for the other QIs. The only difference is that with the risk-adjusted QIs, separate rates are calculated for the different risk-groups for both the individual facility and the comparison group or state.

An example of the indicators included in one set of feedback reports appears in Table 8.2. The report provides feedback to facilities on 24 QIs in 11 different care domains or areas. The information in Table 8.2 also provides an indication of whether the indicator is case-mix or risk adjusted. Such QI data will be used, according to the developers, to

> . . . identify facilities that may have more serious or particular types of care problems, on the basis of a comparison with their peers" and ". . . [within facilities] identify particular areas of care that might warrant a more in-depth review during the survey or other type of visit" (Zimmerman et al., 1995, p. 117).

TABLE 8.1   Reporting Format for Quality Indicators

Quality indicator	Numerator	Denominator	Facility rate	Comparison group rate	Percentile ranking
Prevalence of falls	15	100	15%	20%	25
Prevalence of falls					
• High risk	8	80	10%	20%	20
• Low risk	1	20	5%	10%	10

As one can see, the QIs cover a range of important areas of resident care. Some domains are, of course, covered better than others. Attention to the two indicators under the Quality of Life domain provides ample evidence that it is not through the MDS and the QIs, at least in their current forms, that quality of life in its broadest sense will enter meaningfully into state regulatory activities.

QIS AND THE SEARCH FOR FACILITIES PROVIDING BETTER QUALITY OF CARE

Ideally, one would have some interval metric for measuring the quality of care in a facility. In reality, probably the best that one can do at this point is create ordinal schema that places facilities into some gross classification schema that identifies better, average, and worse facilities. Much of the history of the regulation is a recitation of the attempt to identify "bad" facilities. Ignored until recently was the search for "good" facilities (Zimmerman, 1998). However, this search is an important complement to the attempt to rid the industry of its worst element. It is the operations in these better facilities that can serve as "best practice" models for the industry as a whole. One can also argue that it is the effect of reimbursement changes and levels on these good facilities that may provide us with the most useful information about the adequacy of reimbursement and the effects of restructuring reimbursement methods.

One of the current issues surrounding the use of the QIs is whether they can, in fact, identify higher quality facilities. Recent research has shown that the QIs are relatively stable over relatively short (e.g., 3–6 months) periods of time (Karon, Sainfort, & Zimmerman, 1999). This finding gives one some confidence in the QI's ability to capture information that represents the dynamics of facility operation in specific areas, rather

TABLE 8.2 QIs Used by Ohio Department of Health

Domains/quality indicators	Risk-adjusted
Accidents	
1. Incidence of new fractures	No
2. Prevalence of falls	No
Behavior/emotional patterns	
3. Prevalence of behavioral symptoms affecting others	Yes
4. Prevalence of symptoms of depression	No
5. Prevalence of symptoms of depression without antidepressant therapy	No
Clinical management	
6. Use of 8 or more different medications	No
Cognitive patterns	
7. Incidence of cognitive impairment	No
Elimination/incontinence	
8. Prevalence of bladder or bowel incontinence	Yes
9. Prevalence of occasional or frequent bladder or bowel incontinence without a toileting plan	No
10. Prevalence of indwelling catheter	No
11. Prevalence of fecal impaction	No
Infection control	
12. Prevalence of urinary tract infections	No
Nutrition/eating	
13. Prevalence of weight loss	No
14. Prevalence of tube feeding	No
15. Prevalence of dehydration	No
Physical functioning	
16. Prevalence of bedfast residents	No
17. Incidence of decline in late loss ADLs	No
18. Incidence of decline in ROM	No
Psychotropic drug use	
19. Prevalence of antipsychotic use, in the absence of psychotic or related conditions	Yes
20. Prevalence of antianxiety/hypnotic use	No
21. Prevalence of hypnotic use more than 2 times in last week	No
Quality of life	
22. Prevalence of daily physical restraints	No
23. Prevalence of little or no activity	No
Skin care	
24. Prevalence of stage 1–4 pressure ulcers	Yes

than "random" perturbations in resident outcomes and care. However, these results neither tell one about how much of "universe of quality" that the QIs capture nor do they tell one about the interrelationships among the QIs.

Some investigations using a factor analytic approach have had some measure of success in creating some aggregations of the QIs based on their interrelationships. In analyses attempting to use the QIs to investigate the Structure-Process-Outcome model in nursing homes (Sainfort, Ramsay, & Monato, 1995), QI data from 142 nursing facilities were factor analyzed (Ramsay, Sainfort, & Zimmerman, 1995). The research team couldn't extract a meaningful single factor to summarize the QI results. Instead, they divided the measures into four categories: risk-adjusted process measures, non-risk-adjusted process measures, risk-adjusted outcome measures, non-risk-adjusted outcome measures. Separate analyses were performed within each category of indicators. The results were then based on the risk-adjusted process QIs and the non-risk-adjusted outcome QIs. The reported factor analyses identified four process quality factors and three outcome factors. However, the bulk of the factors derived in these analyses could lay little claim to conceptual cohesiveness or clarity. For example, a diagnosis of diabetes and no foot care program loaded well on the Poor Preventive/Restorative Care Practices factor, while visual impairment and no corrective action loaded equally well on the Poor Care Planning factor. Conceptually, these indicators could have fit under either category, but "correlationally" they truly appeared to be different. And, in the end, the hypothesized relationships between these factors and a set of structural quality indicators for the same facilities were disconfirmed (Ramsay et al., 1995).

The inability to develop useful aggregations of the QIs is somewhat puzzling, since all of the QIs have relatively strong face validity as measures of nursing home quality (Zimmerman et al., 1995). Thus, one feels that the QIs should exhibit considerable coherence and that one should be able to use them in some aggregated form to identify general differences in quality among facilities. This belief has at its base the assumption that one is applying something like classical test theory to the case of nursing home quality and the QIs (Bollen & Lennox, 1991). Such a model implies the relationship that appears in Figure 8.1. In such a model, the intercorrelations among and internal consistency of the indicators (i.e., QIs) will be high. All the indicators are being "moved" in concert by the changes in the latent construct "nursing home quality." Bollen and Lennox (1991) identify such a model as an "effect indicator measurement model" and the indicators themselves as "effect indicators."

In reality, with nursing home quality and the QIs one probably has something much more analogous to Bollen and Lennox's (1991) "causal

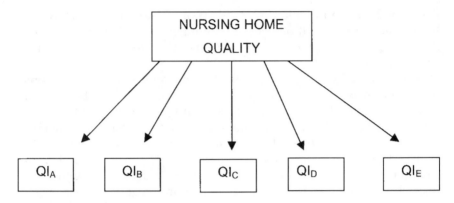

FIGURE 8.1   Classical measurement model and nursing home quality indicators.

indicator measurement model." This model appears in Figure 8.2. In the causal indicator model, the individual indicators can independently influence the latent construct. Quality may go up or down as the result of the movement of a limited number of the total universe of indicators. This also means that the intercorrelations among indicators can be high or low, positive or negative.

Table 8.3 illustrates the types of correlations one finds among the QIs constructed from facilities operating in Cleveland, Ohio in late 1997. Obviously, this illustration includes only two of the indicators, but one would see little difference if they were replaced with other QIs. And, these results probably differ significantly from those obtained by Ramsay et al. (1995).

In our illustration, the prevalence of falls was correlated with 24 other QIs. Seven of the 24 correlation coefficients were negative. Eight of the coefficients were positive and greater than .10. The average correlation between the prevalence of falls and other indicators is .06. One sees little difference with the prevalence of urinary tract infections (UTIs). The average correlation between UTI prevalence and the other indicators is .09. However, only one of the correlations is negative, and seven of the 23 correlations was positive and greater than .10. As Table 8.3 indicates, the correlation between the two chosen indicators themselves is .15.

These are not the types of correlations one hopes for when using an effect indicator measurement model. However, such correlations are perfectly reasonable under a causal indicator measurement model. When each of the indicators themselves has good face validity, low correlations such as those in Table 8.3 are likely to mean that the latent construct is multidimensional and that the various indicators are tapping different dimensions of the construct.

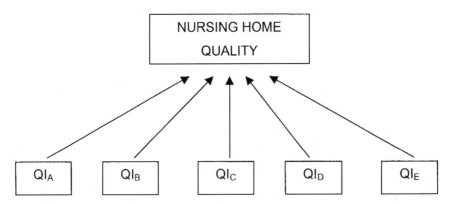

FIGURE 8.2 A causal model of measurement and nursing quality indicators.

However, identifying a measurement model as a causal indicator model is not, as Bollen and Lennox (1991, p.312) indicate, just a "handy excuse for low internal consistency." Instead, the use of a causal indicator measurement model takes one from addressing issues of internal consistency to issues of wrestling with potentially more difficult issues of validity. One must, when dealing with causal indicators, seek validation for any aggregation of indicators in terms of their predictive validity. When the linear combination of the indicators moves, does it push other variables farther along in some causal chain?

For example, one might develop some construct from the QIs and test its correlation with resident satisfaction, family satisfaction, state survey results, ombudsmen reports, or expert assessments. Rantz and her colleagues did that with 14 nursing homes in Missouri. Using an algorithm based on a facility's percentile rankings across 14 QIs, they identified both good and poor facilities. They then did site visits to these facilities. The survey deficiency data and the observers' evaluations of the facilities matched relatively well with the classification of the 14 facilities based on the QIs (Rantz et al., 1997). Such validation is exactly what is required when one uses a causal indicator model of measurement.

Other validation efforts have not provided such promising results. The author and his colleagues used 32 of HCFA's QIs in an attempt to identify higher quality facilities in Cleveland, Ohio. First, the research team identified a subset of all Cleveland facilities that had lower than expected per diem costs (Phillips & Rose, 1999). Within this subset of facilities, the research team used three linear combinations of different sets of QIs (e.g., one with all 32 indicators, another with 13 QIs, and another with 11 QIs) in its attempts to identify higher quality facilities. We found 14 "higher" quality facilities were identified based on their scoring on these aggregates,

TABLE 8.3   Correlations Among Selected QIs—Ohio, 1997

Domains/quality indicators	Prevalence of falls	Prevalence of urinary tract infection
Behavior/emotional patterns		
Prevalence of symptoms of depression	.17	.14
Prevalence of symptoms of depression without antidepressant therapy	.11	.10
Clinical management		
Use of eight or more different medications	.04	.19
Cognitive patterns		
Incidence of cognitive impairment	.19	.08
Elimination/incontinence		
Prevalence of bladder or bowel incontinence		
• high risk	−.02	−.02
• low risk	.17	.07
Prevalence of occasional or frequent bladder or bowel incontinence without a toileting plan	−.07	.03
Prevalence of indwelling catheter		
• high risk	−.06	.13
• low risk	.07	.19
Prevalence of fecal impaction	.06	.13
Infection control		
Prevalence of urinary tract infections	.15	—
Nutrition/eating		
Prevalence of weight loss	.19	.09
Prevalence of tube feeding	−.12	.18
Prevalence of dehydration	.06	.18
Physical functioning		
Prevalence of bedfast residents	−.10	.10
Incidence of decline in late loss ADLs		
• high risk	.14	.00
• low risk	.15	.08
Psychotropic drug use		
Prevalence of antipsychotic use, in the absence of psychotic or related conditions		
• high risk	.06	.00
• low risk	−.06	.05
Prevalence of antianxiety/hypnotic use		
Prevalence of hypnotic use more than 2 times in last week	.05	.04

TABLE 8.3   Correlations Among Selected QIs—Ohio, 1997 *(Continued)*

	Correlations	
Domains/quality indicators	Prevalence of falls	Prevalence of urinary tract infection
Quality of life		
Prevalence of daily physical restraints	−.004	.04
Prevalence of little or no activity	.04	.04
Skin Care		
Prevalence of stage 1–4 pressure ulcers		
• high risk	.08	.15
• low risk	.09	.05

as were 14 facilities with "poorer" quality. These classifications were then compared with a scale based on survey deficiencies and resident advocate ratings of these 28 facilities. Disappointingly, while there was a moderate positive correlation between the survey-based indicator and the advocates' ratings, the classifications based on the QIs displayed small negative correlations with both the advocate and survey-based measures.

These disparate results raise the important issue of how well survey and advocate rankings can serve as a "gold" standard to which any QI-based measure of nursing home quality is compared. Probably a better set of measures would derive from an in-depth on-site observation protocol that evaluated residents' quality of care and life in the facility. This is the model used by Rantz et al. (1997). However, there is no widely agreed on nursing home quality measurement tool based on observation. In addition, this validation strategy is also quite costly to implement.

Faced with these circumstances, in our search for better facilities in Cleveland, the authors chose only those facilities that scored well on any one of the QI aggregations, and on the survey-based measure, and in the resident advocate ratings as higher quality facilities. In essence, if one sees each of these different measures of quality (i.e., QI-based, survey-based, advocate-based) as presenting one with a set of good facilities, we chose the intersection of those three sets as our criterion for identifying better quality facilities in the Cleveland area. Instead of 14 higher quality facilities among the lower cost facilities, eight of these facilities were classified as higher quality.

Given current circumstances, it may be that searching for the intersection of information from multiple sources offers the best currently available resolution to the issue of how one identifies better facilities and better care. In epidemiological terms, this approach focuses on minimizing false positives. One used multiple approaches because of a lack of faith in the "fidelity and bandwidth" provided by any single set of indicators or signals (Bollen & Lennox, 1991).

CONCLUSION

The preceding discussion has moved through relatively abstract discussions of quality of life and quality of care in nursing homes to very focused discussions of HCFA's QIs and how one might use them to identify higher quality facilities. As broad as this span may be, it exposes the reader to the range of issues at the forefront of quality measurement and quality assurance in nursing homes today.

Choosing a measurement strategy and the specific items that will capture well the quality of life in a facility are major challenges. Previous research has given us some reasonable sense of the components of quality of life. Taking that sense and turning it into an operational system of quality measurement and assurance is, however, a challenge that will be an important part of state and federal efforts to improve their monitoring of nursing homes.

Moving the quality assurance process away from simply identifying the worst facilities in operation toward an approach also focusing on identifying the best facilities is currently underway. The use of HCFA's QIs is an early indication of movement in that direction, or at the least, it is an indication that a structure may exist for that movement. But, as the earlier discussion of HCFA's QIs indicates, this task will also be difficult to accomplish. We currently lack the type of "gold standard" against which one would hope to validate that combination of indicators that will lead us to the better facilities. At present, all that we may be able to do is use a combination of more or less flawed sets of indicators to triangulate on and identify better facilities.

As daunting as these issues may seem, we are, in fact, at a very promising point in the evolution of quality measurement and assurance in nursing homes. The Nursing Home Reform Act of 1987 laid a strong foundation for progress with its demand for implementation of a uniform database for all nursing homes and all residents. The changes in emphasis in the survey process and the elevation of resident rights and quality of life to important aspects of the survey process are major steps in the right direction. However, the degree to which these developments become meaningful parts of the quality assurance process, which is driven by public policy, will remain a political issue.

One must have good tools and the "will" to implement and evaluate those tools. The current era is one in which there has been considerable effort by the industry to "throw off the yoke of regulation" (Edelman, 1998; Hawes, 1998; Latimer, 1998). At the same time, the industry itself has shown little real enthusiasm, though it has paid some lip service to, developing a meaningful process of internal monitoring and self-improvement. Discussions within the industry are abuzz with terms like Total Quality Management (TQM), Continuous Quality Improvement (CQI), and customer service. However, as Kane (1998) points out, in nursing homes too often the implementation of Continuous Quality Improvement models means addressing those problems easiest to resolve, while the implementation of a "customer service" focus simply means defining residents' families as the "customer" to be served. Thus, it will in the end be the responsibility of public entities responsible for monitoring nursing home quality and reimbursing them for care to develop the needed tools and to summon up the will to put those tools to good use.

REFERENCES

Arling, G., Karon, S. L., Sainfort, F., Zimmerman, D. R., & Ross, R. (1997). Risk adjustment for nursing home quality indicators. *Gerontologist, 37*(6) 757–766.

Berlowitz D. R., Ash, A. S., Brandeis, G. H., Brand, H. K., Halpern, J. L., & Moskowitz, M. A. (1996). Rating long-term care facilities of pressure ulcer development: Importance of case-mix adjustment. *Annals of Internal Medicine, 124*(6), 557–563.

Bernabei, R., Gambassi, G., Lapane, K., Landi, F., Gatsonis, C., Dunlop, R., Lipsitz, L., Steel, K., & Mor, V. for the SAGE Study Group (1998). Management of pain in elderly patients with cancer. *Journal of the American Medical Association, 279*(23), 1877–1882.

Blaum, C. S., Fries, B. E., & Fiatarone, M. A. (1995). Factors associated with low body mass index and weight loss in nursing home residents. *Journal of Gerontology: Biological Sciences and Medical Sciences, 50A*(3), M162–M168.

Bollen, K., & Lennox, R. (1991). Conventional wisdom on measurement: A structural equation perspective. *Psychological Bulletin, 110*(2), 305–314.

Braden, B. R., Cowan, C. A., Lazenby, H. C., Martin, A. B., McDonnell, P. A., Sensenig, A. L., Stiller, J. M., Whittle, L. S., Donham, C. S., Long, A. M., & Stewart, M. W. (1998). National health expenditures, 1997. *Health Care Financing Review, 20,* 83–127.

Cella, M., Gabay, M., Teitelbaum, M., Walker, A., & Kramer, A. (1996). *Evaluation of the long-term care survey process: Final report.* Cambridge, MA: Abt Associates.

Edelman, T. S. (1998). The politics of long-term care at the federal level and implications for quality. *Generations, 21*(4), 37–41.

Goffman, E. (1961). *Asylum: Essays on the social situation of mental patients and other inmates.* Garden City, NY: Doubleday Anchor.

Hawes, C. (1998). Regulation and the politics of long-term care. *Generations, 21*(4), 5–9.

Hawes, C., Morris, J. N., Phillips, C. D., Fries, B., Murphy, K., & Mor, V. (1997). Development of the nursing home resident assessment instrument in the USA. *Age and Ageing, 26*(2), 19–26.

Hawes, C., Morris, J., Phillips, C. D., Mor, V., Fries, B., & Nonemaker, S. (1995). Reliability estimates for the Minimum Data Set for nursing facility resident assessment and care screening (MDS). *Gerontologist, 35*(2), 172–178.

Hawes, C., & Phillips, C. (1986). The changing structure of the nursing home industry and its impact on cost, quality, and access. In B. Gray (Ed.), *For-profit enterprise in health care* (pp. 492–542). Washington, DC: National Academy Press.

Johnson, M. F., & Kramer, A. (1998). Quality of care problems persist in nursing homes despite improvements since the nursing home reform act. Paper prepared for the Institute of Medicine Committee on Quality in Long-Term Care. Denver, CO: University of Colorado Health Sciences Center.

Kane, R. L. (1998). Assuring quality in nursing home care. *Journal of the American Geriatrics Society, 46,* 232–237.

Karon, S. L., Sainfort, F., & Zimmerman, D. R. (1999). Stability of nursing home quality indicators over time. *Medical Care, 37*(6), 570–579.

Krauss, N. A., & Altman, B. M. (1998). Characteristics of nursing home residents - 1996. Rockville (MD): Agency for Health Care Policy and Research. *MEPS Research Findings No. 5.* AHCPR Pub. No. 99–0006.

Latimer, J. (1998). The essential role of regulation to assure quality in long-term care. *Generations, 21*(4), 10–14.

Lawton, M. P. (1997). Measures of quality of life and subjective well-being. *Generations, 21*(1), 45–47.

Morris, J., Hawes, C., Fries, B., Phillips, C. D., Mor, V., Katz, S., Murphy, K., & Drugovich, M. (1990). Designing the national resident assessment instrument for nursing homes. *Gerontologist, 30*(3), 293–307.

Mukamel, D. (1997). Risk-adjusted outcome measures and quality of care in nursing homes. *Medical Care, 35,* 367–385.

Phillips, C. D., & Rose, M. (1999, July). *Cost and quality in nursing home care in Cleveland: Interim report.* Cleveland: Myers Research Institute.

Porell, F., & Caro, F. G. (1998). Facility-level outcome performance measures for nursing homes. *Gerontologist, 38*(6), 665–683.

President's Advisory Commission on Consumer Protection and Quality in the Health Care Industry (1998). *Quality first: Better health care for all Americans.* Washington, DC: U.S. Government Printing Office.

Ramsay, J. D., Sainfort, F., & Zimmerman, D. (1995). An empirical test of the structure, process, and outcome quality paradigm using resident-based, nursing facility assessment data. *American Journal of Medical Quality; 10*(2), 63–75.

Rantz, M. J., Popejoy, L., Mehr, D. R., Zwygart-Stauffacher, M., Hicks, L. L., Grando, V., Conn, V. S., Porter, R., Scott, J., & Maas, M. (1997). Verifying nursing home care quality using Minimum Data Set quality indicators and other quality measures. *Journal of Nursing Care Quality, 12*(20), 54–62.

Rudder, C., & Phillips, C. D. (1998). Citations and sanctions in the nursing home enforcement system in New York state: Their use and effects. *Generations,* 21(4), 41–44.

Sainfort, F., Ramsay, J. D., & Monato, H. (1995). Conceptual and methodological sources of variation in the measurement of nursing facility quality: An evaluation of 24 models and an empirical study. *Medical Care Research and Review,* 52(1), 60–87.

Zimmerman, D. R. (1998). The power of information: Using resident assessment data to assure and improve the quality of nursing home care. *Generations,* 21(4), 52–56.

Zimmerman, D. R., Karon, S. L., Arling, G., Clark, B. R., Collins, T., Ross, R., & Sainfort, F. (1995). Development and testing of nursing home quality indicators. *Health Care Financing Review,* 16(4), 107–127.

PART III

Design and Delivery of Long-Term Care

9

The Pioneer Challenge: A Radical Change in the Culture of Nursing Homes

Wendy Lustbader

*I*magine this—you live in a nursing home. You wake up when you feel like it. You summon help to get out of bed when you're ready to face the day. You wheel yourself a few yards down the hall to a family-style kitchen for some freshly poached eggs, your favorite breakfast. You sit at a normal kitchen table with a few of your neighbors, and then take your coffee mug back to your room with the morning newspaper. After some quiet time with your coffee and newspaper, you let your assistant know that you will soon be needing her help getting dressed. You know each other well, because she is with you almost every day. You glance at the events calendar, but decide that you would rather stay put the rest of the morning after you stop in at the community meeting. Your assistant promises to remind the afternoon staff that later you'll need help getting over to the child care center, as today is your day to read stories to the children. Right before dinner, you'll have a glass of wine with a friend who visits from another floor and with whom you've had this daily ritual for the past year. At night, you're likely to get caught up in a novel and read past midnight, glad that you'll be able to sleep in the next day if that happens.

Spontaneity. Self-direction. Relationships. Community. Privacy. Meaning. Why do these qualities not describe a typical nursing home in America? Why must we forfeit the basic freedoms of life when we become frail and need assistance? Instead, the acute care model has been dominant in nursing homes for decades. This model is essentially a control model; for example, the providers of care do what they see fit to ensure residents' health and safety. Instead of addressing the meaning of the lives of those who become frail, we have narrowly limited our society's resources to address only the physical concerns of residents. We have centered our efforts on quality of care, largely to the exclusion of quality of life.

In places where care is provided on a short-term basis, taking control over someone's life may make some sense. Acute conditions require intensive management, and doctors and nurses possess specialized knowledge that people need in critical situations. Under these circumstances, we surrender a certain degree of our right to self-determination in the hope of getting better and returning to our lives in the community. The error was to transfer this model of care to a setting where it is not necessary and where people then experience a fundamental and ongoing loss of control over their lives.

Enacting a radical change in nursing homes means challenging the very attitudes and social structures which have made these institutions the places they are. In October of 1995, the National Citizens Coalition for Nursing Home Reform (NCCNHR) convened a panel of people already engaged in pioneering efforts to change the control-oriented culture of nursing homes: Barry and Debora Barkan of Live Oak Living Center, El Sobrante, California; Charlene Boyd of Providence Mount St. Vincent, Seattle, Washington; Joanne Rader of Benedictine Institute for Long Term Care, Mt. Angel, Oregon; and Judy and Bill Thomas, M.D. of the Eden Alternative Foundation, Sherburne, New York. Carter Catlett Williams, a social worker who was a leader in the national effort to bring about restraint-free care in nursing homes, chaired the panel. These pioneers discovered they had much in common and expressed a wish for further dialogue. In March of 1997, they gathered in Rochester, New York along with 28 other invited participants from the fields of regulation and law, nursing home administration (administrators, directors of nursing, and social workers), as well as advocates. As ideas were exchanged and approaches were compared, an exciting convergence of values and principles emerged. A movement was conceived, and what was to become the Pioneer Network was initiated (Lustbader, 2000a; Williams, 1997).

The Pioneer Network serves as a focal point for designing and implementing diverse approaches that hold to a common set of values and principles. Pioneers demonstrate respect for residents and staff by beginning decision making with the person in need of care; seeking to respond to spirit as well as mind and body needs; seeking to enjoy residents and staff as unique individuals; acting on the belief that as staff are treated so will residents be treated; putting the person before the task; accepting risk-taking as a normal part of adult life; acting on the belief that each person can and should make a difference (Fagan, Williams, & Burger, 1997).

This chapter first presents the key elements of culture change proposed by the Pioneers. Then, the current shortage of nursing assistants is examined from the perspective of the working conditions they must endure in traditional nursing homes. The last section explores why change is so difficult, and details specific strategies to support a life of quality for older people in need of care.

KEY ELEMENTS OF CHANGE

Every nursing home has an existing culture, expressed in its traditions, style of leadership, social networks, patterns of interaction, relations with the outer community, degree of connectedness to the natural world, use of language, and ways in which the community celebrates and mourns. The word "culture" holds within it many dimensions of life and thereby conveys the all-encompassing depth of change being proposed. Pioneers believe that the culture of traditional nursing homes must be replaced by a new culture which vitally alters the way of life for residents and staff (Fagan et al., 1997).

The following elements of change are concrete expressions of the values and principles of culture change as defined by the Pioneer Network. There can be no single recipe or set of prescriptive practices which will succeed at all facilities, but these elements, when employed on all three levels depicted here, have been found to promote the well-being of both staff and residents as nursing homes move into the process of change.

Returning the Locus of Control to Residents

Residents retain fundamental control over their lives when they determine their own daily schedules, enjoy choices about eating, select among varied options for keeping clean, and are assisted with maintaining continence as long as possible. Accomplishing this shift back to ordinary self-determination is easiest when staff decision making is placed as close to residents as possible. Other remaining capacities for self-care and mobility can then be supported as the need for assistance arises, rather than in accordance with pre-set orders. Spontaneity and flexibility are thereby returned to both residents and those who assist them.

Assist Residents in Determining Their Own Daily Schedules

In a nursing home where everyone wakes of his or her own accord, staff must be able to decide how they are going to meet the preferences of each person. Nursing assistants must be fully empowered to work out each resident's preferred daily routine and to respond to their spontaneous wishes. They must be affirmed when they respect residents' independent actions and are careful not to intrude in any way. Those who exhibit special sensitivity to residents' needs must be appreciated and supported, rather than penalized by a task-oriented system that puts institutional schedules before individuals' needs (Williams, 1990, 1998).

Restore Choices About Eating

Eating is a complex biological, social, cultural, behavioral, and symbolic act. The food we eat and when, where, and how much we eat are decisions based on individual choices and lifetime habits. Many residents have multiple physical, sensory, and cognitive impairments that make eating difficult, such as having problems getting the food from plate to mouth (Kayser-Jones, 1996). Nursing homes which restore the basic freedoms and pleasures of eating, along with providing individualized assistance, have found that residents eat with more gusto, waste less food, and express greater satisfaction with their lives as a whole. Food carts can be transported up to each unit or neighborhood's kitchen where residents dine family-style. Residents can then decide on the quantity of their own servings from platters, and are at liberty other times of day to get a snack from the refrigerator (Boyd, 1994; Rimer, 1998).

Provide Options for Keeping Clean

In the traditional nursing home, staff determine the times and methods of bathing. These methods are often experienced by the resident as an assault, even a sexual assault. In their own homes, people have the right to set their own standards for cleanliness, and to choose how to keep clean. In nursing homes, we tend to think of bathing options as limited to two: a sitting shower or a bath. This thinking is very much a product of our own time and culture, and it does not reflect the broad range of methods that people historically have used to keep clean. Other methods of bathing which may be more familiar to people are showering standing up or taking a sponge bath at the sink. These methods must become acceptable options in nursing homes. People who are fearful, frail, or low in endurance might be better served by a towel bath in bed (Rader, Lavelle, Hoeffer, & McKensie, 1996). Additionally, after a skillful approach has been made and it is clear that a resident is not in the proper mood for a bath, nursing assistants need to be assured that supervisors and co-workers will not view their acceding to the refusal as an attempt to get out of work (J. Rader, personal communication, January 5, 2000).

Support Continence As Long As Possible

It may take more time to offer help with toileting than to have someone wear incontinence pads, but the person may achieve continence as a result of such prompting. Prior to changes mandated by the Nursing Home Reform Act, treatments for incontinence were estimated at $3.26 billion annually (National Citizens' Coalition for Nursing Home Reform, 1995). When residents are assisted in maintaining continence, there is a lowered incidence of skin breakdown and reduced use of urinary catheters. This is one of many instances where poor care costs more over the long run than good care. Beyond the significant cost savings, the benefit in self-esteem and dignity from retaining such capacity may be immeasurable.

Promote All Remaining Capacities for Self-Care and Mobility

Encouraging someone to participate in getting dressed often takes more time than simply putting the person's clothes on. But when nursing assistants elicit such participation, even from someone with severe dementia, the person becomes calmer and often ends up needing little help besides encouragement (Rogers et al., 1999). Similarly, it may take more time to assist someone with walking to the dining room than to wheel the person over in a wheelchair, but excess disability is reduced and the person retains control over basic areas of life as long as possible.

Enhancing Front-Line Staff's Capacity to be Responsive

By flattening a facility's administrative structure, independent teams or neighborhoods can be created that truly empower residents and those who assist them. When nursing assistants are consistently assigned to the same small group of residents, they get to know these individuals well and can contribute what they learn to the team. Involving nursing assistants in care planning and care conferences flows naturally from recognizing this knowledge. Enabling nursing assistants to set their own schedules and to be actively involved in team development gives them further control over their daily lives, which in turn enhances their capacity to ensure that residents remain decision makers in their own care.

Eliminate Middle Layers of Management

Like other complex organizations, most nursing homes are hobbled by interdepartmental tension and conflicts between layers of management. A fruitful alternative to hierarchical departments is a network of unit-based teams serving groupings no larger than 15 to 20 residents. These independent teams manage their own budgets and evolve solutions to care dilemmas particular to the circumstances and preferences of those who live and work in their small community. Facility-wide, standardized procedures are replaced by team-centered, individualized responses.

Commit to Consistent Assignment

With continuity of assignment, residents and staff can get to know each other. Their understanding of each other gradually builds. Individual preferences are learned. Friendly greetings are exchanged. Residents start looking forward to seeing certain staff, and these workers begin to sense that their presence is becoming especially important to some. After a day off, they know that these people are waiting for them and welcoming their return to work. Warmth develops, and care is given and received with greater ease. This consistency also enables nursing assistants to trust one another enough to spell each other when patience or stamina flags. Greater emphasis throughout is on relationships, rather than tasks (Williams, 1999).

Involve Nursing Assistants in Care Planning and Care Conferences

Nursing assistants quickly gain personal knowledge of the residents they assist on a daily basis. Care plans should be informed by what nursing assistants learn firsthand about residents' needs and preferences, including sufficient detail to ensure that the plan is fully individualized, realistic, and comprehensive. On an ongoing basis, nursing assistants must have their own voices as resident advocates and always be an integral part of care conferences. Providing a means by which nursing assistants can share information across shifts, such as an informal logbook, helps those on day shift present a more complete picture of residents' needs at care conferences.

Enable Nursing Assistants to Set Their Own Schedules

When front-line workers have more control over their work, they respond with an increasingly vibrant and durable commitment to providing the best possible care. They come to understand which staffing patterns are necessary and begin to consult with one another to ensure that each team will have an anchor person to guide intermittent workers who come to the unit. The skills of independence gradually accumulate, as do the habits of trust and cooperation. Managing their own schedules is not only an example of autonomy for nursing assistants, but it becomes a vote of confidence repaid many times over and gives them the same experience of self-direction they are providing to residents (Thomas, 1994, 1999).

Support Team Development

When nursing assistants understand their role as part of a team, they take that responsibility seriously. They realize that their judgment and input has value, because they do not have to climb a ladder to be heard. When a nursing assistant tells her team that a particular resident is not doing well, she knows they all share the responsibility and all have the power to make life better for that person (Boyd, 1994; Thomas, 1994).

Establishing a Homelike Environment

Implementing cross training for all staff levels helps establish a welcoming environment throughout the facility. Including family members in decision making and promoting a sense of community keeps connections growing among family members, staff, and residents. Creating a human habitat instills a feeling of being at home in a place of vibrance, as does re-designing traditional structures to make them less institutional. Developing pro-active relationships with surveyors gives facilities room to experiment with other strategies for giving the environment a homelike feel.

Implement Cross Training for All Staff Levels

Cross-trained, highly capable staff are essential for supporting residents' independence and exercise of choice. In particular, the needs of people with dementia become much easier to meet when all staff are seen as capable of helping out and have been trained in ways to respond with sensitivity and flexibility. With this philosophy, any staff member encountering the person with dementia is ready to render assistance, if needed (Rader, Doan, & Schwab, 1985). Similarly, all staff should be required to get food handler's permits to put them in compliance with state and federal regulations when they want to help a resident make a snack, such as a sandwich or a slice of toast to go with an afternoon cup of tea (Boyd, 1994). Housekeeping staff should be cross-trained as nursing assistants so they can assist with toileting and bathing when residents prefer such help, rather than according to an institutional schedule.

Include Family Members in Decision Making

Inviting family members into the decision-making process is especially important when risks must be taken to promote their relative's autonomy and freedom of expression. In the name of safety, many family members insist that their loved one be restrained, unaware that this subjects the person to the unseen and cumulative dangers of becoming immobilized. The very cautions intended for protection end up causing harm. Family members often need help viewing the situation through the eyes of their relative, rather than through their own fear, guilt, and anxiety. Once they feel fully informed, most family members become willing to take calculated risks in the interest of improving their relative's quality of life. Others need to be reminded that life cannot be made risk-free and that their relative's well-being may be more important than perceived safety (Rader, 1991).

Promote a Sense of Community

The need for community must be recognized. Members of a community define themselves in relationship to one another. It is difficult to have a meaningful role in a socio-cultural vacuum. The life of the community itself provides a structure for belonging, a collective voice, and a place for individuals, on whatever level is appropriate, to tell their personal stories. Through daily gatherings, a community celebrates life. New members are welcomed, teachings are shared, the events of the world are discussed, and the passing of friends is mourned. Questions of life, death, meaning, and philosophy can be discussed. Residents and family members have a forum to talk about what is happening to them and to each other. They address problems within their community. Sometimes they reach solutions, or it may be enough that they have had the opportunity to be heard (Barkan, 1981, 1999).

Create a Human Habitat

A nursing home is a human habitat. As such, it must be inspired by the natural habitats that surround and nurture us all. Dogs, cats, birds, plants, children, and gardens accessible to everyone can transform a sterile monoculture into a human habitat worthy of a home. In addition to being maintained, this new diversity must be connected directly to residents' needs for companionship, for the opportunity to care, and for variety and spontaneity in their surroundings (Thomas, 1994, 1999). We must develop environments where individual differences gain expression, rather than resorting to homogenized activities which result in a one-size-fits-all social environment (Kane, 1996). We must also make nursing homes more permeable to the community at large, bringing the outside world in and creating living linkages to other domains. A child care center located on the premises, theater groups holding open rehearsals, and gardens jointly maintained with outside volunteers are examples of this kind of active connection.

Redesign Traditional Structures

Traditional nursing homes afford little privacy with their double rooms, insufficient personal storage space, and lack of accessible locked spaces where treasured possessions can be secured. Private communication with the outside world may be difficult to obtain, particularly if the person needs assistance making a phone call, writing a letter, or getting to a telephone where she will not be overheard (Kane et al., 1997). Architectural renovation can allow for both privacy and community. Instead of long hallways and a closed-off nursing station, individual resident rooms can be grouped around a common area. A homelike kitchen and living area can be open to the nursing station, making it an integrated whole (Contemporary Long Term Care, 1997). Ideally, the entire building becomes the person's home. For instance, residents who happen to be visiting elsewhere at mealtime do not have to return to their units but can be welcomed to stay so long as their needs can be met (C. Boyd, personal communication, January 20, 2000). Even facilities that are unable to undertake major renovation can establish homelike features in selected areas, make adaptations, and institute practices which create a feeling of being at home.

Develop Pro-Active Relationships with Surveyors

The survey process is experienced as such a threat by many nursing homes that they devote considerable energy to eliminating as much risk as possible (Freeman, 1990). Often this translates into depriving residents of choice and spontaneity for the sake of "safety." A middle ground must be found, even though this takes more time than following rote procedures. What might be seen as neglect or a violation of rules may actually result from a provider's respect for autonomy. In striving to reduce or eliminate restraint use, for example, more falls and minor injuries may occur, but serious injuries are reduced. Performing a mobility/fall risk assessment and sharing the outcome with the resident, family, and staff is important. Communicating the steps that need to be taken to improve each resident's margin of safety is also necessary (Donius, 1999). Surveyors can then be invited to review these assessments and interventions, rather than simply counting the number of falls and seeing this as a measure of a facility's proficiency. Enhanced surveyor training, along with such collaborative discussions, alters the local regulatory climate. Facilities engaged in culture change then feel secure enough to improve their problem-solving methods in the direction of greater resident autonomy (Kane, Freeman, Caplan, Aroskar, & Urv-Wong, 1990).

These elements of change are connected by the primary principle: returning the locus of control to residents. It follows that those who spend the most time with residents, nursing assistants, must be given the capacity either to carry out residents' wishes directly or to convey these wishes to those who do have the power to respond. No longer are the needs of the institution to come before the needs of the individual. But turning this overarching principle into actual practice runs squarely into the reality of human limitations. If nursing assistants have too many people needing their help, they will not be able to respect individual preferences as to the timing and manner of their assistance. They will be rushing from one room to another, seeing people in terms of the tasks their bodies impose. No matter what top management declares about the quality of care offered in a particular facility, kindness and respect do not flourish when there is little time for human engagement (Lustbader, 1991; Lustbader, 2000b). The next section shows why culture change in nursing homes hinges upon the working conditions faced by nursing assistants.

WORKING CONDITIONS FACED
BY NURSING ASSISTANTS

Nursing homes have become a microcosm of social and economic problems in America. Frail elders living there often feel powerless, and bemoan an existence devoid of meaning. The staff who have the greatest impact on their lives, nursing assistants, receive low pay, insufficient training, and minimal respect for the vital work they do. To change nursing homes into places where no one is demeaned will require a radical societal shift both in how frail elders are viewed and how those who do direct care are paid, trained, and respected.

We now have over 2 million nursing assistants. It is estimated that another half million will be needed in the next 2 years, and that this need will increase geometrically as the baby boom generation reaches old age. Presently, staff shortages are being reported in many parts of the country, with facilities claiming that they can barely meet even the most minimal staffing standards. Annual staff turnover rates nationally approach 100% and represent a major cost in the running of such facilities.

At nursing homes where cost-efficiency is the overriding goal, front-line workers are viewed as unskilled and replaceable. The supervisory focus is on getting them to work as quickly as possible, not on ensuring that they meet residents' personal preferences in a kind and decent manner. Levels of stress among workers are high, and this leads to workers fending for themselves rather than working cooperatively. Those who become emotionally attached to certain residents often try to conceal their feelings amidst an ethos which puts efficiency first. Nursing assistants are not given information to assist them in making important judgments, and their input in care decisions is not solicited. High turnover, low commitment, and low quality of care are the results of this approach (Eaton, 1998).

Increasing the wages and benefits paid to nursing assistants is crucial, but we must also transform the ways that nursing assistants are oriented and trained, and how they are supervised over the long run. Nursing homes have, by and large, inherited a style of management practice that is excessively regimented and prescriptive. A rigid, hierarchical command-and-control management structure does not promote the kinds of bonds between people that lead to good care (Unsino, 1998). Many of the challenges in this work are made easier through good communication in well-established relationships, but conventional nursing homes generally do not promote such working environments (Diamond, 1992).

Typically, new staff are talked at and lectured to during long days of orientation. They are inundated by a steady stream of tasks, to all of the mandated subjects and to "the way we do things here." Instructors tend to offer little warmth in what must be a daunting first few weeks on the job. Relationships are scarcely mentioned. No reference is made to workers' own background, ideas, and values which will have great bearing on how well this experience will go and how workers will integrate what they are taught with what they already know (Unsino, 1998).

After orientation, nursing assistants are often assigned to a unit which is understaffed. Evening or night shift can be especially isolating and difficult. Nursing assistants may not have a supervisor who possesses interpersonal skills or is experienced in long-term care. Even skillful, experienced supervisors may be excessively burdened by the demands of being the only nurse for as many as 40 people and coping with the high acuity of many residents, along with daunting paperwork. Staff on such units may not function well, or at all, as a team. New nursing assistants often quit after a few such experiences, feeling too overwhelmed and unsupported to continue through the first month on the job (Unsino, 1998).

One of the most damaging aspects of traditional service delivery is the view that staff should separate their feelings from the work. If the environment is to be caring, staff must be able to care, rather than being held in frozen compliance to institutional prerogatives. If it is assumed that residents are still learning and growing, then such regeneration must be assumed of those who work in nursing homes (Barkan, 1981). Nursing assistants should be encouraged to seek true engagement with the people who count on them in utterly personal ways, but they must also be given the same regard we hope they will bestow on others (Unsino, 1998).

Currently, the transmission of knowledge in nursing homes is organized from the top down. The hierarchical structure of the environment conveys little respect to those at the bottom. There are few opportunities for nursing assistants to exchange what they know with each other or to pass on to superiors what they have learned from experience and their own cultural background. Many have extensive knowledge about the healing arts, with a sure sense of what works for people and what does not. They have devised ways to motivate people to get out of bed, and many understand how to offer solace when the people in their care endure loss. They know what goes on during all hours of the day while someone is involved in the process of dying (Barkan, 1981).

Finally, American tendencies toward class separation and racism are often echoed in nursing homes. In many cities, the majority of nursing assistants are people of color still caught in the cycle of poverty, while the residents are overwhelmingly European Americans who have been more or less advantaged economically and socially. The compassion and caring that nursing assistants ought to offer all residents is sometimes strained by reactive anger at injustices long endured. Similarly, it is not unusual for nursing assistants to experience racially oriented verbal abuse from white nursing home residents whose inhibitions have frayed with age and dementia (Johnson, 1999).

Addressing these dilemmas is critical if staff shortages are to be resolved and if best practices are to be supported. The next section suggests approaches that help reduce many of the problems that currently cause nursing assistants to leave their jobs, and that can improve the working environment for all nursing home staff.

STRATEGIES FOR CHANGING THE CULTURE OF NURSING HOMES

Culture change cannot be declared by administrative fiat. What has been common to all nursing homes that have made strides toward the new culture is the understanding that such transformation happens gradually. Ways to overcome some of the deepest sources of resistance and the most challenging obstacles to change are suggested in the following discussion.

Communicating a Clearly Defined Alternative to the Status Quo

A vision of a better future must be revealed in words and deeds over and over again. Staff who have invested decades in the traditional culture may find it especially difficult to acknowledge that "the way things are done here" has not promoted a good life for residents, despite generous intentions. Culture change seeks to overturn the very circumstances which led to these mistaken approaches, but staff often need to hear portrayals of the vision from many angles before it begins to take hold (Thomas, 1994, 1999).

Recognize that the Process of Change Is Often Painful

A sense of urgency must be tempered by a sense of why people are so reluctant to surrender routines that have made their world a predictable, understandable place. Staff who have been immersed for years in the control model need time to recognize that they have been carrying out arbitrary practices which are not grounded in fostering quality of life for residents and quality of work life for staff. One nursing home administrator experienced considerable pain as she confronted over 30 years of having maintained strict control over both residents and staff. As she slowly let go of these old routines and replaced them with approaches that emphasized resident and staff autonomy, she celebrated the many benefits, but had to face regret at not having instituted such changes earlier (Brecanier, 1998).

Beware of Superficial Changes that Conceal Underlying Problems

One of the seductions in this process is to make superficial changes and then to rest assured that one's nursing home has been transformed. Birds may be chirping in residents' rooms, but do the nursing assistants feel they have a voice in the care plans of the people they assist? Is enthusiastic lip service being given to respecting those who provide direct care, while their training and supervision is still regimented? Are relationships still secondary to the completion of tasks? Many nursing home administrators claim to heed their front-line staff, while at least some of their nurse supervisors continue to impose the control model's ethos of silent obedience (Thomas, 1999).

Ensure that Change Agents Practice What They Preach

Some nursing homes have begun the change process by initiating a culture change committee comprised of representatives from each department. Others have opened the committee to all interested parties. No matter how it is comprised, the committee itself must model the kind of honest and respectful ethos the group hopes to establish. It is not enough to preach the values of culture change; these values must be lived at all levels of the institution.

Encouraging Frank Dialogue

Negative reactions must be welcomed as a sign that real grappling has begun. As long as the process is approached with integrity, there is no need to play a defensive game and to suppress those who wish to take issue with the changes being enacted. Frank dialogue is a healthy and essential aspect of transformation of this magnitude (Barkan, 1981).

Keep Negativity Out in the Open

Making it safe for doubts and anxieties to be expressed keeps negativity out in the open, rather than driving it underground. An anonymous survey can be circulated that allows staff to voice their concerns without fear of displeasing their supervisors. Sorting out which objections have validity and which merely express the fear of change often requires considerable listening and debate. Substantive concerns can be heard and integrated, without losing forward momentum (Thomas, 1999).

Help Each Individual Cultivate a Heightened Awareness

Culture change is a step-by-step, incremental process which requires a commitment to self-examination. The process is more inward than outward, because the culture to be changed resides within each person. Making it safe for staff to help each other discover the vestiges of the control model in their own work becomes a central aspect of the process. Habitual practices tend to keep resurfacing. Over time, many subtle but pervasive institutional assumptions will be identified and brought into question. Front-line staff, all disciplines, and all levels must be involved in this process of confronting the minutia of institutional practice which negatively impact on the quality of residents' daily lives (Unsino, 1998).

Supporting Staff in Developing New Models of Supervision

Staff at all levels need support as they engage in ongoing dialogue and self-examination, but nurses and nursing assistants tend to bear the greatest weight of change. The process of developing new models of supervision can be an area of particular impatience and strain as some staff move further ahead on the path of culture change than others. Conflict can be reduced by actively recognizing and affirming the risks individuals take as they try out ideas that are initially uncomfortable for them.

Encourage Nurse Supervisors to Create New Approaches

Collaborative models of supervision may go against years of practicing within a hierarchical model. Such new methods may also conflict with a nurse's basic professional training. Developing supervisory techniques which nurture rather than intimidate nursing assistants often requires considerable brainstorming with fellow nurses. Those who supervise these nurses must also be careful not to subject them to arbitrary, rule-bound control, or these nurses may reflexively pass on the tyranny to nursing assistants in order to protect themselves from possible censure. As nursing assistants are treated, so will be the residents who depend on them.

Identify and Examine Scope-of-Practice Issues

Scope-of-practice issues may be particularly vexing as nurses simultaneously try to extend front-line staff's capacity to respond to residents in a flexible manner and prevent them from making dangerous errors. Care delegation that is both prudent and informed differs greatly from dumping tasks on nursing assistants due to time pressures and other exigencies. For example, having professional staff on hand at mealtimes to assist those residents with the most complex problems and to serve as role models for nursing assistants is often critical, yet often gets cast aside due to other demands on nurses' time (Kayser-Jones & Schell, 1997).

Create a Forum for Discussing Practice Dilemmas

Nurses should be encouraged to identify areas where nursing assistants need more support, and not censured when their recommendations are perceived as a potential strain on the facility's budget. An open forum for airing these dilemmas raises staff morale as well as residents' level of safety, even if budget realities lead to interim improvements that are still less than ideal. Making the situation better than it was before should be affirmed, while keeping the vision of the path ahead clear and well-defined.

Establish Ongoing Team Development

Mentoring programs for new nursing assistants are especially helpful during their first few months on the job. A small group of experienced people serve as a resource to strengthen new staff and help them surmount difficulties. Problems can then be resolved directly and solutions instituted without delay. The seasoned mentor also identifies systemic problems which may be contributing to poor performance. Weekly meetings promoting a free exchange of ideas become an arena where the best possible quality of life is promoted for each resident. New staff remain excited about both contributing and learning. Unlike classroom-based "in-service training" which offers fixed products of information to be passively memorized and followed, this process encourages active problem-solving and creativity (Unsino, 1998).

Institute Practices to Reduce Staff Turnover

Finding ways to inspire nursing assistants to stay on the job may have to take priority over all other changes. One nursing home chain is experimenting with nursing assistant career paths in which higher pay is tied to work performance, longevity on the job, and the willingness to acquire new knowledge and skills. The career paths offer front-line workers a means of personal and professional growth within their work life as a nursing assistant, rather than having to leave this work in order to advance their status. Holding a title signifying one's advanced knowledge and carrying out responsibilities commensurate with this achievement leads to deep satisfaction on the job (Misiorski, 1999).

Communicating a clearly defined vision, encouraging frank dialogue, and supporting staff through the process of developing new supervisory models often requires several years of determined effort. The Pioneer Network aims to support change agents by putting them in touch with each other and fostering an exchange of best practices and ideas. Nationwide dialogue of this nature may supply external momentum and accelerate the process, especially for facilities just getting started or still mired in resistance.

CONCLUSION

Restoring basic freedoms to those who live in nursing homes improves the morale of both the giver and receiver of care. Front-line workers become advocates for those they assist, rather than emissaries of oppressive schedules. Ensuring that residents themselves decide when to wake up, when to eat, which food to put on their plates, how they wash, and what they do each day begins to undo the control model and makes room for dignity to prevail. Sometimes residents resist the changes designed to restore their self-efficacy. People long institutionalized cannot instantly drop the passive mindset that served them in the traditional nursing home. Participation in worthwhile roles, such as the hiring of new staff, may reawaken previous confidence. A few key successes in expressing their preferences and feeling heard may begin to inspire assertiveness in relating to staff. Once people experience autonomy in one aspect of their lives, they tend to seek it in other contexts, but the shift may be gradual and need considerable encouragement (Williams, 1998).

Enacting the changes proposed by the Pioneer Network requires that major systemic change be underway at all levels of the institution. There must be an overall shift to flexibility—away from expecting the resident to make all the accommodation. One family-style meal a day, while an agreeable thing to do, does not represent the underlying change in attitude that creates a life-affirming environment. Nor will a new decorating job by professionals do it, or several of the latest therapies—aroma, horticultural, rocking-chair, or light therapies. None touch the greatest meaning in residents' lives: relationship. The depth of changes that must take place is profound if people who live in nursing homes are to thrive to the fullest extent possible (Williams, 1998).

Those who fear that culture change will lead to chaos or that quality of care and quality of life will be compromised find that the opposite occurs. Units are transformed into communities where residents and staff know each other and matter to each other. The joy of discovering better responses to residents' needs helps to create a humane environment in which staff feel energized to be fully contributory and engaged (Unsino, 1999). Nursing assistants flourish when they no longer feel stifled by narrowly prescribed task sequences. They enjoy a spirit of teamwork, which flows from co-workers being familiar with each other's strengths and feeling united in caring for people they know well.

Persons with dementia become more fully known by neighboring residents and staff, resulting in their calmer and happier embrace by others. A feeling of belonging arises as they are continually greeted and recognized. Being part of a community becomes a felt, rather than occasionally remembered, reality. An open, central common area gives them a place to be with others without a need to know why they are there, just that it seems right to be there. The status of personhood is bestowed on them by others in a context rich in relationships (Kitwood, 1997).

Emphasizing and supporting relationships requires a careful rearrangement of facility budgets toward the goal of improving the wages for nursing assistants and lowering the number of residents each must serve. Finding ways to ensure that increased funding is actually used for direct care is essential. The National Citizens Coalition for Nursing Home Reform has found that some owners increase their profits by making cuts in housekeeping, laundry, or dietary staff, leaving nursing staff to cope with additional duties without additional help (Burger, Fraser, Hunt, & Frank, 1996). Increasing reimbursement to facilities in accordance with their direct-care staffing levels may be the best way to ensure that enough hands-on caregivers are available.

Forming local partnerships among the major stakeholders in long-term care—residents, families, resident advocates, staff, and surveyors—has enabled some facilities to realize both the spirit and the letter of The Nursing Home Reform Act (OBRA 1987). The present system strives for good outcomes, encouraging facilities to achieve more than just paper compliance. Further exploration is needed to produce a valid measurement tool that identifies the best facilities through intensive on-site observation. In the meantime, such facilities benefit greatly from such stakeholder partnerships which enable them to try new approaches toward both quality of care and quality of life.

Human beings are capable of surviving and flourishing despite difficult circumstances—when their lives have meaning. Those who can find no reason to fight for their continued existence are easy prey for diseases of the body and mind. This is especially true for frail older people. In the traditional nursing home, reasons to live are usually confined to the residual contacts with family and community, or simply a deeply ingrained life force. Loneliness, helplessness, and boredom prevail (Thomas, 1994). Daily life tends toward cultural and spiritual sterility. Because the current model has evolved from acute care, the greatest emphasis is on pathology (Barkan, 1981). Human beings need an emphasis on health and continued growth of mind and spirit.

The transmission of a new nursing home culture is beginning. The vision is clear. One day every nursing home will be an open, diverse, caring community, providing those who live there individualized care based on their choices and personal control, unlimited opportunities for growth in spirit, mind, and body, and continued involvement with family, friends, and the outside world.

REFERENCES

Barkan, B. (1981). The Live Oak Regenerative Community: Reconnecting culture within the long term care environment. *Aging Magazine, 2*(7), 321–322.

Barkan, B. (1999, March). *Pioneering efforts in the nursing home reform movement.* Presented at the annual meeting, American Society on Aging, Orlando, FL.

Boyd, C. (1994, September). Residents first: A long-term care facility introduces a social model that puts residents in control. *Health Progress,* The Catholic Health Association of the United States.

Brecanier, P. (1998, January). Views presented at the Pioneer Network Retreat, Seattle, Washington.

Burger, S. G., Fraser, V., Hunt, S., & Frank, B. (1996). *Nursing homes: Getting good care there.* San Luis Obispo, CA: American Source Books/Impact Publishers, Inc.

Contemporary Long Term Care (1997, August). Providence Mount St. Vincent, Seattle, Washington; Renovation, Architecture and Interior Design Award Winner, 46–47.

Diamond, T. (1992). *Making gray gold: Narratives of nursing home care.* Chicago: The University of Chicago Press.

Donius, M. (1999). Unpublished fall prevention program instituted at Benedictine Nursing Center, Mt. Angel, Oregon.

Eaton, S. (1998, August). *Beyond unloving care: Linking work organization and patient care quality in nursing homes.* Presented at the Academy of Management Annual Meeting, San Diego, CA.

Fagan, R. M., Williams, C. C, & Burger, S. G. (1997, October). *Meeting of Pioneers in nursing home culture change: Final report.* Lifespan of Greater Rochester.

Freeman, I. (1990). Developing systems that promote autonomy: Policy considerations. In R. Kane & A. Caplan, (Eds.), *Everyday ethics: Resolving dilemmas in nursing home life.* New York: Springer Publishing Company.

Johnson, T. J. (1999, May). Subtle, hidden woes of nurse's aides. *Democrat and Chronicle,* Rochester, NY.

Kane, R. A. (1996). Transforming care institutions for the frail elderly: Out of one shall be many. *Generations, 19*(4), Winter.

Kane, R. A., Caplan, A. L., Urv-Wong, E. K., Freeman, I., Aroskar, M. A., & Finch, M. (1997). Everyday matters in the lives of nursing home residents: Wish for and perception of choice and control. *Journal of the American Geriatrics Society, 45,* 1086–1093.

Kane, R., Freeman, I., Caplan, A., Aroskar, M., & Urv-Wong, E. K. (1990). Everyday autonomy in nursing homes. *Generations,* Supplement.

Kayser-Jones, J. (1996). Mealtime in nursing homes: The importance of individualized care. *Journal of Gerontological Nursing, 22*(3), 26–31.

Kayser-Jones, J., & Schell, E. (1997). The effect of staffing on the quality of care at mealtime. *Nursing Outlook, 45*(2), 64–72.

Kitwood, T. (1997). *Dementia reconsidered: The person comes first.* Buckingham, UK: Open University Press.

Lustbader, W. (1991). *Counting on kindness: The dilemmas of dependency.* New York: Free Press/Simon and Schuster.

Lustbader, W. (2000a). The pioneer challenge: Changing the culture of nursing homes. *Aging Today, American Society on Aging, 20*(8), March/April.

Lustbader, W. (2000b). Thoughts on the meaning of frailty. *Generations, 23*(4), Winter.

Misiorski, S. (1999, July). *CNA Career Paths*. Presented at the conference Quality of Care in Nursing Homes: The Critical Role of the Nursing Assistant, American Society on Aging, Philadelphia, PA.

National Citizens' Coalition for Nursing Home Reform (1995). *The high cost of poor care*, unpublished fact sheet, September.

Rader, J. (1991). Modifying the environment to decrease use of restraints. *Journal of Gerontological Nursing, 17*(2), 9–12.

Rader, J., Doan, J., & Schwab, M. (1985). How to decrease wandering, a form of agenda behavior. *Geriatric Nursing*, July/August.

Rader, J., Lavelle, M., Hoeffer, B., & McKensie, D. (1996). Maintaining cleanliness: An individualized approach. *Journal of Gerontological Nursing, 22*(3), 32–38.

Rimer, S. (1998). Seattle's elderly find a home for living, not dying. *The New York Times*, November 22.

Rogers, J. C., Holm, M. B., Burgio, L. D., Granieri, E., Hsu, C., Hardin, J. M., & McDowell, B. J. (1999). Improving morning care routines of nursing home residents with dementia. *Journal of the American Geriatrics Society, 47*(9), 1049–1057.

Thomas, W. (1994). *The Eden Alternative: Nature, hope and nursing homes*. University of Missouri.

Thomas, W. (1999). *The Eden Alternative handbook: The art of building human habitats*. Summer Hill Company.

Unsino, C. (1998). *Staff and organizational development: A process for changing the culture in long term care*. Presented at the annual meeting of the National Citizen's Coalition for Nursing Home Reform, Washington, DC.

Unsino, C. (1999). *A pioneer approach to culture change*, unpublished essay.

Williams, C. C. (1990). Long term care and the human spirit. *Generations, 14*(4), Fall.

Williams, C. C. (1997). Pioneers in nursing home culture change. *Aging and the Human Spirit*, Institute for the Medical Humanities, Galveston, Texas; 7(2); Fall.

Williams, C. C. (1998). *Self-determination in nursing homes: No longer an oxymoron*. Presented at the annual meeting, Gerontological Society of America, Philadelphia.

Williams, C. C. (1999, July). *Relationships: The heart of life and long term care*. Presented at conference Quality of Care in Nursing Homes: The Critical Role of the Nursing Assistant, American Society on Aging, Philadelphia, PA.

10

Better Lives for Elders Through Better Practitioner Judgments

Sidney Katz
Barry J. Gurland

During the last 50 years, problems of growing numbers of chronically ill elders in developing countries have spurred attention to their quality of life. Our explorations concentrate on decision-making judgments that affect quality living—judgments by elders, geriatric practitioners, and other helpers. As essential decision-making bridges, their judgments now integrate poorly understood mixes of intellect, intuition, and heart; and, thereupon, participants convert complex life-quality attributes into workable actions. Although we speak about service transactions, we submit that the chapter's suppositions also bear on health-related self-care, family caregiving, and policy making.

Three premises underlie the chapter's discourse. First, narrow efforts can't manage the complex network of structures and functions that explain life's quality: holistic efforts are needed. Second, decisions and actions that bear on life's quality—whether by those who serve or are served—inescapably draw on an uncertain mix of the following human capacities:

- intellect based on logic-driven experiences through education, training, and active service;
- intuition based on informal subjective and unconscious experiences; and
- values driven by personal-social feelings and conscience.

The third premise is that effective judgments and interactions depend on intelligible language, thought, and communication.

So oriented, we examine the background of attention to health-related quality of life, its complexity, its challenge to practitioners, and the place and power of decision-making judgments in meeting the challenge. We observe that these topics bear directly on *why* and *how* we are persuaded to address judgment uncertainties. Looking to a future when improved judgments deal better with life's quality, we then propose a path to progress.

AGING-INSPIRED ATTENTION TO HEALTH-RELATED QUALITY OF LIFE

Hand in hand with increases in life expectancy, developed countries witness dramatic increases in numbers of elders who are frail and chronically ill (Bright, 1966; Katz, 1983, 1987). This trend carries personal and social burdens that lessen the quality of life of elders and their families—a costly and absorbing, societal problem that Somers labeled *the geriatric imperative* (Somers, 1981).

Scientific advances in cause-effect thinking and progress in managing infections contributed materially to this trend and imperative (Burton & Smith, 1970). In the middle ages, practitioner training lacked scientific discipline. Devastating infections were the leading concerns of medical practice—especially epidemics of plague, syphilis, small pox, diphtheria, tuberculosis, cholera, and typhoid. Poorly prepared practitioners commonly purged and bled their patients. Hospitals were dirty; and poor care reigned.

During the 200 years after that dark period, improved scientific methods enabled the clarification of causes of infections. From Sydenham, Petty, and Graunt, came epidemiological and statistical insight into the prevalence and spread of infections. Virchow described pathogenesis, while Pasteur and Koch used the microscope and tools of microbiology to clarify causes. Such advances showed that contaminated water, crowding, and poor sanitation spread infections—in turn, enabling infection control through hygiene, sanitation, and immunization.

In the last half of the nineteenth century, professional education incorporated scientific methods and discoveries into both clinical training and care. Basic laboratory sciences became partners in practitioner education, and research was introduced as an important mission of training institutions. Scientific fundamentals of human biology, diseases, and treatments became major parts of curricula. Admission requirements and educational standards were raised; and faculties, laboratories, and clinical facilities were strengthened. These advances, along with the introduction of antibiotics in the 1900s, accelerated progress in the treatment and control of infections.

Concurrently, social movements helped to translate scientific and educational progress into health-strengthening activities for citizens at large. For example, social movements in developed countries (e.g., revolutions in America and France) emphasized liberty, equality, and needs of the many. Fostering public responsibility for the welfare of all citizens, these movements laid the foundation for the field of public health—a potent force in the fight against infections.

Thus, as a result of interacting scientific, educational, and social forces, the first half of the twentieth century witnessed infection control in developed countries—especially among infants and children. Life expectancy and number of elders increased. Longer lives and increasingly effective therapy for acute conditions fostered the accumulation of morbidities over time. In turn, chronic diseases replaced infections as leading causes of death and as major societal burdens. Understandably, a prominent health-related question of today is: "If treatments prolong life, do they also make for better lives?" More than in prior times, practitioners openly face the need to attend to whole-person influences of chronic illnesses—to personal, interpersonal, and external challenges to quality living.

Long life spans and large number of elders only partly explain growing attention to the broad effects covered by the phrase *health-related quality of life* (Katz & Gurland, 1991). Other factors include technological and social changes that affect persons of all ages—for example, new communication technologies that spread information widely and sensitize people to life quality threats. People have learned that new products and production methods can harm (as well as benefit) health and the environment. They worry about harmful effects of industrial wastes, radiation, and pesticides: they worry about risks of organ transplants, life support devices, and genetic manipulation. Well-informed, they are better fitted to oppose harmful effects and seek satisfactory lives.

Regarding the influence of chronic illnesses on quality living, the Commission on Chronic Illness (1956) outlined definitive illness-related attributes that underlie burdensome problems of life and living:

- permanent deviation from normal health;
- residual disability;
- nonreversible pathology;
- need for special patient training;
- need for prolonged supervision, observation, or care.

In terms of sensed and expressed experiences, these attributes commonly signal reduced life quality through worrisome events:

- dependence with prospects of helplessness;

- dislocation from home;
- transitions from parental and other meaningful, decision-making roles;
- blows to dignity and self-esteem;
- loss of respect and affection from others;
- stresses on self and family due to changes in physical, mental, social, and economic status;
- needs for subsistence, safety, and comfort; and
- needs for costly services that are in limited supply.

Material and moral burdens that accompany these events commonly reduce personal resilience (i.e., solidity, vitality, competence, and adaptiveness of life processes) to internal and external threats (Bertram & Katz, 1981). Intimately tied to human capacities to survive and thrive, that resilience is a prime determinant of elder capacities to live satisfying lives.

COMPLEXITY CHALLENGES ELDERS, PRACTITIONERS, AND HELPERS

Elders, and their families, use integrated objective and subjective abilities to manage their lives—abilities that are shaped by biological and psychosocial processes. In addition to their inner selves, they take account of the external world—a living and nonliving world that can either help or hinder one's ability to thrive and survive. For example, a daughter who chooses a nursing home for her mother considers body and mental needs, personal-family values and beliefs, life experiences, physical and social surroundings, type of staff, and financial requirements. Practitioner decisions and actions are expected to take the same web of matters into account.

The following abstract reports experiences with that web by practitioners in two hospitals (Stroud, Katz, & Gooding, 1985a):

> Most of the patients in these hospitals struggled with stroke, fracture of the hip, arthritis, cancer, neurological conditions, or leg amputation. Struggles related to life's quality centered in dysfunctions that limited their abilities to live as they once had: to move about, take care of themselves, use their hands, prepare meals, drive cars, and socialize. They feared invalidism and worried about lengthy illness, costly medical care, and financial security. Depression and eroded self-images often hampered service efforts.
>
> Faced with multifaceted problems, interdisciplinary teams with medical, psychosocial, and rehabilitation skills sought to bring diseases under control and restore capacities for normal living. They provided continuous comprehensive services and directly involved patients and families in rehabilitation. In making decisions, practitioners used judgments rooted in

intellectual and intuitive experiences gained through formal training and service. Values and conscience played important roles in service; and judgments and predictions were uncertain.

At the same time, undetected patient experiences influenced patient responses to services—shown by events in the life of Rachel, a patient whose deep anchorages to home, family, and church were only partly detected in the hospital. Rachel had been a constant nurturing center for her husband and children. She had also collected food and clothes for the poor. Through such relationships, she had thrived and found satisfaction.

When crises of family and illness occurred (her bout with cancer and her husband's death), she became severely depressed and inactive. She was hospitalized and, with comprehensive medical and rehabilitative help, regained the ability to take care of herself. At home, she received informal support from family, pastor, and friends.

Rachel's story shows the effects of basic anchorages (Bennett, 1970; Cath, 1963) on the health of elders—also on services and service outcomes. Parallel experiences, widely encountered by practitioners, support the idea that chronic diseases generate structural and functional deficits. These deficits underlie *whole-person*, life-quality problems—problems grounded in linked attributes of:

- body, mind, values, beliefs;
- life experiences in space and time (perceived, real, anticipated); and
- the living and nonliving environment.

In this sense, the degree to which life is satisfying is a function of irreducibly interwoven attributes; and efforts to address life's quality must take the whole into account (not one part alone). In accord, theorists have observed that life and its dynamic powers derive from the intrinsic wholeness of life parts. Accepting the need to study parts, they call for parallel efforts to know what happens when parts are put together.

Need for attention to wholeness—human and ecological—is not a new concept. It is manifest in centuries of diligent philosophic, theologic, and scientific reasoning about the essence of a good life (Birch, 1988; Katz & Gurland, 1991; Lovejoy, 1936; Schumacher, 1977). Most conceived the search for a better life as an elemental attribute of life; and theorists reasoned that *mobility* and *self-awareness* extend the sphere of human actions, helping to shape the self, environment, and personal futures in pursuit of a better life. Observing the complex web of attributes that explain chronic illness and life-quality, current scholars face the need to clarify wholeness.

Attention to wholeness currently focuses on functional capacities—human powers and abilities to adapt and cope. Freud (Krech & Crutchfield, 1958), Havighurst (1968), Kuhlen (1959), and Lawton (1972) conceived that mobility, locomotion, and other self-maintenance functions are organized behaviors that one needs in surviving and adapting. Co-workers and I described ordered recovery of self-maintenance functions in sick elders, noting that the order of recovery paralleled the ordered development of these functions in children (Katz, Ford, Moskowitz, Jackson, & Jaffe, 1963). Gurland, Wilder, and Berkman (1988) reported determinant roles of mental problems in dysfunction, while Andrews and Withey (1974) conceived that social roles and values are determinants of quality of life. World Health Organization reports (1947, 1957, 1984) have repeatedly stressed the need to attend to personal functioning in matters of health.

Accordingly, elder care calls for an expanded orientation to health and illness—one that integrates concepts of human ecology, disease management, and health care sciences (Gregg, 1956). This orientation attends to: wholeness and connections; objective-subjective linkages; psychosocial factors such as inner strength, motivation, lifestyle, and preferences; and broadly defined cost effects of immediate treatment and long-term care. Experts in prestigious academies (National Academy of Sciences, Institute of Medicine, National Research Council, New York Academy of Science) now endorse the need to assess services in terms of their "broad health outcomes and long-term social, economic, and ethical consequences"—as well as in terms of disease-related results (Katz & Gurland, 1991). Besides attending to survival and changes in blood tests, practitioners are asked to pay heed to overall well-being, adaptive abilities, and the quality of life's remaining years. They are challenged, in sum, to make judgments that help elders: meet living needs; respond to external stresses; overcome or manage incapacities; act freely; and enjoy life.

PRACTITIONER JUDGMENTS IN PURSUIT OF QUALITY LIVING

Based on prevailing service paradigms, geriatric practitioners seek to help healthy elders avoid health-related adversity. Faced with sickness or disability, they attempt to promote independent living through restored physical, mental, and social functioning. If complete recovery isn't possible, they seek adaptive resolutions and alternate life purposes. They always undertake to comfort and to alleviate symptoms. Despite a dearth of information about the intricately interlaced attributes that explain quality living, practitioners must exercise judgments that integrate scattered facts, untested suppositions, and obscure intuitions (Feinstein, 1967). Understandably, professional whole-person judgments are uncertain and fallible—as, in turn, are their decisions and actions in behalf of quality living.

Clinical training maintains that judgments should be evidence-based, yet little evidence on hand validates life-quality judgments—to a large degree, because reliable information about objective matters exceeds that about subjective matters. Relatedly, practitioners in training learn more about objective causes, pathogenesis, and treatments than about subjective equivalents; more about physical than mental abilities; and more about acute diseases than chronic conditions. Since these imbalances neglect subjective matters vital to quality living, training cannot assure credible judgments that bear on life's quality. As a practical result, practitioner judgments about short-term and clearly objective matters are more acceptable than judgments in behalf of quality living. Worrisome geriatric imperatives and a sophisticated public require strong whole-person judgments.

Effective interdisciplinary decisions and actions in behalf of satisfactory living also demand strong whole-person judgments. Where quality of life is involved, the power of service judgments depends on practitioner partnerships that converge on integrated decisions and actions. Differences in concepts and training now foster disciplinary divergences that reduce the integrative power of judgments. Each discipline builds its own paradigm of service, research, and education: each has its own way of defining and solving problems. Given incomplete evidence, these practitioner insularities predispose to reductionistic judgments and weak collaboration—advocating and entrenching narrow actions that miss whole-person stresses.

Strengthening judgments that influence quality of life is a complex venture and requires clear guidance. Since these judgments deal with *composites* (not separate parts), *composite insights* that reflect life's wholeness should guide the venture. Early composite insights (not available from academia) could come from practitioners whose whole-person responsibilities directly engage the health-related harmonies and disharmonies of whole-person structures, functions, and interventions. Their algorithmic descriptions of assessments; their grounds for judgments and services; and their perceived outcomes would provide such insights.

Figure 10.1 portrays grounds for a model system of iterative observation, testing, and self-correction—one designed to improve professional judgments in pursuit of quality living. The system would focus on multidimensional issues: that is, quality of life complexity, diverse practitioner frames of reference, and ill-defined service effects on life quality (Katz, Halstead, & Wierenga, 1975; Stroud, Katz, & Gooding, 1985b). Service-based, the system would merge audit, feedback, and evidence-guided self-analysis in continuously iterated, judgment-correcting loops. In so doing, it would look to incrementally strengthen record-keeping, life-quality research, and clinical judgments.

Working through unified structures and processes, practitioners in the envisioned system would seek to interweave disparate whole-person

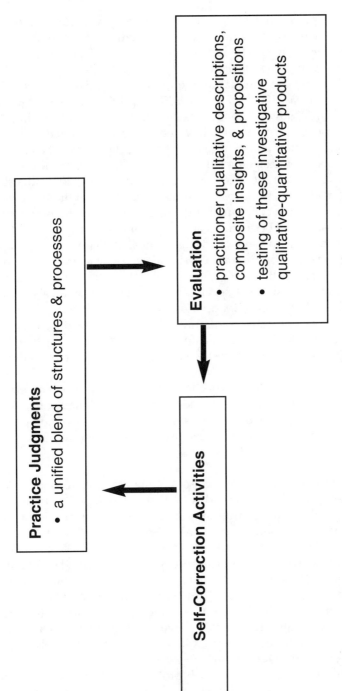

FIGURE 10.1   Improving practice judgments that bear on the quality of life.

211

insights and propositions. Drawing on audit-derived observations and disciplinary evidences (qualitative and quantitative), they would reconcile divergent insights, methods, and strategies through negotiating activities. Given *diverse professional languages and taxonomies* (a "Tower of Babel" phenomenon), successful negotiation requires *qualitatively clear common language and taxonomies* (Hedrick, Katz, & Stroud, 1980/81; Jones, 1973; Katz et al., 1975; U. S. National Committee on Vital Statistics and Health, 1980).

Although equivalent systems have not yet been activated, holistically oriented practitioners and investigators have introduced seed components that set the stage for designing whole-person, judgment-correcting systems. As prime examples of such seeds, we cite: 1) judgment-guiding algorithms that convert assessments into service plans; and 2) multidimensional taxonomies grounded in conceptual and empiric understandings of daily living functions, mental orientation, and physical impairments.

Among those who developed algorithms, Williams (1983) outlined care requirements appropriate to geriatric needs: *needs* in terms of qualitative classes of "health and/or functional status" and *care types* in terms of "health and/or support services" and "settings or levels of care." He highlighted the central importance of physical and psychosocial functioning, need changes, and family and financial resources. As such, Williams (1983) and others (Eastman, 1983; Katz & Falcone, 1980) devised seed sources of composite insights for whole-person, judgment-correcting systems.

With regard to information needed by judgement-correcting systems, multdimensional taxonomies grounded in common language have been developed that converge on whole-person descriptions and comparisons. These taxonomies have already been used to produce useful information for life-quality judgments. In sum:

- Descriptions that use clear classes of hierarchically ordered profiles (covering disability, morbidity, and selected functions) have dealt successfully with complexities and heterogeneities of diagnosis, prognosis, and outcome appraisal (Brorsson, 1980; Commission on Chronic Illness, 1957; Gurland, Katz, & Chen, 1997; Katz, 1983; Katz et al., 1963; Katz, Downs, Cash, & Grotz, 1970; Katz, Ford, Chinn, & Newill, 1966; Katz, Ford, Downs, & Adams, 1969; Katz, Hedrick, & Henderson, 1979; Spector, Katz, Murphy, & Fulton, 1987).
- In service delivery, these profiles have been used to document, display, and monitor functional changes, and use of common language has eased interdisciplinary collaboration (Fretwell & Katz, 1985; Katz et al., 1975; Katz & Stroud, 1989).
- In clinical research, use of such profiles has produced multidimensional information about causal webs, pathogenesis, illness burdens,

and treatment effects (Katz, Vignos, Moskowitz, Thompson, & Svec, 1968; Katz et al., 1969; Katz, Ford, Downs, Adams, & Rusby, 1972; Papsidero, Katz, Kroger, & Akpom, 1979; Stroud et al., 1985c).

Applying this knowledge to geriatric services, practitioners have developed better insights into process elements that explain geriatric team care behavior (i.e., team structure, management, leadership, and interactions) for service assessment, goal-setting, evaluation strategies, and patient education (Katz et al., 1975; Papsidero, Kroger, & Rothert, 1980; Stroud et al., 1985b; Zimney, McClain, Batalden, & O'Connor, 1980). Using new tools to evaluate the effects of geriatric team care, practitioners and investigators have also strengthened the evidence base for judgment-correcting activities. These recent advances now allow the launching of practical, judgment-correcting systems.

PARTICIPATORY JUDGMENTS BY ELDERS, FAMILIES, AND CAREGIVERS

To this point, we have focused on improving practitioner judgments in pursuit of better lives for elders. As a *sine qua non* in that pursuit, we stress that long-term treatment and care are participatory processes that give due weight to understandings and judgments of those who are served, as well as those who serve. Since services presently lack proper ways of incorporating elders, families, and caregivers as participants, new strategies are needed that:

- take proper account of elder, family, and caregiver values;
- recognize their personal initiatives and roles; and
- strengthen their judgments.

Inceptively, such strategies must systematically illuminate the *grounds* for judgments and actions by elders and their helpers.

Gadamer (1976) reasoned that lifelong experiences establish absorbing personal grounds of relevance, that is, "horizons," for judgments and actions. He explained that, in complex situations, horizons ". . . are not immediately understandable but require interpretive effort." In today's world of services, horizons of elders, practitioners, and long-term caregivers are poorly illuminated through informal biographical comments and personal behavior—a situation that makes for weak interpretations and divergent judgments. Applied to judgments in pursuit of quality living, this leads elders and their caregivers to make judgments of uncertain meaning, based on murky mixtures of intellectual and subconscious experiences.

About the place of horizons in meaningful interactions, Gadamer explained,

- *meaning* is not ". . . what [words] 'seem' to say [but] what is recovered by disciplined reconstruction of the historical situation in which it originated";
- *understanding* is ". . . a translation of past meaning into the present situation . . . movement of history [where] past and present are constantly mediated";
- the *past* has a ". . . pervasive power in the phenomenon of understanding";
- the *present* is a ". . . fluid moment, productive and disclosive, but like all others will be fused with future horizons";
- *complexity* obscures meaning and fosters ". . . lax practice of understanding [which] assumes that understanding arises naturally: more rigorous practice assumes that *mis*understanding arises naturally."

Cath (1963), relatedly, described ". . . basic anchorages that people form throughout life: an intact body and body image; an acceptable home; a socioeconomic anchorage; and a meaningful purpose to life." Observing that these factors shape inner identity and influence functional development and health, Bennett (1970) wrote,

> These four anchorages provide the structure within which the individual performs required developmental tasks at various stages of life; and the degree of success with which tasks are performed, and crises met, spells the difference between good and impaired health.

To Bateson (1979), biographical and environmental experiences are *realities of context*—realities essential for meaningful understanding and communication. He reasoned,

- "Without context, words and actions have no meaning";
- ". . . all communication necessitates context"; and
- ". . . contextual shaping [promotes] common understanding and meaningful communication."

Gubrium (1993) linked horizons to quality comprehension. He found that elders in nursing homes expressed horizons through narrative linkages that each made with personal experiences. What they said was understandable in relation to these linkages; and linkages attached subjective meaning to quality interpretation. He wrote, ". . . quality of life and quality of care are not so much rationally assessable conditions, as they are horizoned, ordinary, and biographically active renderings of lifelong experiences."

Life stories of elders reveal a multiplicity of horizon patterns—commonly taking the form of:

- dyadic relationships (marital, parent-child, sibling);
- family nurturing (by woman and man—at home and work);
- transcending stances (spiritual, intellectual, philosophic);
- skills and behavioral styles (talents and attitudes);
- kin, neighbor, and confidante relationships;
- social participation (leisure, group, voluntary); and
- long-standing illness and disability.

Clearly, horizons of meaning vary markedly—each to each. Just as trees, each comes from its own seed. Each grows in its own soil; and each produces its own overarching foliage.

Offering practical guidance, Good and Good (1995) conceived a "meaning-centered approach." They wrote,

- "All illness is a meaningful phenomenon . . . a personal and social reality."
- "A meaning-centered approach views any illness as a concurrence of configurations of meanings and experiences [whose] complex relationships can be analyzed appropriately only if prior attention is given to the meaningful experiential aspects of health and healing."
- A meaning-centered approach calls for ". . . translation of subjective realty, not merely interpretation of objective data . . . [i.e.,] hermeneutic engagement."

Based on these tenets, they launched a service-based program that ". . . expands the range of antecedent conditions believed to cause disease; incorporates multifactorial views of causation; and conceptualizes the relationship between culture and disease." Emphasizing hermeneutic skills that elicit the meanings of illness for patients, they embedded questions about personal experiences and values into history-taking and service—questions that focused on cultural and psychosocial experiences. They introduced seminars, readings, lectures, role-playing, and videotaped interviews that enhanced understandings and judgments.

CONCLUDING COMMENTS

In this chapter, we have discussed service-based judgments that influence quality living—shared, decision-making judgments by elders, practitioners, and caregivers. After reviewing events that inspired health-related

attention to quality of life, we described challenges posed by weak understandings of life-quality complexities for participatory judgments in service transactions. We observed that participants faced with these weak
understandings use judgments of uncertain meaning based on a clouded
amalgam of intellectual, intuitive, and emotional forces.

Drawing on available conceptual and empiric understandings, we
proposed a service-based system of interactive observations, testing, and
self-correction designed to improve presumptive judgments that bear on
quality living. That system would use insights from detailed qualitative
descriptions of whole-person encounters—also their effects—as sources
of questions for qualitative and quantitative study. Evidence-based feedback, self-analysis, and negotiation would generate judgment-correcting
actions; and iterated testing, shaping, and application would generate
incremental corrections. As aids to implementation, we cited existing models of *multidisciplinary service algorithms; multidimensional assessment tools,*
and *hierarchical taxonomies* grounded in common language; and interactive learning strategies.

Looking to relieve reductionistic disciplinary bonds and improve practitioner collaboration, we marked the need to:

- include matters of whole-person well-being and integrative judgments within training and research; and
- incorporate strategies that transcend disciplinary differences within
  service programs.

Relieving reductionistic bonds can also be expected to counteract contextual pressures that incite makeshift service approaches.

We stressed that service efforts to attend to life's quality are participatory processes, where success calls for reconciled understandings and
judgments among elders, families, aides, and personal helpers—as well as
with practitioners. We noted:

- conventional services do not properly heed the values, judgments,
  and drives of elders and personal caregivers; and
- designing corrective strategies calls for knowing the biographical
  experiences that establish absorbing grounds of relevance for elders
  and caregiver judgments and actions.

As a model for corrective strategies, we introduced a recently proposed
"meaning-centered approach" to services.

In sum, for a future where services seek better lives for elders through
better judgments, this chapter explored conceptual and empiric understandings that underlie the judgments and actions of directly engaged

participants—that is, practitioners, elders, families, and other helpers. In behalf of harmonious activism, the chapter set the stage for reacculturating *consumer: practitioner,* and *interpractitioner* collaboration.

REFERENCES

Andrews, F. M., & Withey, S. B. (1974). Developing measures of perceived life quality: Results from several national surveys. *Social Indicators Research, 1*(1), 1–26.

Bateson, G. (1979). *Mind and nature: A necessary unity* (pp. 3–22). Toronto: Bantam Books.

Bennett, L. L. (1970). Protective services for the aged. In *Working with older people: Volume III: The aging person: Needs and services* (DHEW Publication (PHS) No. 1459) (pp. 52–57). Washington, DC: U.S. Government Printing Office.

Bertram, K., & Katz, S. (1981). A preliminary examination of the differentiating power of profiled predictor variables. In S. Katz, *Improved information for quality assurance in long-term care* (Appendix B, Vol. II of A data archive for use in long-term care policy analysis, final report, DHHS Grant No. HS 03760-02) (pp. 1–44). Washington, DC: National Center for Health Services Research.

Birch, C. (1988). Eight fallacies of the modern world and five axioms for a post-modern worldview. *Perspectives in Biology and Medicine, 32,* 12–30.

Bright, M. (1966). Demographic background for programming chronic diseases in the United States. In A. M. Lillienfeld & A. J. Gifford (Eds.), *Chronic diseases and public health* (pp. 5–23). Baltimore: Johns Hopkins University Press.

Brorsson, B. (1980). *ADL-index: Sammanfattande matt pa individens formage att klara det dagliga livets aktiviter.* (Medicinska forskningsradet Tech. Rep. ISBN 91-85546-16X). Stockholm, Sweden.

Burton, L. E., & Smith, H. H. (1970). *Public health and community medicine* (pp. 3–34). Baltimore: Williams & Wilkins.

Cath, S. H. (1963). Some dynamics of middle and later years. Smith College Studies in Social Work, 33(2), 97–126. Commission on Chronic Illness. (1956). *Chronic illness in the United States: Vol. II. Care of the long-term patient* (p. 586). Cambridge: Harvard University Press.

Commission on Chronic Illness (1956). *Chronic illness in the United States: Vol. II. Care of the long-term patient* (p. 586). Cambridge: Harvard University Press.

Commission on Chronic Illness (1957). *Chronic illness in the United States: Vol. IV. Chronic illness in a large city* (pp. 375–376). Cambridge: Harvard University Press.

Eastman, P. (1983, November/December). The case for functional assessment. *Geriatric Consultant, 26*–29.

Feinstein, A. R. (1967). *Clinical judgment* (pp. 12, 24–30, 102, 125–127). Baltimore: Williams & Wilkins.

Fretwell, M. D., & Katz, S. (1985). Functional assessment: Its use in the teaching nursing home. In E. L. Schneider, C. J. Wendland, A. W. Zimmer, N. List, & M. Ory (Eds.), *The teaching nursing home* (pp. 129–136). New York: Raven Press.

Gadamer, H. G. (1976). Editor's introduction. In D. E. Linge (Ed. and Trans.), *Philosophical hermeneutics* (pp. xi–xl). Berkeley: University of California Press.

Good, B. J., & Good, M. D. (1995). The meaning of symptoms: A cultural hermeneutic model for clinical practice. In M. D. Good (Ed.), *American medicine: The quest for competence* (pp. 165–196). Berkeley: University of California Press.

Gregg, A. (1956). The future health officer's responsibility: Past, present, and future. *American Journal of Public Health, 46,* 1384.

Gubrium, J. F. (1993). *Speaking of life: Horizons of meaning for nursing home residents* (a: pp. xv–xvi) (b: pp. 1–76). New York: Aldine De Gruyter.

Gurland, B. J., Katz, S., & Chen, J. (1997). Index of affective suffering: Linking a classification of depressed mood to impairment in quality of life. *American Journal of Geriatric Psychiatry, 5*(3), 192–210.

Gurland, B. J., Wilder, D. E., & Berkman, C. (1988). Depression and disability in the elderly: Reciprocal relations and changes with age. *International Journal of Geriatric Psychiatry, 3,* 163–179.

Havighurst, R. J. (1968). A social-psychological perspective on aging. *Gerontologist, 8,* 67–81.

Hedrick, S. C., Katz, S., & Stroud, M. W., III (1980/1981). Patient assessment in long-term care: Is there a common language? *Aged Care & Services Review, 2*(4), 1–19.

Jones, E. W. (1973). *Patient classification for long-term care: User's manual.* (DHEW Publication (HRA) No. 74-3107). Washington, DC: U.S. Government Printing Office.

Katz, S. (1983). Assessing self-maintenance: Activities of daily living, mobility, and instrumental activities of daily living. *Journal of the American Geriatrics Society, 31,* 721–727.

Katz, S. (1987). Editorial: The science of quality of life (Special issue). *Journal of Chronic Diseases, 40,* 459–463.

Katz, S., Downs, T. D., Cash, H. R., & Grotz, R. C. (1970). Progress in development of the Index of ADL. *Gerontologist, 10*(No. 1, Part 1), 20–30.

Katz, S., & Falcone, A. R. (1980). Use of assessment data for long-term care planning, program decisions, and statistical accounting. *Proceedings of the 18th National Meeting of the Public Health Conference on Records and Statistics: New Challenges for Vital and Health Records* (DHHS/NCHS Publication (PHS) No. 81-1214) (pp. 39–44). Washington, DC: U.S. Government Printing Office.

Katz, S., Ford, A. B., Chinn, A. B., & Newill, V. A. (1966). Prognosis after strokes: Part II. Long-term course of 159 patients. *Medicine, 45,* 236–246.

Katz, S., Ford, A. B., Downs, T. D., & Adams, M. (1969). Chronic-disease classification in evaluation of medical care programs. *Medical Care, 7,* 139–143.

Katz, S., Ford, A. B., Downs, T. D., Adams, M., & Rusby, D. I. (1972). *Effects of continued care: A study of chronic illness in the home.* (DHEW Publication (DHM) No. 73-3010). Washington, DC: U.S. Government Printing Office.

Katz, S., Ford, A. B., Moskowitz, R. W., Jackson, B. A., & Jaffe, M. A. (1963). Studies of illness in the aged: The Index of ADL: A standardized measure of biological and psychosocial function. *Journal of the American Medical Association, 185,* 914–919.

Katz, S., & Gurland, B. J. (1991). Science of quality of life of elders: Challenge and opportunity. In J. E. Birren, J. E. Lubben, J. C. Rowe, & D. E. Deutchman (Eds.), *The concept and measurement of quality of life in the frail elderly* (pp. 335–343). San Diego: Academic Press.

Katz, S., Halstead, L., & Wierenga, M. (1975). A medical perspective of team care. In S. Sherwood (Ed.), *Long-term care: A handbook for researchers, planners, and providers* (pp. 213–252). Holliswood, NY: Spectrum Publications.

Katz, S., Hedrick, S. C., & Henderson, N. S. (1979). The measurement of long-term care needs and impact. *Health & Medical Care Services Review, 2*(1), 1–21.

Katz, S., & Stroud, M. W., III (1989). Functional assessment in geriatrics: A review of progress and directions. *Journal of the American Geriatrics Society, 37,* 267–271.

Katz, S., Vignos, P. J., Jr., Moskowitz, R. W., Thompson, H. M., & Svec, K. H. (1968). Comprehensive outpatient care in rheumatoid arthritis: A controlled study. *Journal of the American Medical Association, 206,* 1249–1254.

Krech, D., & Crutchfield, R. S. (1958). *Elements of psychology.* New York: Alfred A. Knopf.

Kuhlen, R. G. (1959). Aging and life-adjustment. In J. E. Birren (Ed.), *Handbook of aging and the individual* (pp. 852–897). Chicago: University of Chicago Press.

Lawton, M. P. (1972). Assessing the competence of older people. In D. Kent, R. Kastenbaum, & S. Sherwood (Eds.), *Research, planning and action for the elderly* (pp. 122–143). New York: Behavioral Publications.

Lovejoy, A. O. (1936). *The great chain of being: A study of the history of an idea.* Cambridge: Harvard Press.

Papsidero, J. A., Katz, S., Kroger, M. H., & Akpom, C. A. (1979). *Chance for change: Implications of a chronic disease module study.* East Lansing, MI: Michigan State University Press.

Papsidero, J. A., Kroger, M. H., & Rothert, M. (1980). Preparing health assistants for service roles in long-term care. *Gerontologist, 20,* 534–546.

Schumacher, E. F. (1977). *A guide for the perplexed* (pp. 1–8, 15–25, 26–60, 120–128). New York: Harper & Row.

Somers, A. R. (1981). The geriatric imperative. In A. R. Somers & D. R. Fabian (Eds.), *The geriatric imperative: An introduction to gerontology and clinical geriatrics* (pp. 3–19). New York: Appleton-Century-Crofts.

Spector, W. D., Katz, S., Murphy, J. B., & Fulton, J. P. (1987). The hierarchical relationship between activities of daily living and instrumental activities of daily living (Special issue). *Journal of Chronic Diseases, 40,* 481–489.

Stroud, M. W., III, Katz, S., & Gooding, B. A. (1985a). *Rehabilitation of the elderly: A tale of two hospitals* (pp. 18–37). East Lansing, MI: Michigan State University Press.

Stroud, M. W., III, Katz, S., & Gooding, B. A. (1985b). *Rehabilitation of the elderly: A tale of two hospitals* (pp. 146–168). East Lansing, MI: Michigan State University Press.

Stroud, M. W., III, Katz, S., & Gooding, B. A. (1985c). *Rehabilitation of the elderly: A tale of two hospitals* (pp. 12–16, 113–121, 169–209). East Lansing, MI: Michigan State University Press.

U.S. National Committee on Vital and Health Statistics (1980). *Long-term health care: Minimum data set.* (DHHS/NCHS Publication (PHS) No. 80-1158). Hyattsville, MD: U.S. Government Printing Office.

Williams, T. F. (1983). Assessment of the geriatric patient in relation to needs for services and facilities. In W. Reichel (Ed.), *Clinical aspects of aging* (2nd ed., pp. 543–548). Baltimore: Williams & Wilkins.

World Health Organization (1947). The constitution of the World Health Organization. *WHO Chronicle, 1*(29).

World Health Organization (1957). *Measurement of levels of health: Report of a study group.* (WHO Tech. Rep. Series, No. 137). Geneva, Switzerland.

World Health Organization (1984). *Uses of epidemiology in aging: Report of a scientific group.* (WHO Tech. Rep. Series, No. 706). Geneva, Switzerland.

Zimney, L., McClain, M. P., Batalden, P. B., & O'Connor, J. P. (1980). Patient telephone interviews: A valuable technique for finding problems and assessing quality in ambulatory medical care. *Journal of Community Health, 6*(1), 35–42.

11

Assessing Consumer Satisfaction with Long-Term Care Services

Farida Kassim Ejaz
Georgia J. Anetzberger
Alice J. Kethley

T his chapter takes a unique perspective of a long-term care agency that struggles with assessing the consumer's perspective on quality of care set in the context of the individual client's quality of life. The majority of chapters in this book have examined approaches to defining and conceptualizing quality of care and quality of life in long-term care. Definitions may differ from Lawton, arguing that conceptions of quality of life that do not adequately represent both the subjective and objective aspects of quality are deficient, to Phillips who debates the relationship between quality of care and quality of life and which of these is a subset of the other. However, the message is clear: definitions of quality are evolving as we move to the 21st century and reflect upon the historical role of how long-term care services have emerged in this country (Noelker & Harel, chapter 1). It is a similar historical course of events that has affected how The Benjamin Rose Institute (BRI) defines and measures quality of life and care with the services provided to its nursing home residents and to community-based clients in their homes or in other community settings.

This chapter begins by detailing the history of BRI in relation to its continuing mission to improve the quality of life for older persons by offering them high quality services that are routinely monitored to assess consumer satisfaction. Next, issues and methods for assessing satisfaction with care and services among residents and their family members in BRI's nursing home are discussed. Lastly, the model and procedures for assessing consumer satisfaction for home- and community-based clients are explicated.

HISTORICAL ROOTS

The Benjamin Rose Institute (BRI), founded in 1908, is a nonprofit, non-sectarian organization. In its first year of operation it served 79 clients with a $20,000 budget. By 1999, the budget grew to about $23 million, enabling BRI to directly serve more than 1,600 clients with home- and community-based services, 689 long- and short-term residents in its nursing home and conduct a variety of applied aging studies, with research grants totaling $860,995. The magnitude of BRI's operations reflect the complexity and diversity of our times with regard to providing quality care with compassion and dignity while respecting client self-determination and autonomy in a highly regulated health care market.

Yet, life was not so complicated when BRI started serving its clientele in the early 1900s. The decision by Benjamin Rose, a Cleveland businessman turned benefactor, to establish The Benjamin Rose Institute grew out of the experience of witnessing the plight of his friends. While preparing his will, Mr. Rose was reported by his lawyer as expressing grief over the number of his friends who worked hard and contributed to the community but outlived their savings and were reduced to poverty and shame. His concern over the quality of life of his friends became as much a part of his legacy as the approximately $3 million bequested to establish his Institute. Today the mission of The Benjamin Rose Institute reflects this original concern for quality of life; it is: "To improve the quality of life for older people, their families, and their caregivers through community-based and residential care, research, education, and advocacy."

The challenge to the trustees and employees of the Institute over the years has been to define and measure the Institute's success in providing quality care to improve the quality of life of its clients. During the initial years of operation, the Institute provided pensions to applicants whom the trustees deemed as being deserving based on their application and recommendations from clergy and friends. As described by Noelker and Harel (chapter 1), charitable care was characterized by a paternalistic stance that expected passivity and submissiveness from recipients. The average pension was $17.34 a month and was often considered the difference between death and survival. In order to evaluate the effectiveness of the pensions, trustees called on recipients in their homes. Records from these visitations report: ". . . it has been a pleasure to see the real good that the monthly allowance does, not only in affording material relief, but in freeing the mind from anxiety and worry . . ." (The Benjamin Rose Institute, 1998).

The signing of the Social Security Act by Franklin D. Roosevelt in 1935 marked the beginning of the complex system of health and social services which BRI offers today both in the homes of clients and in residential care settings. As the trustees continued to follow-up personally with the agency's beneficiaries, they became convinced of two things that altered the course of the Institute. First, the trustees recognized that quality services for older persons were not available even if the funds to purchase such services were there. Second, there was a need for professional staff who were well-trained to provide high quality services. This led to the hiring of Margaret Wagner, a social worker, in 1930 as the first executive director. She guided the Institute to develop a program of quality care that would serve as a model for other agencies. The tradition of improving the quality of life through financial assistance shifted to a broader definition of improving clients' quality of life through comprehensive services, a goal that is reflected in today's mission and programs.

In 1941, BRI purchased Belford House and formed a group home, departing from the Institute's practice of supporting the aged in their own homes because it recognized that some older persons are best served in a group setting. Belford House served 10 women with physical disabilities who benefited from housing with supportive services and socialization. According to Ms. Wagner: "The home was operated on the basis of what we had learned older people wanted, not on what we thought they wanted or should have." (The Benjamin Rose Institute, 1998). These early reflections demonstrate the agency's shift in philosophy to move away from serving "well deserving," passive clients (Noelker & Harel, chapter 1) to respecting individual autonomy and quality of life.

As the number of home- and community-based clients grew along with those seeking residential services, the Institute's service system expanded in response. Sometimes services were provided by in-house staff. Other times, contracts were developed with other agencies in the area, thereby creating a network of services to which clients had access. For example, the Institute started its own Home Aide Program, a service that did not exist elsewhere, but contracted with the Visiting Nurse Association for nurses to supervise them.

As the clientele of the Institute increased, it became impossible to continue the tradition of "calling on" recipients to judge if the care provided improved the quality of their lives. The trustees and the growing staff became convinced that more comprehensive service and client information was essential if sound decisions were to be made concerning program growth and development as well as evaluating and measuring the effectiveness of services. They also recognized that the financial resources of the Institute could never keep up with the increasing number of requests for services. It was imperative that they have information to monitor program effectiveness, make decisions concerning program expansion and development, and measure client satisfaction. The concept of quality which the early trustees had measured by in-person interviews with clients in their homes had been expanded to include the performance of the Institute's service programs and its decisions concerning the best allocation of limited resources.

The need for information led to the establishment of the research department in 1961, that became the Margaret Blenkner Research Center, bearing the name of its first research director. The presence of researchers on the staff of a long-term care agency has been an asset and served as a model adopted by other service organizations. The Center has contributed greatly to gerontological literature with landmark studies in protective services, post-hospitalization home care, relocation trauma, family caregiving, and case management. More importantly, it has provided the leadership for computerization, information networking, planning, and evaluation. It is the presence of trained researchers working with clinical staff that guides the organization to ask questions which lead to meaningful answers based on empirical evidence and to use the information to improve the quality of services.

Over the years, computers and electronic advancements have increased the ability of public agencies to impose more stringent regulations and at the same time have increased fragmentation of funding and services. Each responsible funding authority, such as Medicare Home Care, Mental Health, and PASSPORT (the State of Ohio's home- and community-based Medicaid waiver program), has developed its own measures, guidelines, and reporting systems, none of which has the capacity to communicate electronically with the others. The impact on agencies such as the Institute has been the creation of multiple databases for reporting and billing purposes that do not have the capacity to track client change over time, service impact, or cost of services for an individual with multiple problems and service needs. Regulatory compliance has also resulted in expenses related to purchasing hardware and software, hiring additional staff dedicated to developing and implementing information systems, and training clinical staff in correct documentation.

It is clear from the nature of the regulations imposed on the agency that any attention given to quality long-term care has focused on quality of care. Phillips (chapter 8) cites three reasons why government regulation and oversight of quality care became widespread in long-term care: the large amounts of public funds spent (of the $82.8 billion expended in 1997 on nursing home care, over 62% was derived from public funds), the presence of a vulnerable population, and the abdication of responsibility for quality care by providers. These reasons have prompted quality of care to become the primary focus of state-sponsored quality assurance and quality measurement (Cella, Gabay, Teitelbaum, Walker, & Kramer, 1996). An example of this has been the use of the Minimum Data Set (MDS) in nursing homes for development of quality indicators that are primarily focused on outcome measures of quality of care (Zimmerman et al., 1995). In the Medicare-sponsored home care industry, similar efforts at understanding quality of care are emerging with the recent adoption of the Outcomes and Assessment Information Set (OASIS) (Shaughnessy, Crisler, Schlenker, & Hittle, 1998).

It has become apparent to the trustees and staff of the Institute that such trends, although time-consuming, have moved the industry toward a better understanding of the quality of care provided to our clients. However, what is also apparent is that the regulations have not made similar advances with regard to assessing the subjective perspective of quality of care and its link to the quality of life of individual clients. Since BRI's mission from its inception was to understand how services helped in improving the lives of its clients, the Institute is faced with the struggle of defining and measuring the subjective perspective of the quality of care received by clients and its impact on their quality of life. Lawton (1991) has argued that both objective and subjective realities must be taken into consideration when defining quality, because objective realities may not fully capture how a person defines his/her perception of that reality. Each individual has internal standards and evaluations of life (and care) that are idiosyncratic and do not totally correspond with external standards (Lawton, 1991).

The remainder of this chapter describes how BRI attempts to evaluate one aspect of the subjective component of the client's reality: clients' satisfaction with the quality of care and services in the agency's two service divisions: Kethley House, its nursing home, and the Community Services Division. The results from this evaluation are applied to the quality assurance programs that BRI has established. Toward that end, the goal is to improve not only the quality of services and care that clients receive but to set it in the context of their quality of life.

Although BRI has the same overall goal for all its services, the two divisions have used varying procedures to assess consumer satisfaction. The varying procedures result from three major factors that influence the provision of long-term care services: a) long-term care in this nation has not been carefully planned, but has evolved haphazardly and has been geared toward institutional care; b) historical landmarks that spurred the consumer satisfaction movement had different effects on institutional- and community-based care; and c) each division at BRI has substantial latitude to implement the overall goals of the Institute in the context of its unique system of service delivery.

ASSESSING CONSUMER SATISFACTION IN BRI'S NURSING HOME

Historical Trends in the Industry

The movement to assess consumer satisfaction in the nursing home industry was spurred by several historical landmarks. In the mid-1980s, the National Citizens' Coalition for Nursing Home Reform (NCCNHR, 1985) held focus groups with over 400 nursing home residents from 70 facilities nationwide and its report (published in 1985) widely disseminated what residents believed were the quality markers for life and care in a nursing home. Another study conducted by Institute of Medicine (1986) found that the opinions of residents were often overlooked in long-term care (LTC) facilities. As a result, the Omnibus Budget Reconciliation Act (OBRA) was implemented in 1991, spearheading the residents' rights movement and paving the way for nursing homes to become focused on improving their overall quality. To ensure attention to resident rights, OBRA mandated that nursing home routine inspections must include direct contact with a sample of cognitively alert residents to gain their subjective perceptions of quality.

However, assessing consumer satisfaction with LTC services did not entirely stem from such ideological roots. A more practical reason for monitoring the consumer perspective reflected the trend set by some nursing homes to apply for accreditation by the Joint Commission for Accreditation of Health Care Organizations (JCAHO). JCAHO requires a facility to have a formal complaint management system, including methods to assess resident satisfaction with the quality of care and services provided to them. Another reason for the growing attention to consumer satisfaction stems from the competition for managed care contracts for subacute patients and the consequent need for marketing nursing home services. One method of proving to managed care companies that nursing home residents are satisfied with the care they receive is to conduct nursing home satisfaction surveys.

The trend to conduct consumer satisfaction surveys has become so popular that a recent survey of 81 randomly selected nursing homes in Ohio found that almost 80% were conducting them (Noelker, Ejaz, & Schur, 2000). Although Ohio may be unique in this regard, it is clear that assessing the subjective perspectives of nursing home residents has become a popular movement in the nursing home industry.

BRI's Use of Consumer Satisfaction Surveys in Residential Care

The first formal nursing home consumer satisfaction survey at BRI was conducted in 1994. By 1995, an organized system was developed to undertake this task. BRI's nursing home currently has 184 beds with 134 LTC beds and 50 beds for short-term, subacute, Medicare residents (in 1999, 430 short-term residents were served). With such a large consumer base, management became increasingly aware of the industry-wide trend to recognize the consumer's perspective on care and services and initiated the survey process by allocating staff time and resources. A staff person from the research division at BRI was named as the project coordinator and assigned the task of working with key nursing home staff to develop and implement the survey. The nursing home representatives on the project were comprised of social service, nursing and administrative staff.

The Survey Committee began the process by reviewing the pilot work carried out by the research division in 1994, along with satisfaction instruments used by a variety of agencies providing similar services, and relevant journal articles and magazines in long-term care. The Survey Committee identified key questions and issues while developing its own survey. (See Ejaz, 2000 for further details on conducting consumer satisfaction surveys in nursing facilities.) Through the years, the research staff along with nursing home staff have refined the survey and used it for implementing quality assurance programs aimed at improving the quality of care provided to residents.

Defining the Consumer in the Nursing Home

Three types of nursing home consumers are surveyed by BRI: 1) cognitively alert LTC residents, 2) family members of all LTC residents, and 3) subacute patients. Since the majority of BRI's LTC residents have some form of dementia, only those who are defined as cognitively alert by the social workers on the LTC units are surveyed. Based on current MDS+ records, just 20% of BRI's LTC residents meet the criteria for cognitive competence. Therefore, families or responsible parties of all LTC residents are also surveyed. Although the literature suggests that often families present very different perspectives from residents when evaluating care (Aharony & Strasser, 1993; Kleinsorge & Koenig, 1991; Lavizzo-Mourey, Zinn, & Taylor, 1992; Strasser, Schweikhart, Welch, & Burge, 1995), families surveyed by BRI have provided valuable insights regarding their relatives' care.

The third group of consumers who are surveyed are the subacute, short-term patients, discharged from an acute care setting. The instrument designed for such patients focuses on similar issues as those for LTC residents but also includes items on discharge planning. Since the subacute patients typically do not suffer from the same degree of dementia as LTC residents, they are directly surveyed. However, almost 40% in the last survey reported that they did not fill out the survey themselves but had help from family or friends.

Lessons Learned from Conducting the BRI Nursing Home Consumer Satisfaction Surveys

Lessons that BRI staff has learned from conducting consumer satisfaction surveys are summarized as follows:

- Responses to a mailed survey of LTC residents are very poor (only 26% in the first year). By changing the approach to a one-on-one interview with residents, using student interns from local universities who are trained by research staff, the response rate has increased to 70–80% over the years.
- It is possible to survey the families of LTC residents and subacute patients using a mailed questionnaire approach. However, in the first year, the response rates were 31% and 26% for LTC families and subacute patients, respectively. A reminder postcard increased the response rates for LTC families to 46%.
- Consumer satisfaction can best be assessed by using instruments that cover a wide range of service areas and include multiple items that are more sensitive to identifying differences between services (DeVellis, 1991; Spector, 1992; Stewart & Ware, 1992). For example, many LTC residents with length of stays ranging between 2 and 4 years, find it difficult to answer questions about their admission or about billing services and some rarely go for physical or occupational therapy. Yet, rehabilitation services are very important in the short-term, sub-acute population, although they do not participate as much as LTC residents in activities or eating their meals in the dining room.
- Questions in each area generally deal with the quality of the care provided as well as the manner (e.g., compassionate and respectful) with which the care is provided, thereby linking the concepts of quality of care and quality of life together. In fact, the literature suggests that respect and compassion by staff are critical elements of how quality care can be defined (Brannon, Cohn, & Smyer, 1990; Duncan & Morgan, 1994; Heiselman & Noelker, 1991; Spalding & Frank, 1985).
- Certain key service areas are divided to distinguish between the quality of care provided by professional staff versus that provided by direct-care staff. For example, significant differences exist between

the care provided by professional nurses versus that provided by nursing assistants. Such distinctions have led to in-service training focused on nurse assistants. The literature has also emphasized the distinct role played by nurse assistants in providing the majority of care to nursing home residents, and the importance of the quality of that care (Duncan & Morgan, 1994).

- Since acquiescence response bias is a problem in most consumer satisfaction surveys (LaMonica, Oberst, Madea, & Olf, 1986), there is more variation in responses when the following three response categories are used: "no improvement needed," "some improvement needed," and "a great deal of improvement needed" than using "strongly agree" to "strongly disagree" statements. Adding a fourth response category ("not familiar with") distinguishes between missing data and the respondent's unfamiliarity with the services or staff.
- Although closed-ended responses are used for most questions, providing consumers with the opportunity to include open-ended comments has helped to address immediate problems and to have a better understanding of some of the findings from the closed-ended questions. If consumers sign their names on the survey forms and seek urgent attention to a problem, the complaints are forwarded to the nursing home administrator for immediate action.
- Using bar graphs to report the results, especially with regard to changes from previous years, is more comprehensible and "user-friendly" for administrative and direct-care staff.
- Significant changes over time have been tracked to boost staff morale in areas where quality assurance programs proved to be successful. When an area significantly declines over time, staff have focused on that particular area to examine why such a decline occurred and to develop a quality improvement project to address the concerns.

Examples of Some Quality Improvement Projects in the Nursing Home

Several quality improvement projects that have proved highly successful in our nursing home relate to the dietary department. Since many residents were complaining of the taste and variety of the food offered to them, the administrative staff had a college student majoring in nutrition conduct a more in-depth survey of residents and families to examine the critical issues around such complaints. Based on the survey results, key administrative staff worked with the Director of Dietary to improve the food services. The nursing home also added more variety in beverages and snack foods, upgraded the ambiance in the dining room with new tablecloths and flowers on the tables, offered a printed menu the evening before to make meal selections for the next day, and hired more staff to help with the serving and feeding of food, if necessary. Such changes had a major impact in improving the dining experience of the residents and the families who visit them during meal times.

Another area of focus has been on improving the quality of care provided by nursing assistants (NAs) and the compassion and respect shown by them to residents. Key to improving NA care is reorienting and retaining competent, nurturing NAs. Although high turnover in this population is still a problem industry-wide including BRI, the agency has increased wages to become more competitive, offered more training on sensitivity in how care is provided, and increased permanent assignments on the units to try to create ongoing relationships between staff and residents. In addition, the research division has undertaken a number of studies to examine issues of respect between NAs, the residents, and their families. As a result of these studies, 289 NAs, 133 family members, and 114 residents have been interviewed from various nursing homes in the area to identify factors related to job satisfaction among the NAs and resident and family satisfaction with care (Ejaz, Noelker, Schur, Whitlatch, & Looman, in review; Noelker, Schur, Looman, Ejaz, & Whitlatch, in revision; Schur, Noelker, Looman, Whitlatch, & Ejaz, 1998; Whitlatch, Schur, Noelker, Ejaz, & Looman, in revision).

Some of the negative findings identified in these studies included issues of racial discrimination (treating NAs as servants), misunderstandings of the workload of NAs, the guilt faced by family members about institutionalizing their relative, and their lack of knowledge as to what to do when they visit. The positive findings included families' appreciating the work that nurse assistants do for residents, the bond that is created between NAs and residents, and the NAs' empathy with the family members' situation (Looman, Noelker, Schur, Whitlatch, & Ejaz, 1997).

In addition, a series of focus groups were conducted by BRI staff with NAs and also with their supervisors to specify ways to improve their initial education, orientation to the job, continuing education, recognition programs, and supervision. Some areas consistently identified for improvement were fostering teamwork, flattening the hierarchy, greater respect for staff, and better staffing (also stated by Lustbader, chapter 9). Such efforts have had a tremendous impact on improving the quality of care for consumers of our nursing home services, thereby improving their overall quality of life.

ASSESSING CONSUMER SATISFACTION IN BRI'S COMMUNITY SERVICES DIVISION (CSD)

Historical Trends in the Industry

The historical movement to address consumer satisfaction with community services can be seen from the early 1970s, when the Older Americans Act required consumer participation in the development of state or area planning. Further, during the 1970s, the independent living movement of younger disabled adults also stressed the importance of consumers having the right to hire or fire formal caregivers. In the 1990s, expert panels making recommendations for quality home care concluded that consumers must participate in defining and evaluating quality (Kane, Illston, Eustis, & Kane, 1991; Riley, 1989).

Despite such trends, the movement to assess satisfaction with home- and community- based care (HCB) has been slow. This is due to a variety of reasons including the fact that the consumers of HCB services are typically persons of advanced age with chronic illnesses, suffer from multiple disabilities, and are low income (Smith & Longino, 1995). As such, their service needs may be far-ranging, including health monitoring, personal care, social services, and daily money management. Measuring consumer satisfaction in light of consumers' functional limitations and other deficits as well as the diversity of services provided can be difficult (DiMatteo & Hayes, 1980). In addition, relationships between formal caregivers and consumers who are socially isolated may become so personal and interdependent that any objective assessment of service delivery is severely compromised. Besides the limitations related to client characteristics, governmental regulations and funding cuts have resulted in a shortage of service providers with the closing of home health agencies nationwide leaving consumers with fewer choices ("More HHAs To Close," 1999).

Despite the problems faced in assessing satisfaction with HCB services, concerns about consumer satisfaction are widespread and the commitment to client autonomy and self-determination ensure a continuing investigation of service satisfaction. Kane (1995, p. 7) suggests that "only the individuals receiving home care are able to comment on whether. . . . they are comfortable when bathed and the water temperature suits them, whether the cleaning is done to their satisfaction or whether the comportment of home-care personnel is satisfactory." Toward that end, the monitoring of consumer satisfaction among HCB clients requires an approach that is consumer-sensitive and varied. Its function should be perceived as empowering consumers and as essential to improving the operations of service providers.

BRI's Community Services Division Formalizes
the Assessment of Client Satisfaction

Since its early days of service delivery, BRI conducted assessments of client satisfaction, and in the early 1990s began to formalize the process using a multifaceted approach. Although each method used has its advantages and limitations, collectively they provide an effective means for understanding consumer preferences and concerns as well as for identifying areas of needed change in program design or implementation.

CSD offers numerous types of services to older people, their families, and their caregivers, including social services, nursing, adult day care, housekeeping, personal care, respite, senior companion, transportation, and shopping. Services are arranged by the social worker or nurse assigned to the case, who acts as both assessor and case manager. In this context, she/he helps the client to identify service needs and then select appropriate resources to address these needs. Services not available through CSD but needed by the client are obtained through referral to other community agencies.

CSD case managed services are offered to persons 60 and over who reside in Cuyahoga County, Ohio, with priority given to individuals who are vulnerable or disadvantaged. The typical service recipient is a woman over age 75 with multiple chronic illnesses and functional incapacities. She is low income, lives in Cleveland's inner city, and has minimal family support. Approximately 1,600 clients were served in 1999 by CSD using agency endowment funds, grants, gifts, and third-party reimbursement under Medicare, Medicaid, or private insurance.

Measuring consumer satisfaction at CSD is a function of the Quality Improvement (QI) Council which has as its goal to assess quality of care and make recommendations for change. This is accomplished through four major activities: 1) overseeing the annual QI plan; 2) setting goals and priorities for QI; 3) insuring appropriate staff education and support for QI; and 4) selecting aspects of care for monitoring (Schweikhart & Strasser, 1994). The QI Council at CSD meets regularly throughout the year, is chaired by the CSD Director, and is comprised of administrative and clinical staff, consumer representatives, and a member of the agency Board of Trustees. In addition, a quarterly report of QI activities is made to the Board's Operations Committee, with an annual summary given to both the Board as a whole and select funders.

The methods used to ascertain consumer satisfaction in CSD reflect several assumptions:

- Clients must be given sufficient opportunity to offer their opinions about services received.

- In order to be comprehensive consumer satisfaction measures must be administered frequently, be representative of diverse forms, and applied objectively in a manner that respects client function and ability.
- There can be no adverse consequence for negative opinions expressed by clients.
- Opinions offered by clients must be given serious consideration for program development and operations improvement.
- Clients who refuse to offer an opinion must be respected in that decision.

The four primary methods used by CSD for determining consumer satisfaction with services are: 1) client response cards; 2) consumer forums; 3) telephone surveys of clients; and 4) consumer representation on advisory councils. Besides the four primary methods, consumer satisfaction with CSD services is ascertained through periodic special studies and the formal client complaint or grievance process.

Self-addressed, stamped response cards are given to clients by case managers at their initial and annual assessments and include space for clients to comment either anonymously or by name about services received. Their advantages are that clients can provide any manner of comment, they are inexpensive to use, and clients control when they are used. Their disadvantages are that they are easily lost or misplaced, the client must be capable of reading and writing, and specific dimensions of service provision cannot be examined. As an example of how this method led to service improvement, billing statements were reformatted based on clients' written complaints about a change in billing format that made them more difficult to read.

Annually, all clients are invited to consumer forums. Those wishing to attend are provided with transportation, if needed. The forums, which include refreshments and entertainment or education, provide staff with opportunities to describe QI procedures and for clients to voice their opinions about services and their delivery. The advantages of the forums are that clients who are unable to read or write can attend, promoting interaction between clients and program managers, and the casual atmosphere fosters free expression for comment. Their disadvantages are that homebound clients cannot attend, clients must be comfortable speaking in public, they are more costly in terms of time and resources, and they do not confer anonymity, thus clients may fear reprisals. As an example of how this method led to service improvement was when a client complained that he was not notified that he was assigned to a different case manager, CSD policies were changed to ensure that all clients are given advance, written notification of any change in staff.

The telephone survey method involves structured telephone interviews with clients by the QI coordinator to explore specific dimensions of care. Clients who are surveyed every quarter include all those who no longer receive services and a random sample of 5% of the current client population. The advantages of this method are that it consistently yields information on specific dimensions of services, probes can be used to elicit details, and clients who no longer receive services can be candid without fear of reprisals. The disadvantages are that not all clients have telephones or can use them, some are reluctant to respond to phone surveys, and this method is dependent on the skills of the interviewer to establish rapport quickly, which is often difficult if clients have mental health or other problems. Here is an example of how this method led to service improvment. Two clients had complained that they were deprived of homemaker services once they no longer had a need for case management. Therefore, a change was made to enable paraprofessional services to be provided without professional oversight in certain select cases.

The fourth method, inclusion of consumer representatives on all CSD advisory councils, ensures that the clients' perspectives on program planning, policy development, operations, and community outreach are elicited. The advantages are that clients can comment in a broader context, staff hear their perspective and can explore it in detail, and it gives staff a different perspective of clients as leaders and not simply service recipients. The disadvantages are that only some clients are capable of serving and their perspective may not be representative, only a limited number can participate, and there is a tendency to select the same clients to serve on the advisory councils, thereby limiting the richness of available perspectives. As an example of how this method led to service improvement, the caregiver of an Adult Day Program participant requested expanded hours of program operation. Thus, the program was opened an hour earlier and closed a half-hour later.

In addition to the above four methods, CSD also has a formal client complaint and grievance process that in part reflects the requirements of funding and regulatory sources. Clients who are dissatisfied with services have the opportunity to call or write expressing their concerns. If they call, the concerns are handled as complaints that are logged, investigated, and resolved, if possible. If the concerns are expressed in writing, they become grievances and follow a formal process of review and handling that is linked hierarchically within the organization and dealt with in a timely manner. Complaints can be received and handled by any CSD staff. Grievances are initially the responsibility of the Client's Rights Officer who also is the QI coordinator. Complaint logs and grievances are compiled quarterly for review by the CSD director and the QI Council.

Like the other consumer satisfaction methods employed by CSD, client complaints and grievances have brought about changes in policy and practice that, in turn, have helped improve the quality of life for consumers. For instance, several CSD clients complained that there was no continuity in service between CSD and BRI's nursing home. This was evidenced by the infrequent and complicated admission of a CSD client into the nursing home. Consequently, staff of the two BRI divisions met and developed processes and procedures to improve client placement.

Lessons Learned From Conducting Consumer Satisfaction at CSD

CSD has found that with varied services, funders, and client characteristics, multiple and diverse methods are needed to adequately measure consumer satisfaction. No single method captures the attention, responds to the abilities, and is sensitive to the comfort level of all clients. Most methods also require considerable staff time to implement. Those that do not, such as the client response cards or consumer representation on advisory councils, typically tap the opinions and comments of only a small number of respondents. Nonetheless, comments received through these methods have often revealed critical aspects of service delivery and therefore, have resulted in important changes at CSD.

CONCLUSIONS AND FUTURE DIRECTIONS FOR ASSESSING CONSUMER SATISFACTION AT BRI

Although BRI staff believe that significant progress has been made in our effort to examine consumer satisfaction, there are numerous limitations. One of these includes low response rates and hence potential for biased results because people who do not respond to surveys may have systematic differences in their opinions than those who do. Other limitations include the use of different approaches by the two divisions making cross-division comparisons difficult, the limited extent to which multivariate analyses can be conducted because of small sample sizes, and the inability to benchmark results with those from similar organizations. However, the latter is changing because BRI as a member of HealthRays Alliance, which is an alliance of 23 long-term care facilities, has partnered with other facilities to have an outside consultant conduct satisfaction surveys for members. BRI research staff are serving a key role in the quality committee of the HealthRays Alliance and are working closely with the consultant to help design and pretest the consumer satisfaction tools for nursing home residents, their families and sub-acute clients. The advantage to BRI will be the ability to benchmark our nursing home consumer satisfaction survey results with the aggregate results of other facilities. Similarly, the HealthRays Alliance membership also contracts with an outside consulting firm to use the MDS data on long-term care residents to develop outcome indicators of quality of care that also benchmark each nursing home against the others in the alliance. Such approaches will, perhaps, help identify industry-wide strengths and limitations in northeast Ohio. The alliance membership has also agreed to develop best practice models from those facilities that have higher than average satisfaction levels in certain service and staff areas, and better quality of care outcomes, thereby providing pertinent information to implement quality improvement projects throughout the alliance.

BRI is also concerned with linking its objective measures of quality (those that are required by funding agencies such as the MDS and OASIS) and the subjective evaluations of care as evidenced in our consumer satisfaction surveys. Hence a goal is to try to connect these different data sets in the future in order to have a more complete picture of quality, thereby enacting Lawton's (1991) belief that quality must be assessed by both objective and subjective measures. For example, some measures in the MDS do lend themselves to quality of life issues, such as depression, involvement in activities, social engagement, dignity, and privacy and could potentially be linked with nursing home residents' satisfaction survey data on similar items or on global measures of satisfaction. Similarly, HCB satisfaction survey data may be linked to the more objective measures in the OASIS. Such links will help glean better information on quality of care and quality of life from the current fragmented measures of state-mandated assessments of quality and the subjective assessments that we have historically espoused.

In conclusion, from its early beginnings, BRI accepted the challenge not merely to provide "material relief" to its clients, but to free their "minds from anxiety and worry." Almost 60 years ago, its first Executive Director expressed a commitment to provide care based on "what we had learned older people wanted, not what we thought they wanted or should have." In the continuing quest to respect such values, BRI staff is committed to facing newer challenges in the 21st century. One such challenge posed by Zimmerman and Bowers (2000) is that unless satisfaction surveys are prepared to take on a more expanded role, their utility will be reduced and their relevance heavily compromised. BRI recognizes that substantial work is needed on both conceptual and methodological arenas in the attempt to link the objective and subjective measures of quality, thereby helping to advance the integration of measures of quality of life and quality of care in a broader, more comprehensive manner.

REFERENCES

Aharony, L., & Strasser, S. (1993). Patient satisfaction: What we know about and what we still need to explore. *Medicare Care Review, 50*(1), 352–382.

The Benjamin Rose Institute (1998, October). *Serving Cleveland's elderly: A history of the Benjamin Rose Institute* [Brochure]. The Benjamin Rose Institute, Cleveland, OH: Author.

Brannon, D., Cohn, M., & Smyer, M. (1990). Caregiving at work: How nurses aides rate it. *Journal of Long Term Care Administration, 181,* 10–14.

Cella, M., Gabay, M., Teitalbaum, M., Walker, A., & Kramer, A. (1996). *Evaluation of the long-term care survey process: Final report.* Cambridge, MA: Abt Associates.

DeVellis, R. F. (1991). *Scale development: Theory and applications.* Newbury Park, CA: Sage.

DiMatteo, M. R., & Hayes, R. (1980). The significance of patients' perceptions of physician conduct: A study of patient satisfaction in a family practice center. *Journal of Community Health, 6,* 18.

Duncan, M. T., & Morgan, D. L. (1994). Sharing the caring: Family caregivers' views of their relationships with nursing home staff. *Gerontologist, 34*(2), 235–244.

Ejaz, F. K. (2000). An overview of the process of conducting consumer satisfaction surveys in nursing facilities. In J. Cohen-Mansfield, F. K. Ejaz, & P. Werner (Eds.), *Satisfaction surveys in long-term care,* 137–165. New York: Springer Publishing.

Ejaz, F. K., Noelker, L. S., Schur, D., Whitlatch, C. J., & Looman, W. (in review). Predictors of family satisfaction with care in nursing facilities. *Gerontologist.*

Heiselman, T., & Noelker, L. S. (1991). Enhancing mutual respect between nursing assistants, residents and their families. *Gerontologist, 31,* 552–555.

Institute of Medicine, Committee on Nursing Home Regulation (1986). *Improving the quality of care in nursing homes.* Washington, DC: National Academic Press.

Kane, R. K. (1995, July/August). The quality conundrum in home care. *Aging Today,* 7–8.

Kane, R. A., Illston, L. H., Eustis, N. N., & Kane, R. L. (1991). *Quality of home care: Concept and measurement.* Minneapolis: School of Public Health, University of Minnesota.

Kleinsorge, I. K., & Koenig, H. F. (1991). The silent customers: Measuring customer satisfaction in nursing homes. *Journal of Health Care Marketing, 11*(4), 2–13.

La Monica, E., Oberst, M. T., Madea, A. R., & Olf, R. M. (1986). Development of a patient satisfaction scale. *Research in Nursing and Health, 9,* 43–50.

Lavizzo-Mourey, R. J., Zinn, J., & Taylor, L. (1992). Ability of surrogates to represent satisfaction of nursing home residents with quality of care. *American Geriatrics Society, 40,* 39–47.

Lawton, P. M. (1991). A multidimensional view of quality of life in frail elders. In Birren, J. E., Lubben, J. E., Rowe, J. C., & Deutchman, D. E. (Eds.), *The concept and measurement of quality of life in the frail elderly* (pp. 3–23). San Diego: Academic Press.

Looman, W. J., Noelker, L. S., Schur, D., Whitlatch, C. J., & Ejaz, F. K. (1997). Nursing assistants caring for dementia residents in nursing homes: The family's perspective on the high quality of care. *American Journal of Alzheimer's Disease,* *12*(5).

More HHAs to close June 1, as cost reports come due (1999, April 19). *Home HealthLine,* 3–4.

National Citizens' Coalition for Nursing Home Reform (1985). *A consumer perspective: The residents' point of view.* Washington, DC: Author.

Noelker, L. S., Ejaz, F. K., & Schur, D. (2000). Use of satisfaction surveys: Results from research in Ohio nursing homes. In J. Cohen-Mansfield, F. K. Ejaz, & P. Werner (Eds.), *Satisfaction surveys in long term care.* New York: Springer Publishing Co.

Noelker, L. S., Schur, D., Looman, W., Ejaz, F. K., & Whitlatch, C. J. (In revision). Impact of stress and support on nursing assistants' satisfaction with supervision. *Journal of Applied Gerontology.*

Riley, P. A. (1989). *Developing consumer centered quality assurance strategies for home care.* South Portland, ME: Human Services Development Institute, University of Southern Maine.

Schur, D., Noelker, L. S., Looman, W., Whitlatch, C. J., & Ejaz, F. K. (1998, Jan/Feb). 4 steps to more committed nursing assistants. *Balance, 2*(1), 29–32.

Schweikhart, S. B., & Strasser, S. (1994). The effective use of patient satisfaction data. *Topics in Health Information Management, 15*(2), 49–60.

Shaughnessy P., Crisler, K., Schlenker, R., & Hittle, D. (1998, June). Oasis: The next 10 years. *Caring magazine,* 32–42.

Smith, M. H., & Longino, C. F., Jr. (1995). People using long-term care services. In Z. Harel & R. E. Dunkle (Eds.), *Matching people with services in long-term care* (pp. 25–47). New York: Springer Publishing Co.

Spalding, J. & Frank, B. W. (1985, July). Quality care from the residents' point of view. *American Health Care Association Journal,* 3–7.

Spector, P. E. (1992). *Summated rating scale construction: An introduction* (Series/ Number 07–082). Newbury Park, CA: Sage.

Stewart, A. L., & Ware, J. E. Jr. (Eds.) (1992). *Measuring functioning and well-being.* Durham, NC: Duke University Press.

Strasser, S., Schweikhart, S. B., Welch, G. E., & Burge, J. C. (1995). Satisfaction with medical care: It's easier to please patients than their family members and friends. *Journal of Health Care Marketing, 15*(3).

Whitlatch, C. J., Schur, D., Noelker, L. S., Ejaz, F. K., & Looman, W. J. (in revision). The stress process of family caregiving in institutional settings. *Gerontologist.*

Zimmerman, D. R., & Bowers, B. J. (2000). Satisfaction surveys and other sources of information on quality of long-term care. In J. Cohen-Mansfield, F. K. Ejaz, & P. Werner (Eds.), *Satisfaction surveys in long term care.* New York: Springer Publishing Co.

Zimmerman, D. R., Karen, S. L., Arling, G., Clark, B. R., Collins, T., Ross, R., & Sainfort, F. (1995). Development and testing of nursing home quality indicators. *Health Care Financing Review, 16*(4) 107–127.

12

Quality of Care and Quality of Life for Isolated Elderly

Zev Harel
Georgia J. Anetzberger

This chapter provides an overview of the characteristics, needs, and service efforts to meet the basic needs of a most vulnerable segment of the older population, the isolated elderly. Concern for the care and life experiences of isolated elderly has evolved in recent decades in response to an increase in vulnerability on the part of the growing numbers of older and disabled persons. Professional concerns, to date, have focused primarily on locating and serving isolated elders; their quality of care and quality of life have received little attention. Isolated older persons, like all isolated persons, are a heterogeneous group. Isolated older persons may include those persons that have never married, or may be widowed, childless, and/or lacking family ties. The state of isolation may be chosen by the individual person or be a consequence of social, organizational, or societal factors (Chappell & Badger, 1989; Rathbone-McCuan & Hashimi, 1982).

Public concern about the isolated elderly began at mid-twentieth century, coinciding with three increasingly widespread phenomena in the United States: First, more and more elderly persons resided outside of extended family households or institutions (Fisher, 1978). Second, a larger number of the elderly lived alone (Michael, Fuchs, & Scott, 1980). Third, younger families moved away from their hometowns in search of economic opportunities, leaving elderly members with seemingly diminished informal support (Litwak, 1960). In and of themselves, however, none of these phenomena foster isolation. Alternative living arrangements can be found, surrogate families formed, and supportive networks developed. Isolation results when the elderly experience inadequate social contact or support and an inability to alter the situation themselves.

In the applied gerontological literature, empirical evidence clearly indicates that isolated elderly who are not integrated into caring networks of related others fare poorly in their mental health and psychological well-being. In the mid-seventies, Lowenthal (1964) and Bennett (1980) documented the adverse mental health consequences of social isolation among the elderly. Rathbone-McCuan and Hashimi (1982) provided an overview of the population groups comprising the isolated elderly and offered direction for practice on their behalf.

A review of related literature reveals that critical challenges faced by aging persons and their family members entail the finding and securing of adequate, effective, and quality care arrangements and the ability to pay for the cost of care (Harel & Dunkle, 1995). For the isolated vulnerable elderly, this challenge is greater. They lack the ability to adequately care for themselves or seek the assistance they need, they are likely not to have the care of an informal support system, and many among them lack needed financial resources. For these reasons, it is the professional community that is faced, first, with the burden and challenge to find them and, second, to secure on their behalf needed resources and services for their survival and security. Unfortunately, legislative initiatives by elected officials at the national and state levels and administrative actions, taken by public officials at the local and state levels, are often guided by concerns about how to curtail rising costs and expenditures for benefits and services rather than expand the resources and services which vulnerable older persons need.

Health and social work professionals have been focusing their efforts on the development of responsive services for all aged in an environment of resource scarcity. They have provided direction for the development of home- and community-based service alternatives for all vulnerable aged, including the isolated elderly, with the general goal of aiding their efforts to maintain as dignified and secure existence as possible (Harel & Dunkle, 1995; Levande, Bowden, & Mollema, 1987). Even though there has been a considerable increase in service availability in recent years, the informal helping networks provide more than 80% of the care for all aged residing in the community (Brody, 1990; Harel & Noelker, 1995). For these reasons, developing innovative approaches in service delivery to this vulnerable segment of the aged population will continue to be of utmost importance. To be effective, these approaches must have the ability to clearly define and access the isolated elderly as well as assure the systematic planning and delivery of quality of care and ongoing evaluation of service delivery effectiveness.

This chapter offers a review and discussion of critical issues in long-term care services needed and/or used by isolated elderly. It reviews, first, defining elements of social isolation in the elderly, discerning between four terms of importance to this chapter: older persons living alone, a demographic term; the socially isolated aged, a sociological term; the lonely aged, a psychological term; and the vulnerable isolated elderly, a professional term in the fields of health and social services. Second, it reviews factors which predispose and/or contribute to the isolation/loneliness of the aged, the consequences of social isolation among the elderly, and the care and services needed to assure the survival, basic security, and dignified quality of life for this segment of the elderly population. Third, current arrangements in service delivery aimed at meeting the needs of isolated aged are reviewed. In the final section, a number of suggestions are advanced, which in the authors' view are needed for the refinement and improvement of the quality of care and services to this most vulnerable segment of the aged population.

THE VULNERABLE ISOLATED ELDERLY

Vulnerability, by definition, entails being at risk. While everyone throughout life is at risk to various contingencies, in later life, one becomes significantly more vulnerable to relocation, institutionalization, and death because of increased morbidity, ill health, injury, acute and chronic illness, impairment or disability (Harel & Noelker, 1995; Townsend & Harel, 1990). Severely vulnerable elderly are considered to be those in poor health and functional status with limitations and deterioration in social, psychological, and physical functioning (Reed, 1990). This severe state of vulnerability may be exacerbated by limitations in economic, social, and psychological resources and by environmentally hazardous living situations (Harel & Harel, 1995; Harel & Noelker, 1995). All isolated elderly are vulnerable; however, the severely vulnerable isolated elderly are at special risk. They are defined as isolated older persons with one or more serious illnesses, chronic conditions, functional limitations, and/or cognitive impairments who do not have the benefit of needed personal, social, and environmental resources and who, on their own, cannot meet their basic needs. They are likely to experience serious physical and mental health problems along with declining functional competence—necessitating greater dependence on others for provision of their basic needs.

In the absence of informal caregivers, service providers are called upon to assure their survival and for the gratification of their basic needs. Furthermore, their severe vulnerability may be exacerbated by personal, social and organizational factors, and environmental hazards. Consideration of social isolation in the elderly may be aided by empirical studies on the elderly who live alone, elderly living in transient unstable environments, the homeless, elderly veterans and the abused, neglected and exploited elderly (Anetzberger, 1995; Chappell & Badger, 1989; Damron-Rodriguez & Cantrell, 1995; Rathbone-McCuan & Hashimi, 1982; Rubinstein, 1995; Rubinstein, Kilbride, & Nagy, 1992).

A review of demographic characteristics of the aged reveals that about 30% among the noninstitutionalized aged lived alone in 1994, the percentage being considerably higher for those in the higher age groups and among women. In the general aged population, elderly men are twice as likely to be married and to live in a two or more person household than women (AARP, 1999). Among elderly living alone, there are clear gender differences. A higher fraction among older men who live alone are likely to have never been married. Women, on the other hand, because of their higher life expectancy and earlier widowhood, are more likely to live alone for longer time duration, after having been married for a significant number of years.

Aging is associated with a progressive, unidirectional, and irreversible set of losses, including declining health and functional status, and reduced resources which, in turn, contribute progressively to vulnerability and severe vulnerability among the elderly (Harel & Noelker, 1995; Townsend & Harel, 1990). As indicated elsewhere (Harel & Noelker, 1995), about 20% of the aged are among the severely vulnerable aged at any point in time. About 5% of the aged, or one of four of the severely vulnerable older persons, are likely to be residing in an institutional setting on any given day. For every person in an institution, however, there are more than two persons in the community, some of whom are homebound in their own dwelling units or in the home of a family member or friend (Doty, Liu, & Weiner, 1985). The remaining 3% to 4% percent include those in various semiprotected and unprotected environmental settings such as assisted living, board and care homes, foster care, single-room occupancy (SRO) hotel rooms, hazardous living situations, and those that are homeless (Harel & Dunkle, 1995). Isolated elderly can be found in institutional settings and in the community. Among those residing in the community, many are likely to live in personally or environmentally secure places while some may be subject to various hazards.

The isolated elderly need to be seen, therefore, on a continuum ranging from the slightly vulnerable, at lesser risk, to the severely vulnerable, at the greatest risk. The least vulnerable are those aged who are in reasonably good health, residing alone in various living situations, with the benefit of a caring social network. At the other end of the continuum are those isolated elderly who experience poor health and functional status, live alone without the benefit of caring others, and have unsuitable and/or environmentally hazardous living environments.

The isolated elderly living alone are at any time in a potential and/or active state of progressive decline, requiring preventive measures first, followed by increasing need for supportive attention, assistance, and care and, finally, protective environments, in the most vulnerable stages of their lives. While still in the community, vulnerable isolated elderly may be faced with involuntary changes in living arrangements including, for a significant fraction, the need for nursing home placement. Lastly, they are at greater risk of death, especially in the absence of needed attention, assistance, and access to adequate health care.

The vulnerable isolated elderly, in this view, include both those living alone without adequate social contacts and those who feel lonely. The severely vulnerable isolated elderly include those who live alone and feel lonely, those who reside alone in unsuitable and hazardous living environments, and the homeless who have poor health and functional status with limited and/or no resources who, on their own, cannot meet their basic needs. For these reasons, it is important to understand in professional practice the characteristics and needs of different groups of isolated elderly (see Table 12.1): a) those who live alone with limitations in social and economic resources; b) those who reside in unsuitable and/or hazardous environments, including the homeless; c) the physically and functionally frail isolated aged; d) the mentally impaired aged, and e) the isolated elderly with multiple impairments and limitations.

Contributory Factors to Social Isolation

Factors which predispose and/or are conducive to isolation in old age include genetic predisposition, lifestyle characteristics, socio-demographic and socioeconomic status on the personal level; social factors such as the absence of adequate social contacts, social resources and social support; organizational forces, like barriers that make access to services difficult; and societal factors such as economic policies and social programs that provide inadequate benefits and funding for needed services (Harel & Noelker, 1995; Townsend & Harel, 1990).

The consequences of severe vulnerability among isolated elderly include the inability to meet, on their own, their basic needs; the necessity to be dependent on others for survival and basic security, defining elements of quality of life for many among them; the possible need for a protective living environment; and, sometimes, untimely death (see Table 12.2). It is important that service agencies have the resources to address the needs of these aged.

Rathbone-McCuan and Hashimi (1982) suggest that elderly persons become isolated because of "situations or events that seem to interfere with the ability of an elder to maintain personal integrity and social involvement" (p. 11). Isolators can be physical (e.g., sensory loss), psychological

TABLE 12.1   Vulnerable and Severely Vulnerable Isolated Elderly

Elderly population		
Isolated	*Vulnerable*	*Severely vulnerable*
• Live alone • Have no social resources	• Are socially isolated • Have limited social and economic resources • Feel lonely • Face environmental hazards	• Cannot meet basic needs • Are homeless • Have poor health and functional status • Have poor cognitive and mental health • Have a configuration of the above conditions

(e.g., mental illness), economic (e.g., inadequate income), or social (e.g., death of family or friends). Their impact is felt when the elderly person is unable to resolve problems or compensate losses resulting from the isolators. It is compounded when isolation provides an additional barrier to receipt of needed help. Rathbone-McCuan and Hashimi (1982) conceptualize the resources required by isolated elderly persons across three systems—neighborhood, social, or self-help groups; age-specific community agencies; and problem-specific agencies—with problems not solved in informal groups being referred to more formal structures.

Case Examples

The following are but a few examples of isolated elderly, ranging from those who are vulnerable to those in states of severe vulnerability. They illustrate the characteristics of isolated elderly as actual or potential service consumers, including their need for attention, assistance, and care. Isolated elders may come to the attention of service agencies, occasionally by self-referral but, most frequently, by referral from agencies or calls from concerned neighbors and/or public service workers.

Mrs. B. characterizes a segment of isolated widowed elderly women who, in addition to declining health and some functional limitations, feels very lonely and is severely depressed. She often does not feel inclined to eat or to care for herself and for her household. Since she has recently relocated to a new community, following the death of her husband, she has very few social contacts and social relations.

> Mrs. B., a 76-year-old European American widow, lives alone in a suburban community in a large urban area. She was referred by a concerned out-of-town son to a geriatric assessment unit of a local hospital. Following evaluation, the

TABLE 12.2 Severe Isolation: Determinants, Status, and Consequences

Determinants	Status	Consequences

• Personal
Genetics
Family history
Lifestyle
Health practices
Socio-demographic
   characteristics
Socio-economic status
	• Decline
	• Deterioration
	• Illnesses
	• Disabilities
	• Functional limitations
	• Personal incompetence
		• Place-bound
		• Cannot meet on their
		  own survival and
		  security needs
		• Dependence on others
		  for care and service
		• Relocation
		• Institutional placement
		• Death

• Social Social network Social support		
• Organizational Access/barriers Strategies Services Programs		
• Societal Policies Programs		

hospital social worker called a local agency that offers mental health services to the elderly. Mrs. B. relocated to this area, following the death of her husband, to be near her only son's family. Her son, however, recently moved away and Mrs. B. became depressed and felt very lonely. She did not feel up to caring for herself or for her home. She spent much time in bed, had no energy and rarely ventured from her apartment. Because her only son's family was at a considerable distance, there was concern on the part of the hospital social worker about how Mrs. B. would manage on her own in her state of depression and severe sense of loneliness.

Mrs. S. characterizes a segment of the isolated widowed elderly women who, in addition to declining health and functional status, also experienced declining mental health and psychological functioning. Because of these limitations, she no longer feels competent to carry out necessary household management activities or to reach out to neighbors and maintain needed social contacts.

Mrs. S., an 82-year-old African American widow, lives alone in a subsidized apartment building in a large urban area. She was referred by the social worker of the psychiatric unit of a local hospital at the time of discharge, following admission for a major depressive episode. Prior to admission, Mrs. S. had been spending most of her time in bed. A reduced appetite had yielded a 20-pound weight loss, leading to her current weight of less than 100 pounds. Having very little energy, she had rarely ventured from her apartment. She indicated that she had no support system, not even acquaintances she could approach in time of need in her building. There was concern on the part of the hospital social worker about how she would manage on her own in her apartment.

Mrs. D. and *Mrs. G.* illustrate another segment of the isolated widowed elderly women. This group experiences declining functional status, including cognitive impairment which, in turn, leads to personally endangering behaviors and an inability to carry out necessary personal care and household management tasks.

Mrs. D., an 88-year-old widow, living alone in her own home, was experiencing increasing degrees of confusion and memory loss. Her cognitive decline resulted in her having difficulty attending to errands and making proper decisions. She was hoarding items resulting in her once spacious rooms becoming narrow passageways. Changes in her judgment and reasoning resulted in her purchase of many unneeded items, inability to use personal transportation, and unwillingness to use public transportation. She reported having no friends or support group and refused to have contact with an out-of-town son.

Mrs. G. is an 88-year-old widow who lives alone in a high-rise apartment and suffers from hypertension and the residuals of stroke. She gets around using a wheelchair, but needs assistance with most daily living tasks and is fiercely independent. Although she once was active in community and social groups, the stroke left her unable to get out much without tiring. It also made communication frustrating except for the simplest of thoughts. Mrs. G. has outlived most of her family and friends. All that remains is a cousin, who handles crises and comes monthly to shop and do errands. Unfortunately, it isn't enough.

Ms. C. characterizes a segment of the isolated never married elderly women who, in various stages of life depended on assistance from others to meet basic needs. When her brother, who was her caregiver, died, she no longer was able to carry out personal care and household management tasks necessary for continued community residence. The consequence of this state of being required the finding of adequate relocation options.

Ms. C., an 85-year-old single woman, had lived her entire life with her parents and bachelor brother in an isolated world. After the death of their parents, the brother became the caregiver in almost every aspect of their lives.

When he died suddenly, Ms. C. had to have immediate placement in a nursing home due to physical frailty and the absence of family or friends.

Mr. P. is an example of a segment of isolated older men in deteriorating living situations. His drinking episodes, which become more frequent with time, lead him to engage in personally endangering activities.

Mr. P., a 75-year-old African American male, was referred to a service agency by a public utility worker after several calls for help by Mr. P. to the utility company. Mr. P. experiences poor ambulation, inadequate hygiene, extreme financial problems, forgetfulness, and complicated grief in a solitary community residence. He is a heavy drinker and reports poor relations with a sister.

Mr. R. illustrates the lifestyle and behaviors of the mentally impaired homeless person who, with his health impairment episode becomes a nuisance to those who previously tolerated his presence and, consequently, finds himself in a life-threatening situation.

Mr. R. is a World War II veteran who has used the premises of an urban industrial complex for his living environment. For years, those working at the complex tolerated his odd behaviors and provided him occasionally with food and money. Following a severe illness which included hospitalization, his poor hygiene and threats towards others became unacceptable to those in the complex. An agency was called to help a situation which was perceived by the referral source as impossible and dangerous to Mr. R.

These are but a few case examples that offer a glimpse into the lives and experiences of isolated elderly, and the challenges they pose for planning and service delivery. It is obvious that each group of isolated elderly requires different resources and program and intervention strategies.

CARE AND SERVICE NEEDS OF ISOLATED ELDERLY

There are clear indications that difficulties performing personal care and household management activities increase dramatically with age (Kane & Kane, 1987; Reed, 1990). Limitations in the performance of activities of daily living are very high among the severely vulnerable aged and are precursors to institutionalization and a defining element of eligibility (Branch & Jette, 1982). Functionally impaired older persons cannot, on their own, meet their basic needs, and therefore, are not able to live minimally secure and dignified lives without assistance or services (Kane &

Kane, 1987). They require ongoing attention and assistance which are the salient elements of long-term care services. States of chronic illnesses/ conditions require a continuum of care that may include a wide spectrum of home- and community-based as well as institutional long-term care services. The concept of continuum of care also recognizes the need for and the importance of an informal social support system. The goal of a system of long-term care for the elderly, including the isolated elderly, ought to be the improvement and maintenance of security and quality of life (Brody, 1990; Harel & Dunkle, 1995; Kane & Kane, 1987; O'Brien & Flannery, 1997).

There are considerable variations in the older population's need for and utilization of health and social services. Evidence indicates that service utilization is affected by a number of factors, in addition to health impairment and functional limitations. These include structural arrangements and barriers in service delivery; values, attitudes, and actions of human service professionals; and the needs, knowledge, access, attitudes, and actions of the aged service consumers themselves and those of members of their informal support networks (Harel, Noelker, & Blake, 1985; Townsend & Harel, 1990).

Physical and mental limitations, coupled with lack of knowledge and/or needed service, may lead to and/or exacerbate physical and mental deterioration which, in turn, will lead to isolation. This isolation may be compounded by limitations in economic and social resources and poor physical environment, and may result in situations where older persons are likely to be homebound, without needed services—and will become candidates for death and/or institutionalization.

Severely vulnerable older persons who have adequate economic resources may purchase the services they need either in the community or in an institutional setting. Persons who are poor enough to qualify for Medicaid are most likely to be found in institutions and/or utilizing publicly available community-based health and social services. Vulnerable persons in need of services who are not poor enough to qualify for Medicaid and who are not rich enough to pay for needed services themselves, have very limited or no choices. In the case of the severely vulnerable isolated elderly, including those in unstable and hazardous living environments and the homeless, their survival and security is contingent on coming to the attention of service providers. Isolated elderly are likely to be among those who are unaware and/or lack access to the home and community-based services that may be available for their use. Service needs for this population have to be seen as requirements for care and organized arrangements that reduce the states of vulnerability and/or the factors that contribute to increased vulnerability on their part. Quality of care, in this view, represents the organized care and service arrangements that reduce and or delay states of vulnerability and aim to reduce and or delay the consequences of vulnerability on the part of isolated elderly persons.

CURRENT EFFORTS TO ASSURE QUALITY OF CARE FOR ISOLATED ELDERLY

Meeting the needs of the vulnerable and severely vulnerable isolated elderly requires a broad continuum of care and support, since many among them are unable, on their own, to provide for themselves. A significant number of these individuals are comparable to a segment of the nursing home population exhibiting a similar degree of vulnerability and functional impairment. However, either because of lack of access or because of choice, they continue to reside in their own living situations. Services have been developed by initiatives of the public and voluntary sectors and, to a lesser extent, by the private sector to enable them to live with some degree of security. The goals of these services may be seen for the most part as preventive and supportive; some of the services, however, also have a protective function, especially from the perspective of professional service providers.

Implicit in the professional objectives of home- and community-based services are: a) a commitment to the promotion of survival, security, and well-being for the aged; b) recognition of the need to enhance the coping resources of the aged person; and c) respect for the preferences of the service consumers and their caregivers (Harel & Harel, 1995). Maintaining these objectives, and the principles they reflect, is crucial to the viability of a service network which aims to meet the service needs of vulnerable isolated elderly.

The risks of severe vulnerability as shown in Table 12.2 include being place bound (morbidity), dependent on others for care and service, relocation, institutional placement, and death. Services have as their primary goal to reduce, to the extent possible, these risks and to foster security and quality of life for vulnerable and severely vulnerable isolated persons. In the process of service initiation and service delivery, the aim is to offer the care needed to reduce the effects of exacerbating factors and capitalize on those resources that are likely to slow down and/or moderate the progression of severe vulnerability, and hence contribute to quality of life.

Federal Initiatives

Public concern initially led communities to develop and test program models for bringing isolated elderly persons to the attention of service providers who could offer needed assistance. These local efforts were supported and then expanded by funding through the Older Americans Act passed in 1965. The Older Americans Act (OAA) was the first federal program to focus on home- and community-based services for elderly persons (National Academy on Aging, 1995). From its earliest days, OAA attempted to address the needs of isolated and vulnerable elderly, beginning in the mid-to-late 1960s with demonstration project grants to public and voluntary organizations for services like friendly visiting, telephone reassurance, homemaking, and senior centers (Binstock, 1991). This commitment to serving isolated and vulnerable elderly grew during the 1970s with amendments to OAA prioritizing access and in-home services and targeting service delivery to elderly persons in "greatest economic and social need." Amendments in 1984 defined social need as "caused by physical or mental disabilities as well as language and problems or discrimination towards racial or ethnic groups." Amendments in 1987 authorized new initiatives for vulnerable elderly persons, including those who were abused or neglected, mentally ill, or frail. The 1990s, however, have brought about a shift away from socially isolated and vulnerable elderly as an OAA focus, with Congress periodically attempting to remove targeting provisions and elder abuse programming (O'Shaughnessy, 1998).

The Social Services Block Grant, which replaced Title XX of the Social Security Act, is another important federal public program that provides home- and community-based services for isolated and vulnerable elderly persons. Title XX was established in 1974, to offer states funding for services which address the goals of self-support, independence, or protection. For isolated and vulnerable elderly persons, this meant the development and expansion of mostly traditional services through the public welfare system, like adult day care, protective services, transportation, and counseling. Title XX represented the first time the federal government made a commitment to fund social services to persons who were typically poor or near poor (Jansson, 1993). It was block granted in 1981 and cut thereafter under subsequent administrations, but more recently cuts have been less severe (Albright & Cohen, 1999).

At the same time that funding through the Older Americans Act and Social Services Block Grant has leveled or declined, Medicaid waivers serving vulnerable elderly persons have been authorized and grown (Applebaum & Austin, 1990). Of particular importance are the Home- and Community-Based Waiver (2176) and PACE (Program of All-Inclusive Care for the Elderly).

Waiver 2176 allows Medicaid to pay for services in the home and community at significantly less than the cost of nursing home care for low income, frail elderly persons considering nursing home care. Key components of the program are assessment, case management, and appropriate service mix. Waiver 2176 has become a key long-term care policy and program (Applebaum & Austin, 1990; Kane, Kane, & Ladd, 1998). It has been implemented throughout the country, expanding significantly from its origins as the National Channeling Demonstration. For example, Ohio, which was site for one of the demonstrations, has witnessed a growth of 200% from 1993 to 1996 in the caseload for PASSPORT (the name given Waiver 2176 locally), while the number of nursing home beds remained essentially the same (Ohio Association of Area Agencies on Aging, 1995). Not surprisingly, Medicaid funding showed significant increase during that period as well, although population projections for disabled elderly persons in the state suggested but a minimal increase (Mehdizadeh, Kunkel, Atchley, & Applebaum, 1990).

PACE is a Medicaid waiver program that allows the pooling of Medicaid and Medicare dollars for captivated managed care of frail elderly persons at risk of institutionalization. Modeled after On Lok in San Francisco, PACE is found in more than a dozen communities nationwide, but is enjoying growing popularity as a model for long-term care, especially in urban settings. Its appeal lies in the comprehensive array of services offered, focus on interdisciplinary intervention, and use of day health centers in most service delivery settings (Eleazer & Fretwell, 1999). Evaluation of PACE has shown it to be essentially cost-effective, with high levels of client satisfaction, while perhaps somewhat limited in growth potential and broad application of the model among nursing home eligible elderly persons (Kane, Illston, & Miller, 1992; Branch, Coulam, & Zimmerman, 1995; Clauser, Kidder, & Mauser, 1996; Eng, Pedulla, Eleazer, McCann, & Fox, 1997).

There is a built-in accountability structure for these federal programs to assure that eligibility requirements are met on the part of service consumers and that service providers deliver the services for which they are reimbursed. These programs can be utilized by severely vulnerable isolated older persons if they apply and are found eligible. The programs, however, do not have the resources needed for outreach efforts needed to identify and facilitate access to services for severely vulnerable isolated older persons. Furthermore they lack a structure to ascertain the quality of these services and their effect of the quality of life of service consumers.

State Initiatives

There are two primary public programs related to isolated or severely vulnerable elderly persons at the state level. The first type offers protection from harm for those at risk of or suffering from abuse or neglect. Adult protective services law has been enacted in 44 states (Tatara, 1995). The second type provides informed consent for those unable to give it because of disability. Conservatorship, guardianship, and various power of attorney laws are found in all states (Homel & Wood, 1990; Kapp & Bigot, 1985). Inherent in both types of state public policy is the intent to preserve the rights of elderly persons (and other adults), recognizing that these rights can be compromised because of isolation, vulnerability, or the stereotypic images associated with old age and disability.

Adult protective services evolved during the 1960s with a broad target population consisting of adults with mental or physical incapacities that limited their ability to protect themselves or their interests (U.S. Senate Special Committee on Aging, 1977). It began to focus on elder abuse (including self-neglect) during the late 1970s as interest in this social problem grew. At that time, states began passing adult protective services and elder abuse reporting laws, thereby codifying public concern about the maltreatment of elderly persons (Traxler, 1986).

Primarily the responsibility of public departments of social services at the local level (American Public Welfare Association & National Association of State Units on Aging, 1986), adult protective services have several important functions which are applicable in service delivery for the vulnerable isolated elderly, particularly those living in unstable and/or hazardous situations (Anetzberger, 1995). These include: a) receiving and investigating reports of abuse or neglect; b) assessing client need; c) providing or coordinating services to correct harm and reduce risk ; and d) seeking legal intervention for incapacitated victims or criminal penalty for perpetrators.

Many victims of abuse or neglect are isolated and vulnerable. In fact, the literature on elder abuse cites these as the most common risk factors for abuse occurrence on the part of victims (Byers & Lamanna, 1993; Johnson, 1991; Kosberg & Nahmiash, 1996; Pillemer, 1985; Reis & Nahmiash, 1998; Wolf, 1996). Yet, isolation and vulnerability can serve as barriers to protective intervention. Isolation can make abuse detection difficult, and victims suspicious of help offered. Vulnerability can reduce care options to only such restrictive forms as institutionalization and guardianship, usually perceived as the ultimate threats to personal autonomy and dignity by victims (Byers & Lamanna, 1993). As a result, the combination of elder abuse, isolation, and vulnerability, while suggesting a need for adult protective services, may limit either its acceptance by victims or its effectiveness as an intervention (Vinton, 1991; Wolf, 1986).

Surrogate decision making is essential for elderly persons with limited capacity for informed consent. Laws to appoint such authority have existed for 2,500 years. However, increasingly their implementation has been called into question as seemingly large numbers of elderly persons are declared incompetent or incapacitated in court, and have guardians or other surrogate decision makers appointed, thus losing individual rights based on inadequate evidence or procedural safeguards (Ahearn, 1987; Budish, 1992; Coleman & Dooley, 1990; Sabatino, 1996).

Isolated and vulnerable elderly persons may have more need for surrogate decision makers than those without these characteristics. Nonetheless, they also are more likely to have their autonomy unnecessarily compromised as a result of perfunctory legal processes or paternalistic attitudes (Schimer & Anetzberger, 1999). Isolation by its very nature suggests the unavailability of others who might advocate for the individual through personal knowledge and concern. Vulnerability, too, implies the existence of inabilities which may limit effective self-advocacy or access to other advocates.

These national and state level programs make it possible for social service agencies to locate and serve vulnerable isolated elderly persons. The approaches used by social workers in locating and accessing care and services for vulnerable isolated older persons reflect salient elements which are essential for effective intervention with persons in general.

Community-based Service Initiatives

Community-based initiatives in service delivery for isolated and vulnerable elderly have declined in recent years as a result of several factors. First, support for service initiatives has eroded with cuts in public funding. For example, in 1996 most of the revenues for Title IV of the Older Americans Act were eliminated in the broader movement to reduce government intervention. Because the intent of Title IV is to foster the development of demonstration, research, and training projects, a key support for service initiatives was lost. In the area of elder abuse alone, from 1978 to 1993, Title IV supported 79 different projects and enabled the testing of related service strategies not otherwise possible. Second, public funding cuts also forced some charitable organizations, such as community foundations and United Way, to divert funding toward the operation of existing services and away from support of program service initiatives. Although understandable, in the long run this approach undermines efforts to improve and expand the service delivery system. Finally, service initiatives and quality of care in service delivery for isolated and vulnerable elderly have suffered in the wake of health care reform (Experton, Li, Branch, Ozminkowski, & Mellon-Lacey, 1997). With its emphasis on cost containment and vertically integrated care, isolated and vulnerable elderly persons represent a high risk population whose care needs often are regarded as too unpredictable and costly. Therefore, they tend to fall outside the focus of hospital chains and health maintenance organizations vying for elderly consumers (Butler, Sherman, Rhinehart, Klein, & Rother, 1996).

In spite of declining support for service initiatives targeting isolated and vulnerable elderly, there are a few programs that deserve mention. In general, they reflect a return to community or neighborhood control and use of volunteers in cooperation with service professionals. Some programs are limited in their focus; most tend to be concerned with both isolation and vulnerability.

With a focus on illness and impairment, St. Mary's Hospital in Milwaukee developed a program to link medically isolated elderly persons with health care. The elderly persons live in a high density area near the hospital and lack either a physician or satisfactory health care connection. A nurse gerontologist was hired to make home visits and serve as the primary link to health services. Within a 6-year period, 750 elderly persons were served and 81% of these persons still live independently in the community as a result of the coordinated health services (Haworth, 1993). Equally successful is the North of Market Older Women's Alcohol Outreach Program in San Francisco. The program develops social support rather than using the traditional approach of "beating down" an alcoholic's defense barriers. It resulted in a 60% rate of complete abstinence for the participants over a 3-month minimum (Fredriksen, 1992).

Other focused service initiatives which address the needs of isolated and vulnerable elderly persons target additional populations. For example, in various locales support groups exist for victims of elder abuse, some of which are ethnically specific in order to reduce language barriers as well as the isolation that victims of violence experience (Neremberg, 1996). In Boston, a mobile unit offers meals and social work services to homeless elders wherever they are found (Tully & Jacobson, 1994). The gatekeeper program is particularly important in rural settings to identify isolated and vulnerable elderly (Florio et al., 1996). Using postal carriers, utility meter readers, and others who make frequent visits to residences, the program is able to link elderly persons with needed services. Lastly, peer counseling has helped elderly with mental health problems learn coping skills at the same time that it offers social support for recovery (Wacker, Roberts, & Piper, 1998).

Grossman (1996) offers a useful summary of recent service initiatives to keep elderly persons at home but connected to needed care. Among the nearly dozen programs she describes are three that deserve mention here because of their emphasis on the broad concerns of isolated and vulnerable elderly. The Living at Home/Block Nurse Program operates in 19 communities in three states. It offers 7-day, 24-hour in-home care from professional service providers and volunteers to maintain frail elderly persons at home. Funded mainly through third-party reimbursement and client fees or charity secondarily, the program is neighborhood-based and run by residents. Similarly, the Faith in Action Program relies on community governance and linkage to participating congregations in order to offer in-home assistance to persons of all ages with severe disabilities, most of whom are elderly. Evolving from the Interfaith Caregivers Project, which is found in 400 communities in 48 states, Faith in Action relies on volunteers from the congregations to extend supportive services in times of need. Finally, the Bay Area Independent Elders Program in San Francisco and surrounding communities uses local coalitions of businesses, religious organizations, public officials, and volunteers to identify isolated elderly and provide them with various formal and informal services. Funded by local foundations, the program has improved the overall responsiveness and resources of the service delivery system.

Loneliness poses a particular dilemma for service initiatives during times of resource scarcity. Although recognized for its adverse effect on health and mental health, service models to address loneliness are usually less able to capture the interest of public or private funders. Therefore, service initiatives tend to rely on enhancing current service arrangements. For instance, loneliness among elderly persons has been alleviated through the creation of surrogate families. Modeled after families forged in the gay community, these relations tend to originate out of caregiving and social need. Surrogate families can consist of friends, neighbors, volunteers, or professional care providers (Genevay, 1992; Thompson & Heller, 1990). For example, sometimes a group of friends will buy an apartment complex, and individuals reside in separate units in the same building. As health or other crises arise, the friends rally to assist one another. Elsewhere neighbors perform the caregiving functions that family members would assume if they were available. Mr. P., described earlier as a case example, relied on his next door neighbor to bring him meals and transport him to doctor's appointments after a recent hospitalization. Finally, social workers and nurses at The Benjamin Rose Institute and other long-term care organizations frequently come to be regarded as "family" by clients. At recent consumer forums clients of the Institute remarked, "I just love my social worker. She is like family to me," or "I wasn't a person until [my nurse] started coming around. I would just sit and cry all day, feeling sorry for myself. She's my savior." Professional relations that have surrogate family qualities require time and flexibility to develop. In the rush toward managed care and limited home visits, this approach may be compromised.

Intervention Strategies

Programs and services for isolated and vulnerable elderly persons may be made available or targeted at this population. The latter approach describes most resources of neighborhood, social, or self-help groups. There are exceptions, however, such as pastoral nursing for homebound parishioners through some churches or bereavement groups organized by membership associations like the American Association of Retired Persons. Age-specific and problem-specific agencies have the richest resource base targeted at isolated and vulnerable elderly persons. Collectively they provide needed access, in-home, community-based, supportive, and therapeutic services (Anetzberger & Palmisano, 1993; Cox, 1993; Herbert & Ginsberg, 1990; Wacker et al., 1998).

Access services connect isolated elderly persons with available resources. They include information and referral programs, outreach, and case management. Access services are essential for isolated elderly persons. Lacking alternatives, they typically have no other way to find out about sources of formal assistance. Unfortunately, each access service is limited in its ability to address the needs of this population. For example, because of their isolation, isolated elderly persons may not be aware of existing information and referral programs. Outreach is staff intensive and therefore often too expensive to offer in times of agency downsizing or cost containment. As a result, it is not available in most communities. Lastly, with their frequent suspicion of outsiders, isolated elderly persons may feel uncomfortable around professional case managers and resent the attempt to include them among their "managed cases."

In-home services address the needs of disabled elderly persons who cannot manage personal or household tasks. They include visiting nursing, personal care, chore services, homemaking, and home-delivered meals. Government funding has increased the availability of in-home services for disabled elderly persons in recent years. However, the nature and scope of service delivery may render these services less than adequate for meeting individual needs. For instance, nursing visits may be more gauged to reimbursement potential than actual need, homemaking may be limited to monthly cleaning, and home-delivered meals may not reflect personal taste or cultural background.

Community-based services facilitate socialization and group interaction. They include adult day care, congregate meals, and senior centers. For lonely elderly persons, they offer structured opportunities for interpersonal contact. They also provide stimulation and group learning with peers of similar interests and abilities. When community-based services fail, it is usually because lonely elderly persons attending their programs have been unable to integrate established social cliques, programming is organized more to meet the needs of staff than participants, and program procedures are rigid and inflexible to individual circumstance.

Supportive services offer isolated and vulnerable elderly persons help in taking advantage of other services or managing living alone. Supportive services, which include transportation, escort, telephone reassurance, and friendly visiting, often are provided by volunteers. As a result, their quality reflects the commitment of individual volunteers and the orientation, supervision, and assistance volunteers are given by their auspice agency.

Finally, therapeutic services are important for addressing the residuals of physical or mental illnesses, injuries, or other problems. They include counseling, alcoholism treatment, and rehabilitation. The stigma attached to mental health interventions among the current older generation may prevent their acceptance of counseling. Also, the relative lack of counselors with expertise in aging may limit the amount of quality service available. Further, rehabilitation tends to be so closely tied to a reimbursement source that services like physical and speech therapy generally cannot be obtained unless allowable under Medicare or Medicaid.

Whether or not isolated older persons avail themselves of services offered will depend on their perceived barriers to service delivery (Anetzberger & Palmisano, 1993; Biegel, Farkas, & Wadsworth, 1992). Personal reluctance may keep them from accepting help. This response results from pride, preference for informal care, wish to be left alone, denial of need, or mistrust of service providers. Agency barriers likewise can keep persons away. These barriers include insufficient promotion of services, inaccessible programs, a cumbersome application process, cultural insensitivity, and inflexible programming.

CONCLUSION—NEEDED IMPROVEMENTS

Rathbone-McCuan and Hashimi's (1982) suggested intervention strategies offer useful guidelines for professional efforts aimed at meeting the needs of isolated elderly. Relying on the principles guiding practice efforts with severely vulnerable elderly (Harel & Harel, 1995), changes are needed at all three levels: policy, planning, and service delivery.

At the policy level, it is essential to assess major federal and state public policies to assure that these provide community service agencies with the resources needed to serve the basic needs of all aged, including the diverse groups of isolated elderly. It is especially important to ensure the resources needed to locate and serve the severely cognitively impaired, mentally impaired, and hard-to-reach older persons in environmentally unstable living situations and the homeless.

At the planning level, it is important for the aging network, and especially area agencies on aging and community offices on aging, to establish viable working relationships with police departments, utility companies, and postal services for the primary purpose of locating the isolated vulnerable and severely vulnerable elderly and referring them to the attention of service agencies. There is also a need to establish viable linkages with television and radio stations along with community resources such as libraries, schools, religious institutions, and civic groups for dissemination

of information concerning the availability of resources and services for all
aged, including the isolated elderly.

At the service delivery level, the intervention strategies advanced by
Rathbone-McCuan and Hashimi (1982) have been used as a point of departure for elements identified and described in Table 12.3. These include

**TABLE 12.3   Critical Elements in Effective Intervention With Isolated
Elderly to Assure Quality of Care**

Element	Specific activities
Outreach and case finding	Worker engages in systematic outreach activities, including interaction with clergy, police officers, postal workers, and utility workers.
Facilitating access and establishing relationships	Worker alleviates suspicions, spends time discussing topics of personal interest and concerns, gradually addressing functional limitations and need for assistance with daily living tasks, access to medical treatment, and other needed resources.
Assessing health and functional status and service need	Worker assesses health status, functional limitations, cognitive functioning, mental status, and resources. Community resources and possible referrals are discussed.
Understanding and utilizing community resources	Worker has a good understanding of health, mental health, and social services available at the agency and in the community. Worker is aware of eligibility criteria and how to access them.
Respecting individual choice	Worker is respectful of person's preferences and choices concerning available options and resources.
Seeking out and involving informal care	Worker discusses with person social contacts and social resources and facilitates the establishment of social contacts and social relations as preferred and possible.
Facilitating and coordinating care	In implementing the care plan, worker arranges services from multiple agencies.
Facilitating change in care arrangements	As it becomes necessary, the worker facilitates access to needed resources and services.
Using a gradual and incremental approach	As it becomes apparent that relocation will be necessary, the worker involves the person in the exploration of living alternatives and in the decision making.

TABLE 12.3 *(Continued)*

Element	Specific activities
Maintaining an ongoing, professional relationship	Worker follows on an ongoing basis a regular schedule of meeting with the isolated person and arranges for emergency contacts as necessary.
Seeking least restrictive alternatives	Worker seeks out least restrictive alternatives. This is of special importance in work with homeless persons and with persons who need protective services.

outreach and case finding activities, facilitating access and establishing relationships, assessing health and functional status and service need, understanding and utilizing community resources, respecting individual choices, seeking out and involving informal care, facilitating and coordinating care, facilitating changes in care arrangements, using a gradual and incremental approach, maintaining an ongoing professional relationship, seeking least restrictive care alternatives, case finding, the establishment of professional relationships, and the delivery of effective services.

Specific attention needs to be placed on case finding and facilitating relations with other service provider agencies. In the service initiation phase, it is important to allay suspicions, reduce agency barriers, and set realistic goals that relate to the maintenance and improvement of their life quality. Efforts also need to be directed towards building an adequate working relationship with isolated older persons and members of their informal support system when they are available.

In the service delivery phase, premium must be given to service consumer mastery of the living situation, right of choice, and self-determination. It is of critical importance to aid in the location and maintenance of appropriate social contacts. In the ongoing process of care coordination it is essential that appropriate professional relationships be maintained with service consumers. Finally, every effort should be made to ascertain on an ongoing basis the quality of care and the effects that care and services have on slowing down/reducing the consequences of severe vulnerability and enhancement of the quality of life for isolated older persons. Quality of life for isolated elders needs to include both the assurance of their survival and basic security, as well as the pursuit and attainment of higher level needs.

REFERENCES

AARP (1999). *A Profile of Older Americans 1999.* Washington DC: AARP.

Ahearn, W. (1987). *Guardians of the elderly: An ailing system.* New York: Associated Press.

Albright, S., & Cohen, A. (1999, January 19). Lawmakers and advocates are working to boost Social Services Block Grants. *Aging News Alert,* p 3.

American Public Welfare Association & National Association of State Units on Aging (1986). *A comprehensive analysis of state policy and practice related to elder abuse.* Washington. DC: APWA/NASUA.

Anetzberger, G. J. (1995). Protective services and long-term care. In Z. Harel & R. Dunkle (Eds.), *Matching people and services in long-term care* (pp. 261–282). New York: Springer Publishing Co.

Anetzberger, G. J., & Palmisano, B. (1993). *The Ohio aging network education project: A core curriculum for senior service providers.* Cleveland, OH: Western Reserve Geriatric Education Center.

Applebaum, R., & Austin, C. (1990). *Long-term care case management: Design and evaluation.* New York: Springer Publishing Co.

Bennett, R. (1980). *Aging, isolation and resocialization.* New York: Van Nostrand Reinhold Company.

Biegel, D. E., Farkas, K. J., & Wadsworth, N. (1992). Social service programs for older adults and their families: Service use and barriers. In P. K. Kim (Ed.), *Services to the aging and aged: Public policies and programs.* New York: Garland Press.

Binstock, R. (1991). From the great society to the aging society—25 years of the Older Americans Act. *Generations, 15*(3), 11–18.

Branch, L. G. Coulam, R. F., & Zimmerman, Y. A. (1995). The Pace Evaluation: Initial findings. *Gerontologist, 35,* 349–359.

Branch, L. G., & Jette, A. (1982). A prospective study of long-term care institutionalization among the aged. *American Journal of Public Health, 72,* 1373–1379.

Brody, S. (1990). Critical policy issues in health and long-term care. In Z. Harel, P. Ehrlich, & R. Hubbard (Eds.), *Vulnerable aged: People, services & policies,* (pp. 223–234). New York: Springer Publishing Co.

Budish, A. D. (1992). Guardianship: Sanctuary or snare? *Modern Maturity, 35*(3), 56–58.

Butler, R. N., Sherman, F. T., Rhinehart, E., Klein, S., & Rother, J. C. (1996). Managed care: What to expect as Medicare—HMO enrollment grows. *Geriatrics, 10,* 35–42.

Byers, B., & Lamanna, R. A. (1993). Adult protective services and elder self endangering behavior. In B. Byers & J. E. Hendricks (Eds.), *Adult Protective services: Research and practice* (pp. 3–31). Springfield, IL: Charles C. Thomas.

Chappel, N., & Badger, M. (1989). Social isolation and well-being. *Journals of Gerontology, 44,* S169–76.

Clauser, S. B. Kidder, D., & Mauser, E. (1996). "The PACE evaluation": Two responses (Letter to the editor). *Gerontologist, 36,* 7–8.

Coleman, N., & Dooley, J. (1990). Making the guardianship work. *Generations, 14* (Supplement), 47–50.

Cox, C. (1993). *The frail elderly: Problems, needs and community responses.* Westport, CT: Auburn House.

Damron-Rodriguez, J., & Cantrell, M. (1995). Veterans and long term care services. In Z. Harel, & R. Dunkle (Eds.), *Matching people and services in long-term care* (pp. 109–132). New York: Springer Publishing Co.

Doty, P., Liu, K., & Weiner, Y. (1985). An overview of long term care. *Health Care Financing Review, 6,* 69–78.

Eleazer, P., & Fretwell, M. (1999). The PACE model (program for all inclusive care of the elderly): A review. In P. R. Katz, R. L. Kane, & M. D. Mezey (Eds.), *Emerging systems in long term care* (pp. 88–117). New York: Springer Publishing Co.

Eng, C., Pedulla, J., Eleazer, Q. P., McCann, R., & Fox, N. (1997). Program of All-inclusive Care for the Elderly (PACE): An innovative model of integrated geriatric care and financing. *Journal of the American Geriatric Society, 45,* 223–232.

Experton, B., Li, Z., Branch, L., Ozminkowski, R. J., & Mellon-Lacey, D. M. (1997). The impact of pay or provider type on health care use and expenditures among the frail elderly. *American Journal of Public Health, 87*(2), 210–16.

Fisher, D. H. (1978). *Growing old in America.* Oxford: Oxford University Press.

Florio, E. R., Rockwood, T., Hendryx, M. S., Jensen, J. E., Raschko, R., & Dyck, D. (1996). A model gatekeeper program to find the at-risk elderly. *Journal of Case Management, 5*(3), 106–114.

Fredriksen, K. I. (1992). North of Market: Older Women's Alcohol Outreach Program. *Gerontologist, 32*(2), 270–272.

Genevay, B. (1992). "Creating" families: Older people alone: What is the role of service providers? *Generations, 17*(3), 61–64.

Grossman, H. D. (1996). There is just no place like home. *Journal of Long-Term Home Health Care, 15*(2), 33–40.

Harel, Z., & Dunkle, R. (1995). *Matching people and service in long-term care.* New York: Springer Publishing Co.

Harel, Z., & Harel, B. (1995). Community and home-based programs and services. In Z. Harel & R. Dunkle (Eds.), *Matching people and service in long-term care* (pp 181–200). New York: Springer Publishing Co.

Harel, Z., & Noelker, L. (1995). Severe vulnerability and long-term care. In Z. Harel & R. Dunkle (Eds.), *Matching people and service in long-term care* (pp. 5–24). New York: Springer Publishing Co.

Harel, Z., Noelker, L., & Blake, B. (1985). Comprehensive services for the aged: Theoretical and empirical perspectives. *Gerontologist, 25,* 644–649.

Haworth, M. J. (1993). Hospital-based community outreach to medically isolated elders. *Geriatric Nursing, 14*(1), 23–25.

Herbert, A. S., & Ginsberg, L. H. (1990). *Human services for older adults: Concepts and skills* (2nd ed.). Columbia, SC: University of South Carolina Press.

Homel, P. A., & Wood, E. F. (1990). Guardianship: There are alternatives. *Aging, 360,* 7–12.

Jansson, B. S. (1993). *The reluctant welfare state: A history of American social welfare policies* (2nd ed.). Pacific Grove, CA: Brooks/Cole.

Johnson, T. F. (1991). *Elder mistreatment: Deciding who is at risk.* New York: Greenwood Press.

Kane, R. A., & Kane, R. L. (1987). *Long-term care: Principles, programs and policies.* New York: Springer Publishing Co.

Kane, R. A., Kane, R. L., & Ladd, R. C. (1998). *The heart of long-term care.* New York: Oxford University Press.

Kane, R. L., Illston, L. H., & Miller, N. A. (1992). Qualitative analysis of the program of all-inclusive care for the elderly (PACE). *Gerontologist, 32,* 771–780.

Kapp, M. B., & Bigot, A. (1985). *Geriatrics and the law: Patient rights and professional responsibilities.* New York: Springer Publishing Co.

Kosberg, J. I., & Nahmiash, D. (1996). Characteristics of victims and perpetrators and milieus of abuse and neglect. In L. A. Baumhover & S. C. Beall (Eds.), *Abuse, neglect and exploitation of older persons: Strategies for assessment and intervention* (pp. 31–49). Baltimore MD: Health Profession Press.

Levande, D., Bowden, S., & Mollema, J. (1987). Home health services for the dependent elders: The social work dimension. *Journal of Gerontological Social Work, 11*(3), 5–17.

Litwak, E. (1960). Occupational mobility and extended family cohesion. *American Sociological Review,* 25.

Lowenthal, M. F. (1964). Social isolation and mental illness, *American Sociological Review, 29,* 54–70.

Michael R. T., Fuchs, V. R., & Scott, S. R. (1980). Changes in propensity to live alone, 1950–1976. *Demography, 17,* 39–57.

Mehdizadeh, S. A., Kunkel, S. R. Atchley, R., & Applebaum, R. A. (1990). *Projected need for long-term care in Ohio's older population.* Oxford, OH: Miami University, Scripps Gerontology Center.

National Academy on Aging (1995). *Facts on the Older Americans Act.* Washington, DC: Author.

Neremberg, L. (1996). *Older battered women: Integrating aging and domestic violence services.* Washington, D.C.: National Center on Elder Abuse.

O'Brien, R. C., & Flannery, M. T. (1997). *Long-term care: Federal, state and private options for the future.* New York: Haworth.

Ohio Association of Area Agency on Aging (1995). *Program: Report Card.* Columbus, OH: Author.

O'Shaugnessy, C. V. (1998, December 1). *Older Americans Act: 105th* Congress Issues. Washington, D.C.: The Library of Congress, Congressional Research Services.

Pillemer, K. (1985). Social isolation and elder abuse. *Response.* Fall, 2–4.

Rathbone-McCuan, E., & Hashimi, J. (1982). *Isolated elders.* Rockville, MD: Aspen.

Reed, W. (1990). Vulnerability and sociodemographic factors. In Z. Harel, P. Ehrlich, & R. Hubbard (Eds.), *Vulnerable aged: People, services & policies.* New York: Springer Publishing Co.

Reis, M., & Namiash, D. (1998). Validation of the Indicators of Abuse (IOA) screen. *Gerontologist, 38*(4), 471–80.

Rubinstein, R. (1995). Special community settings. In Z. Harel & R. Dunkle (Eds.), *Matching people and services in long-term care* (pp. 89–108). New York: Springer Publishing Co.

Rubinstein, R. L., Kilbride, J. C., & Nagy, S. (1992). *Elders living alone: Frailty and perception of choice.* New York: Aldine De Gruyter.

Sabatino, C. P. (1996). Competency: Refining our legal fictions. In M. Smyer, K. W. Schaie, & M. B. Kapp (Eds.), *Older adults' decision making and the law* (pp. 1–28). New York: Springer Publishing Co.

Schimer, M. R., & Anetzberger, G. J. (1999). Examining the gray zones in guardianship and involuntary protective services laws. *Journal of Elder Abuse & Neglect, 10*(3/4), 19–38.

Tatara, T. (1995). *An analysis of state laws addressing elder abuse, neglect and exploitation.* Washington, DC: National Center on Elder Abuse.

Thompson, M. G., & Heller, K. (1990). Facets of support related to well-being: Quantitative social isolation and perceived social support in a sample of elderly women. *Psychology and Aging, 5*(4), 535–544.

Townsend A., & Harel, Z. (1990). Health vulnerability and service need among the aged. In Z. Harel, P. Ehrlich, & R. Hubbard (Eds.), *Vulnerable aged: People, services & policies* (pp. 32–52). New York: Springer Publishing Co.

Traxler, A. (1986). Elder abuse laws: A survey of state statutes. In M. W. Galbraith (Ed.), *Elder abuse: Perspectives on an emerging crisis* (pp. 136–167). Kansas City, KS: Mid America Congress on Aging.

Tully, C. T., & Jacobson, S. (1994). The homeless elderly: America's forgotten population. *Journal of Gerontological Social Work, 22*(3/4), 61–81.

U. S. Senate Special Committee on Aging (1977). *Protective services for the elderly: A working paper.* Washington, DC: US Government Printing Press.

Vinton, L. (1991). Factors associated with refusing services among maltreated elderly. *Journal of Elder Abuse, 3*(2), 89–103.

Wacker, R. R., Roberts, K. A., & Piper, L. E. (1998). *Community resources for older adults: Programs and services in an era of change.* Thousand Oaks, CA: Pine Forge Press.

Wolf, R. S. (1986). Major findings from three model projects on elderly abuse. In K. A. Pillemer & R. S. Wolf (Eds.), *Elder abuse: Perspectives on an emerging crisis* (pp. 138–167). Kansas City, KS: Mid America Congress on Aging.

Wolf, R. S. (1996). Understanding elder abuse and neglect. *Aging, 367,* 4–9.

Index

Page numbers followed by "*t*" indicate tables.